Drug Repurposing - Advances, Scopes and Opportunities in Drug Discovery

Edited by Mithun Rudrapal

Published in London, United Kingdom

Drug Repurposing - Advances, Scopes and Opportunities in Drug Discovery
http://dx.doi.org/10.5772/intechopen.106301
Edited by Mithun Rudrapal

Contributors
John Oluwafemi Teibo, Chioma Ejiro Irozuru, Titilade Kehinde Ayandeyi Teibo, Olabode Ebenezer Omotoso, Ahmad O. Babalghith, Gaber El-Saber Batiha, Mithun Rudrapal, Dipak Chetia, Soumya Bhattacharya, Manisha Kotadiya, Jin-Ho Joo, Kimberly Stieglitz, Gemma Topaz, Dongjun Yoo, Richard Anderson, P. Subash, Kareti Srinivasa Rao, Bhabani Sankar Satapathy, Biswabhusan Biswal, Pralaya Kumar Sahoo, Himansu Bhusan Samal, Snigdha Pattnaik, Sangram Keshari Biswal, Binapani Barik, Shanta Bhar, Xolani Henry Makhoba, Sunil T. Galatage, Arehalli S. Manjappa, Raghwendra R. Waghmode, Swapnil S. Harale, Sujit A. Desai, Swapnil S. Chopade, Kranti S. Bille, Rubina U. Watangi, Shweta N. Kalebere, Aditya S. Hebalkar, Shradhey V. Dhobale, Harshada N. Gunjat, Poonam R. Dhenge, Purva S. Ikke, Saheblal A. Shaikh, Rutuja J. Patil, Sakshi B. Shinde, Rutuja V. Khatavakar, Anuja B. Patil, Prajakta N. Khatavakar, Sourabh S. Hegaje, Rushikesh B. Katkar, Innocent Mary Ifedibalu Chukwu Ejiofor, Christabel Ekeomodi, Kingsley Ifeanyi Obetta, Mmesoma Linus Okolocha, Somto Chukwu Nnacho, Martins Oluwaseun Isijola, Aleksandr Urakov, Natalya Urakova, Evgeny Fisher, Yulia Andreevna Sorokina, Aleksandr Samorodov, Jingjun Huang, Jiayi Chen, Zhifeng Zhao, Xinyu Wang

First published in London, United Kingdom, 2023 by IntechOpen
IntechOpen is the global imprint of INTECHOPEN LIMITED, registered in England and Wales, registration number: 11086078, 5 Princes Gate Court, London, SW7 2QJ, United Kingdom

British Library Cataloguing-in-Publication Data
A catalogue record for this book is available from the British Library

Additional hard and PDF copies can be obtained from orders@intechopen.com

Drug Repurposing - Advances, Scopes and Opportunities in Drug Discovery
Edited by Mithun Rudrapal
p. cm.
Print ISBN 978-1-83768-776-3
Online ISBN 978-1-83768-777-0
eBook (PDF) ISBN 978-1-83768-778-7

For EU product safety concerns:
IN TECH d.o.o., Prolaz Marije Krucifikse Kozulić 3, 51000 Rijeka, Croatia,
info@intechopen.com or visit our website at intechopen.com.

Meet the editor

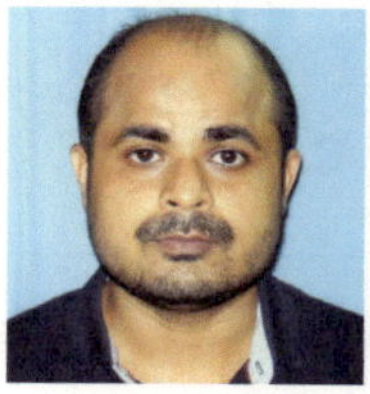

Mithun Rudrapal, Ph.D., FIC, FICS, CChem (India), is an Associate Professor in the Department of Pharmaceutical Sciences, School of Biotechnology and Pharmaceutical Sciences, Vignan's Foundation for Science, Technology & Research (Deemed to be University), Guntur, India. Dr. Rudrapal has been actively engaged in teaching and researching the field of pharmaceutical and allied sciences for more than 13 years. He has more than 100 publications in peer-reviewed international journals to his credit and has filed a number of Indian and international patents. In addition, Dr. Rudrapal is the author of a dozen published or forthcoming books and works in the areas of medicinal chemistry, computer-aided drug design (CADD), drug repurposing, phytochemistry, herbal drugs, and nanophytotherapeutics.

Contents

Preface

Drug repurposing, also known as drug repositioning, drug reprofiling, or therapeutic switching, is the process of identifying new pharmacological indications from old, existing, investigational, or FDA-approved drugs, as well as applying newly developed drugs to the treatment of diseases other than the drugs' original or intended therapeutic use. The drug repositioning approach has the potential to be employed over traditional drug discovery programs because of the reduction of monetary discovery, duration of development, and risk of failure. In recent years, the drug repositioning strategy has gained considerable momentum, accounting for about one-third of new drug approvals corresponding to repurposed drugs and generating around 25% of annual revenue for pharmaceutical industries. The application of computational approaches and techniques for the prediction and exploration of the pharmacological effects of developing drug candidates and/or lead molecules offers significant hope for current drug discovery programs because it is inexpensive, time-saving, and less risky. The use of computational approaches in drug discovery research not only helps in the discovery of new drugs from leads or existing drug molecules but also in the repurposing of existing drugs. This book delivers useful and current information on various computational approaches, biophysical tools, databases, and experimental techniques that can be utilized for repurposing drugs and identifying the uses, novel drug targets, and mechanisms of existing drug candidates for various emerging or deadly diseases. The recent COVID-19 pandemic is a clear indication that there is a dire need for advanced silico tools and computational techniques along with in vitro and in vivo techniques for drug discovery. This volume presents recent advances in drug repurposing and computational approaches for the discovery and development of drugs against certain difficult-to-treat and life-threatening diseases, including microbial infections, parasitic diseases, neurological disorders, cardiovascular diseases, and cancer. In addition, the book examines the challenges of drug repurposing and computational approaches. Chapters present up-to-date and in-depth information in a lucid, constructive, and unambiguous manner with adequate consistency in flow, continuity, and technical clarity. Through this book, readers can enhance their knowledge and skills with modern technologically advanced techniques, computational approaches, and in silico tools available for the discovery of drugs by drug repurposing strategies. The book is designed for graduate students, post-graduate students, doctoral researchers, senior academic researchers, professors, and others in the pharmaceutical, biomedical, and allied (biochemical, biotechnology, bioinformatics, etc.) sciences from higher academic institutions, universities, and pharmaceutical and biotechnology companies. The editors would like to thank all the contributors and reviewers for their invaluable and timely contributions to this edited volume. Feedback and suggestions from prospective readers and other stakeholders are most welcome.

Mithun Rudrapal
Associate Professor,
Department of Pharmaceutical Sciences,
School of Biotechnology and Pharmaceutical Sciences,
Vignan's Foundation for Science, Technology
and Research (Deemed to be University),
Guntur, India

Section 1

Repurposing and Drug Development

Chapter 1

Role of Drug Repurposing in Cancer Treatment and Liposomal Approach of Drug Targeting

Sunil T. Galatage, Arehalli S. Manjappa, Raghwendra R. Waghmode, Swapnil S. Harale, Rushikesh B. Katkar, Sujit A. Desai, Swapnil S. Chopade, Kranti S. Bille, Rubina U. Watangi, Shweta N. Kalebere, Aditya S. Hebalkar, Shradhey V. Dhobale, Harshada N. Gunjate, Poonam R. Dhenge, Purva S. Ikke, Saheblal A. Shaikh, Rutuja J. Patil, Sakshi B. Shinde, Rutuja V. Khatavakar, Anuja B. Patil, Prajakta N. Khatavakar, Sourabh S. Hegaje and Suresh G. Killedar

Abstract

Cancer is the leading cause of death, and incidences are increasing significantly and patients suffering from it desperately need a complete cure from it. The science of using an already-invented drug that has been approved by the FDA for a new application is known as "drug repurposing." Currently, scientists are drawn to drug repositioning science in order to investigate existing drugs for newer therapeutic uses and cancer treatment. Because of their unique ability to target cancer cells, recently repurposed drugs and the liposomal approach are effective in the treatment of cancer. Liposomes are nanovesicles that are drastically flexible, rapidly penetrate deeper layers of cells, and enhance intracellular uptake. More importantly, liposomes are biocompatible, biodegradable; entrap both hydrophobic and hydrophilic drugs. This chapter summarizes various approaches to drug repurposing, as well as drug repurposing methods, advantages and limitations of drug repurposing, and a liposomal approach to using repurposed drugs in cancer targeting. This chapter also summarizes liposomal structure, drug loading, and the mechanism of liposomes in targeted cancer treatment. The lipid-based liposomal approach is emerging as a powerful technique for improving drug solubility, bioavailability, reducing side effects, and improving the therapeutic efficacy of repurposed drugs for cancer treatment.

Keywords: cancer, drug repurposing, liposomes, drug targeting, enhanced permeability effect, Etc.

1. Introduction

During the treatment of cancer in a patient, it is necessary to follow certain principles, such as diagnosing the disease at an early stage, making efforts for its prevention, and completing the eradication of malignant cells. Whereas three modes of treatment are available to treat cancer, including surgery, chemotherapy (also called pharmacotherapy), and radiation therapy [1], Radiation therapy is nothing but the eradication of malignant cells by means of radiation. This technique helps to destroy localized cancer cells (**Figure 1**). In pharmacotherapy, various chemical entities are used to kill and disorganize an uncontrolled cell growth programme in a body [2]. Cancer does not only affect humans; it can also harm wildlife and other life forms. Tumour cells might break out from the initial bulk and begin the unregulated growth cycle all over again. The phenomenon of tumour cells leaving one location and developing cells that travel and proliferate over other body parts is known as metastasis. It was estimated by the WHO that cancer is the foremost cause of death in the world, and in the year 2018, it is expected that 9.6 million people died as a result of it. It is categorized by the development of osteocytes, bone lesions, anaemia, skeletal destruction, renal failure, and hypocalcaemia. It is a bone marrow cancer that affects both the marrow and the bones. It also affects different body locations; hence it is called multiple myeloma. Bone marrow-originating myeloid cells such as myeloid resultant suppressor cells, macrophages, myeloid dendritic cells, monocytes, osteoclasts, and lymphocytes are drafted to tumours, which can either increase anti-tumour immune function or encourage tumour growth [3]. Recent research indicates that anti-resorptive targeted therapies can have an impact on tumour-associated myeloid cells through direct or indirect pathways, indicating that anti-resorptives have an osteoclastin-dependent mechanism of action. As the cancer progresses, the signs and symptoms change dramatically. Symptoms can be entirely dissimilar from

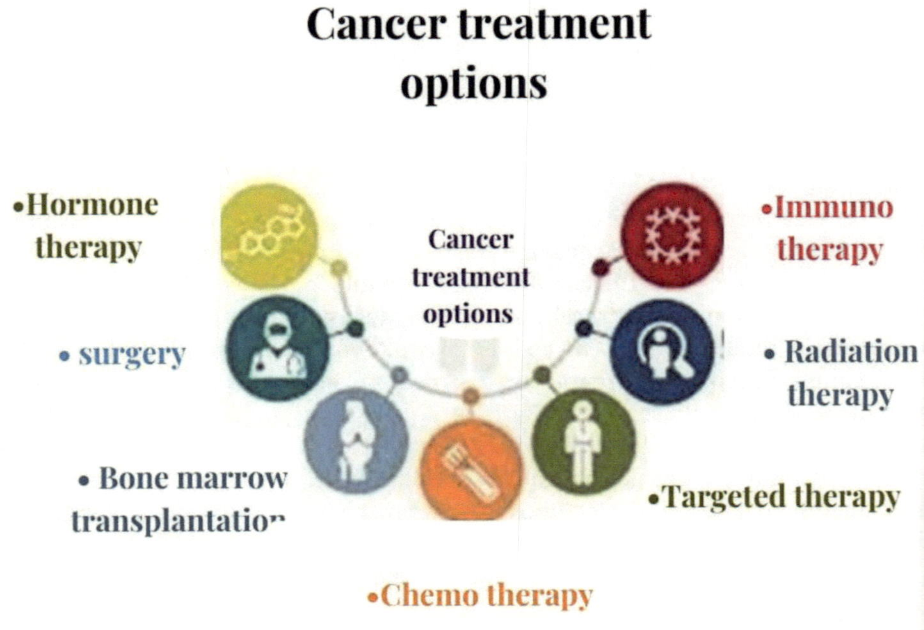

Figure 1.
Schematic representation of cancer treatments.

patient to patient. A few symptoms are most common, like fatigue, bone problems, kidney problems, and low blood counts. Some symptoms become severe; these are: osteoporosis, osteocytes, bone lesions, and skeletal destruction [4].

Targeted cancer treatment, in which the selected cancer cells are eliminated and healthy cells are left alone, is becoming extremely prevalent [5]. The arrival of nanostructures has resulted in the development of advanced materials and channels for cancer treatment targeting [6, 7]. Nanotechnology has opened up new possibilities for biological and biomedical applications, such as improving the targeted administration of anticancer drugs. Nanotechnology has a lot of benefits for treating cancer. In reality, tumour blood vessels are severely disordered, with an ineffective lymph capillary network and loose endothelial cells in comparison with normal tissue. Because of their improved permeability and high body retention, nanoparticles such as liposomes can be transported preferentially to the tumour location [8].

2. Drug repurposing in cancer treatment

This technique helps to destroy localized cancer cells. In pharmacotherapy, various chemical entities are used to kill and disorganize an uncontrolled cell growth programme in a body [8]. Chemotherapeutic agents pose the greatest risk to cancer patients because of the drugs' lethal effects and the possibility of cell damage to their bone marrow, which makes them more susceptible to other diseases. If we have not targeted the malignant cell only, then these chemotherapeutic agents also kill the normal cells in the same host, which creates more damage to the patient's body and its biological structure [9]. Different strategies of drug repurposing are denoted in **Figure 2**.

Extensive research is carried out to investigate and develop new therapeutic entities in the oncology field and drug research to achieve the maximum therapeutic effect with greater patient comfort and a lower toxicity profile. On the other hand it raises the cost of treatment for a patient, making it necessary to exert maximum effort to achieve desired treatment goals at the lowest possible cost of treatment. Drug repurposing is the most effective way to reduce the effort required to develop new drug molecules while also lowering treatment costs. The science of using an already-invented drug that has been approved by the FDA for a newer application is known as drug purposing. Now a day drug repositioning science attracts the more researchers to investigate existing drugs for its newer therapeutic use. The drug being repositioned is already being used to treat diseases in humans, giving the manufacturer access to knowledge regarding its safety, effectiveness, therapeutic, and toxicity profiles. To reposition medications that are already approved for human use efficiently, rigorous selection is required, followed by a detailed demonstration of the treatment's usefulness in new biological contexts. The following methods are used to select drug candidates for drug repositioning [10].

2.1 Repositioning based on therapeutic activity

This method involves testing the therapeutic effectiveness of a drug by performing an in vitro or in vivo study. For the finding of therapeutic entities, comprehensive public library data is used. The therapeutic agent is examined for its protein targets and cellular targets while searching for a suitable drug candidate through activity-based repurposing of the drug (**Figure 3**) [11, 12].

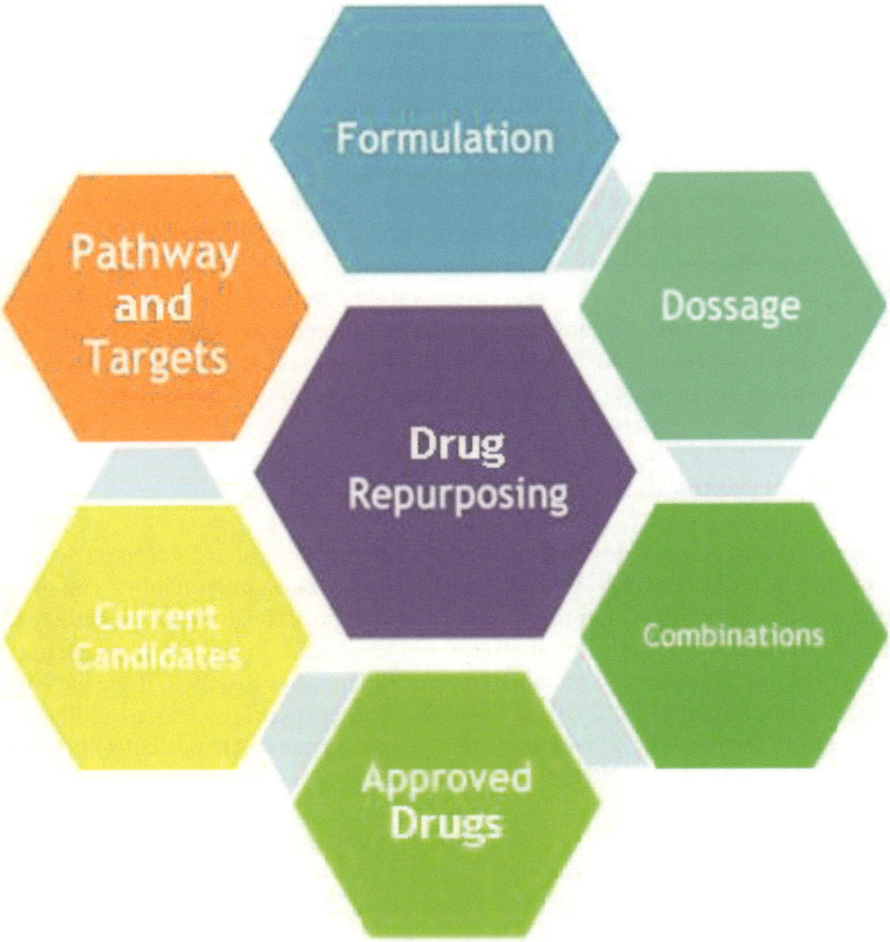

Figure 2.
Strategies to repurpose the drug candidates.

2.2 Drug repositioning through literature evidence

This drug repurposing method involves the selection of a drug based on its published therapeutic evidence. The literature study of such drug databases available on PubMed, ClinicalTrail.gov, Drug Quest, MEDLINE, and other available databases is screened, and the required potential molecules are identified by applying such data in a dynamic way (**Figure 4**) [13].

2.3 In silico method: In this method

Various bioinformatics tools and a public database are used to understand drug protein interactions. For this method, extensive genomic studies and structural evaluations of various proteins are carried out. Most pharmaceutical drug manufacturers adopt the in silico method for drug repurposing. To identify the protein interaction and possible drug candidate, researchers use the science of

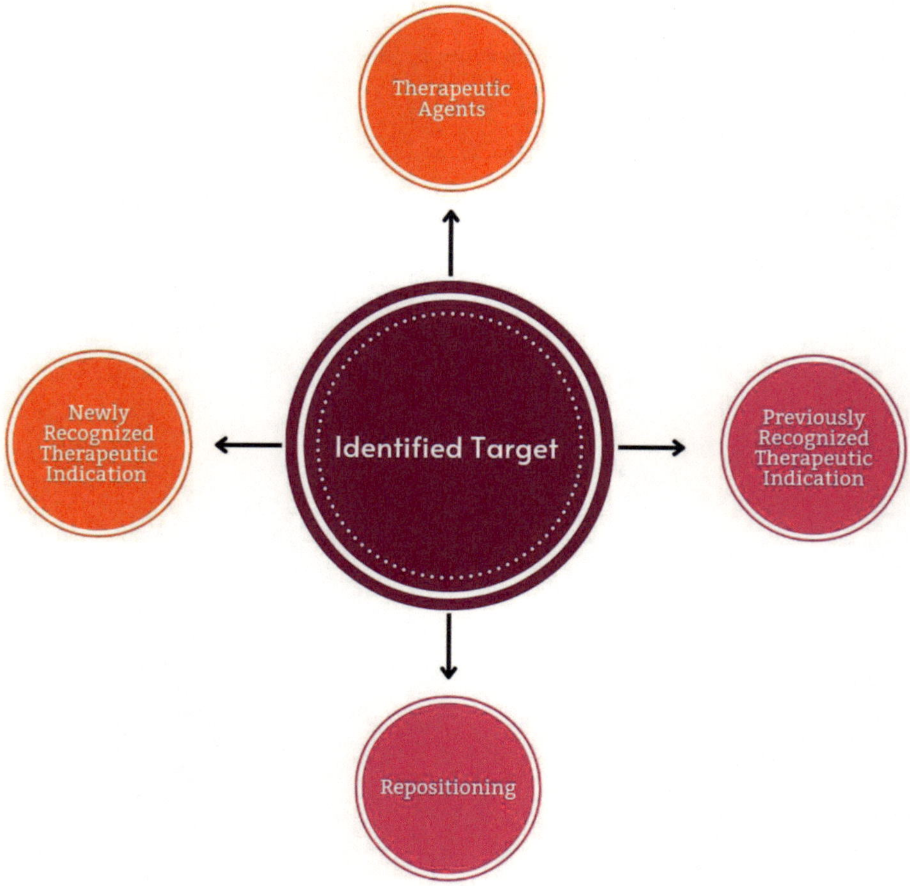

Figure 3.
Diagrammatic representation of Drug Repositioning (Case A).

artificial intelligence, neural network techniques, and other bioinformation tools (**Figure 5**) [11, 14].

2.4 Advantages of drug repositioning

1. Drug repositioning helps to curtail the drug development cost, which leads to an improvement in the economy of the treatment [15].

2. It helps to cut down the risk associated with the task of drug development.

3. Minimize the time requirement in drug investigation as compared to the traditional method of drug development.

4. The availability of extensive data related to drug kinetic and dynamic properties reduces the efforts required to select a suitable dosage form, and assess the safety and toxicity of a drug.

5. Researchers can skip performing preclinical experiments by relocating drugs, which helps reduce the drug development cost.

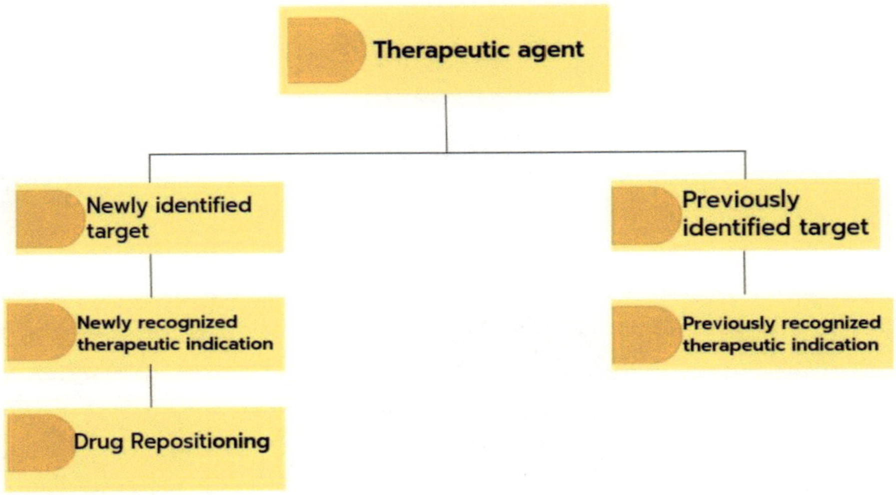

Figure 4.
Diagrammatic representation of Drug Repositioning (Case B).

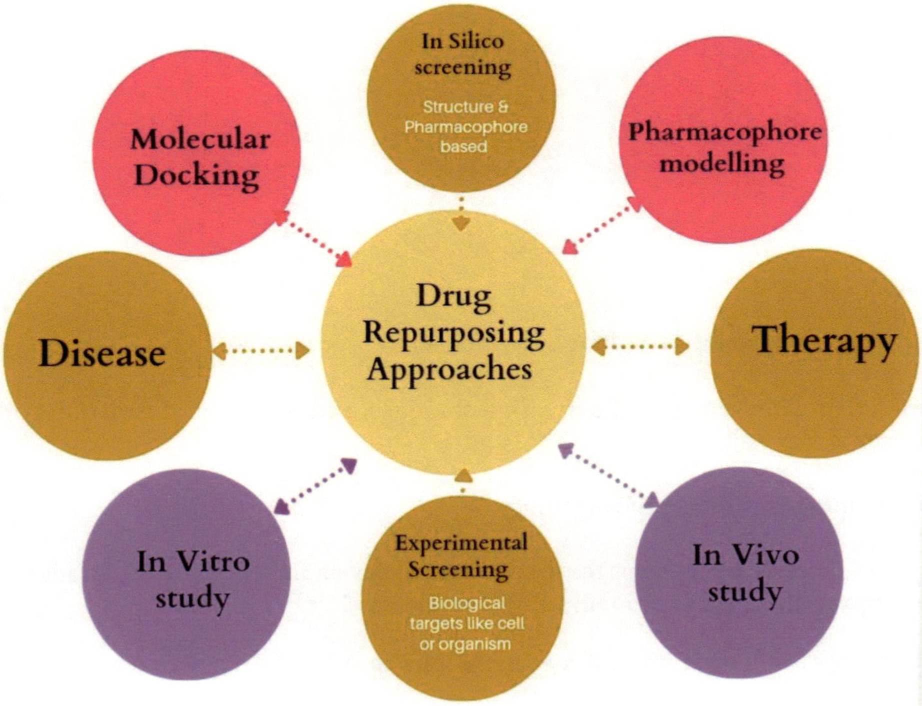

Figure 5.
Diagrammatic representation of drug repurposing approaches.

2.5 Limitations of drug repositioning

1. More money is spent on licensing requirements for drug repositioning to investigate new therapeutic applications of already approved drugs [16].

2. The drug repositioning process includes intellectual property protection for repurposed medications, which is especially important for off-patent drugs.

3. Pharmaceutical industries have shown little interest in repurposing medications because such rights are difficult to grant.

4. Anticancer activity of repurposed medications is more commonly reported when used in conjunction with established cytotoxic drugs rather than as single agents.

3. Repurposed drug targeting

Nanoparticulate drugs (including liposomal drugs) are generally developed for therapeutics developed against cancer to avoid non-specific distribution to healthy cells and tissues that generally causes lethal side effects. Due of the permeable tumour vasculature and decreased lymphatic outflow, the nanomedicines (including liposomes) with prolonged circulation durations preferentially penetrate tumour tissue. This phenomenon is referred to as the "increased permeability and retention (EPR) effect Drug repurposing is a technique for finding new applications for medicines that go beyond their original medicinal indications. On the other hand, drug repurposing is the most effective way to reduce the coast, time and effort required to develop new drug molecules while also lowering treatment costs. The development of nanomedicines (including liposomes) for these repurposed drugs could provide many benefits; increased kinetic, dynamic and biopharmaceutical characteristics, and avoids their primary indications via targeting them to tumour through EPR effect. Furthermore, these nanomedicines could be easily surface modified to passively and actively target tumour cells and cellular components. Therefore, nanomedicines composed of repurposed drug could be preferred over plain drugs or their conventional generic dosage forms currently available in the market.

4. Liposomes (LPs)

An LPs is a spherical vesicle made up of one or more lipid vesicles that is increasingly being used to deliver therapeutic entities. Liposomes are one of several promising drug delivery systems that represent an efficient approach for delivering active compounds to the target site, and various formulations are currently in clinical use. LPs technology has been developed from typical vesicles to second generation liposomes, which are created by changing the lipid composition, length, and charge of vesicle liposomes and can be employed on a regular basis as what the body does to drugs and what drugs do to the body can be controlled. The LPs provide selective passive targeting to tumour tissues, and the encapsulation method contributes to increased effectiveness, therapeutic index, and stability. Reduced polymer toxicity, site evading effect, helping to enhance the pharmacokinetics of the therapeutic moiety, and suppleness to bind ligands at specific sites to achieve active targeting, to name a few advantages [6]. Liposomes were studied for the first time at the Babraham Institute in Cambridge by two scientists who used an electron microscope to examine phospholipids in dry form with negative staining. These two scientists are Dr. Alec Bengham and R. W. Horne, who identified the liposome assembly in 1961 and published their study in 1964. Liposome is the name given to a compound made up of lipids (lipo) and body (soma). So that liposome is nothing but a lipid body in which medicine is to be delivered [17]. Many anticancer medications have been designed to terminate tumour cells that are developing uncontrollably because they divide more quickly than normal cells. However, in this instance, ordinary cells grow fast, and a chemotherapeutic agent might harm such cells, resulting in chemotherapy side effects. Blood cells that create bone marrow, cells in the digestive tract (cells in the mouth, stomach, gut, and oesophagus), and sexual organs and hair follicles are among the fast-growing normal cells that are impacted. Some anticancer medications have the capacity to harm cells in key organs, including the heart, kidney, bladder, lungs, and neurological system. Medication diffusion in solid tumours is hampered by a variety of vascular supply and cellular gravity within tumour cells, particularly in tumour regions. Drug delivery design develops in such a way to ensure that macromolecular medicines are released slowly via the tumour. Advanced technologies are designed to improve tumour tissue permeability. These are triggered by the maladaptive nature of tumorigenesis, which is characterized by structural and physiological abnormalities that lead to hyperpermiability. The medicinal compounds have a larger molecular structure, which leads to the build-up of high-molecular-weight molecules with limited distribution volumes and the ability to circulate for lengthy periods of time through aberrant arteries and concentrate in tumours [18–20].

4.1 Structural features of liposome

LPs are small cell membrane sacs. Because these LPs can be packed with medications, they are a viable option for treating illnesses and cancer. Liposome membranes are composed of phospholipids with a head and a tail group. Because of the length of the hydrocarbon chain, the head part is hydrophilic and the tail part is hydrophobic. Phospholipids are naturally occurring two-layer stable membranes. Because head groups are hydrophilic, they are fascinated by water and arrange in such a way to form a surface-like assembly away from it when there is water present. In a cell with outside water, while the other is fascinated by water within the cell. They resemble tiny spheres that are smaller than a normal cell's size, whether as bilayers or monolayers. Liposomes are created as bilayers, while micelles are formed as monolayers. Phospholipids form the mainstream of the lipids in the plasma membrane; these phospholipids are phosphatidyl ethanolamine and phosphatidylcholine [19–21]. Liposomes have the capability to penetrate cancer in its natural state. Endothelium cells are contained by tight junctions in the endothelial walls of all healthy human blood vessels. These tight connections prevent large blood particles from spilling out of the vessel. In the event of a tumour vessel, this type of arrangement does not exist, making it symptomatically porous. This capacity is known as the enhanced permeability and retention effect (EPR) (**Figure 6**). Liposomes with a diameter of less than 400 nm can enter tumours quickly from the bloodstream, but they are maintained in the bloodstream by the endothelium wall in healthy tissue [23–25].

4.2 Drug loading mechanism into liposome

The drug features and the lipids determine how pharmaceuticals are loaded into liposomes. Hydrophilic medications are confined in the inner watery compartment,

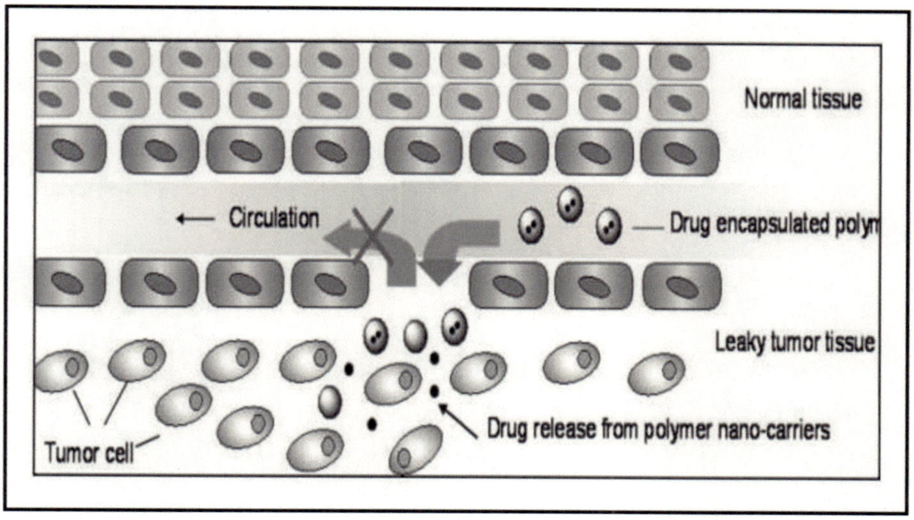

Figure 6.
Diagrammatic representation of EPR effect [22].

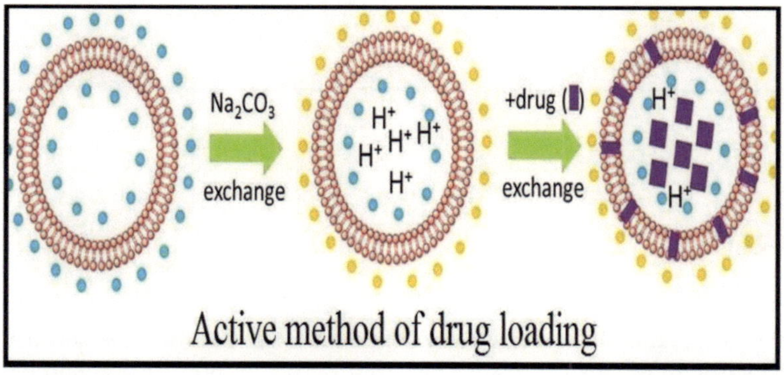

Figure 7.
Active loading of drug into liposome [26].

while hydrophobic pharmaceuticals can screen within the lipid hydrocarbon area. In practice, few medicines may segregate into hydrocarbon or aqueous compartments; for example, Amphotericin-B (Amph-B) binds to hydrophobic lipid membranes. The resulting lipid configuration influences Amph-B parcelling and its rate of exchange outside of the liposome envelope (**Figure 7**). Incorporating a negatively charged lipid improves the stability of the membrane's connection [27, 28].

According to the trans-membrane pH gradient, weak bases can concentrate in liposomes. Liposome formation is dependent on two critical steps: the formation of a pH gradient with a lower intra-liposomal pH and the subsequent loading of the drug. Gradient generation of a trans-membrane proton can be done in a variety of ways. Liposomes are made in citrate buffer, and then transferred to a pH 7.5 buffer by an exogenous buffer exchange. Ionophores, on the other hand, can be employed with action gradients. Ultimately, liposomes developed in the presence of significant amounts of ammonium sulphate (**Figure 8**). The withdrawal of salt solution causes the creation of a pH gradient, which is also accountable for the drug entrapment mechanism [22, 30, 31].

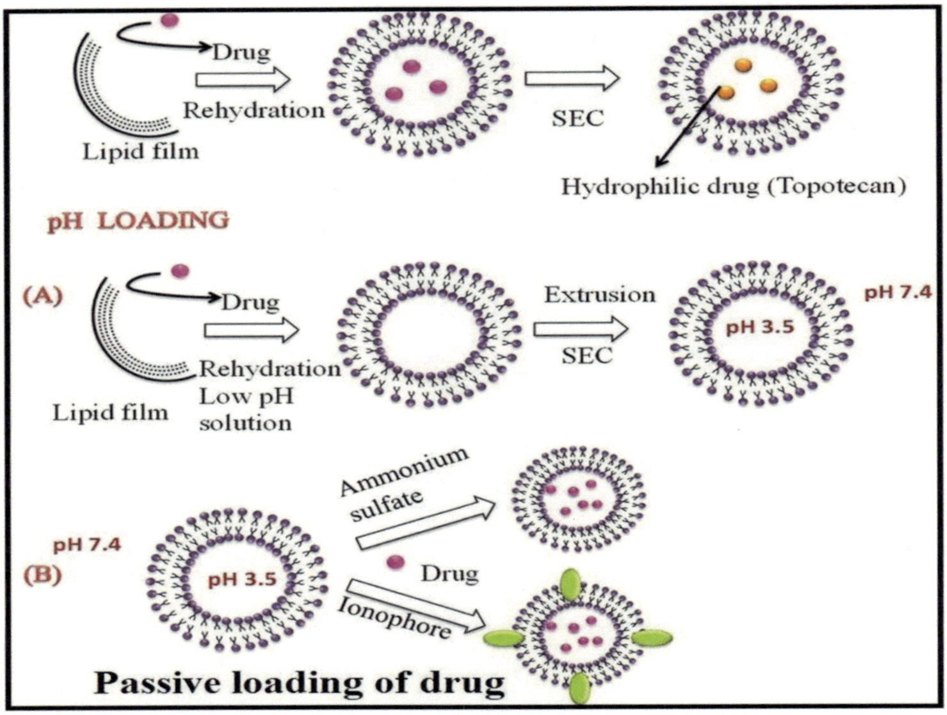

Figure 8.
Passive loading of drug into liposome [29].

5. Drug targeting

Much of the effort in liposome research has been focused on tumour targeting. Liposomes in circulation extravagate through the 'leaky' tumour vasculature; alternatively, attachment of specific antibodies or other proteins to the liposome surface may cause specific targeting. However, the increased clinical efficacy of such targeting in human patients has not been easy to prove. Most of a liposomal drug given intravenously is taken up by phagocytosis into the reticulo-endothelial system, which is extremely efficient at trapping particulate matter circulating intravenously (**Figure 9**). The reticulo-endothelial system may be circumvented by several different methods, such as saturation with large doses of liposome particles or selective macrophage inactivation by pharmacological means However, such a strategy could theoretically further compromise the immune system of cancer patients [33, 34].

Liposomes as a Drug Depot Many drugs are most effective when they are delivered over extended periods of time. For example, agents specific for the division phase of the cell cycle kill cancer cells only when they are dividing. However, even for the most rapidly growing tumours, only a small fraction of the cells are dividing during the drug's residence time. Therefore, depot formulations are needed to maintain therapeutic concentrations for prolonged periods. In contrast to biodegradable polymers or chemical modifications of the standard drug, liposomes and other lipid-based formulations have the advantage of not creating a new chemical entity, and the need for extensive toxicological studies is largely avoided. This is especially the case for the more efficient lipid-based drug delivery systems, where the amount of lipid used is small relative to the amount of drug delivered (**Figure 9**). Even if

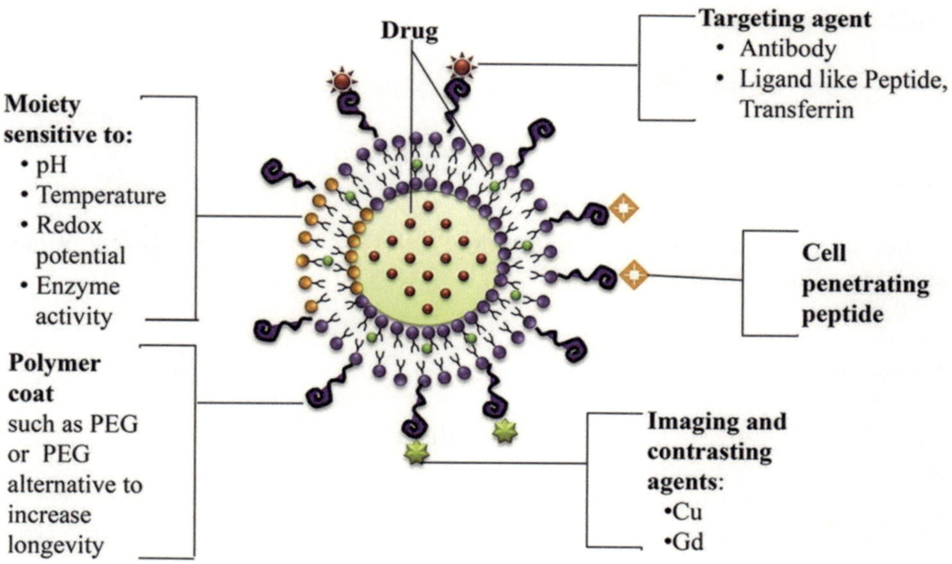

Figure 9.
Liposomal drug delivery to treat cancer [32].

efficacy and toxicity remain unchanged, the convenience and improved patient compliance of fewer painful injections may be sufficient for those drugs that require frequent multiple injections or continuous infusions [35–37].

6. Conclusions

Nowadays drug repurposing and drug targeting through nanoparticulate drug delivery gain significant attention for delivering various APIs in treatment of cancer through oral and topical route successfully. Loading the repurposing drug in to liposomes escalate therapeutic efficacy and residences toxic effects along with patients compliance. Nanomedicines could be easily surface modified to passively and actively target tumour cells and cellular components. Therefore, nanomedicines composed of repurposed drug could be preferred over plain drugs or their conventional generic dosage forms currently available in the market. The advantages of various methodologies and strategies for drug targeting are outlined in the current chapter, along with information on liposomal drug targeting, liposomal structure, mechanism of liposomal drug loading, and liposomal drug targeting. Drug repurposing and liposomal drug targeting are potent methods for enhancing solubility and bioavailability, minimizing side effects, and developing innovative drug delivery systems to increase the therapeutic effectiveness of drug repurposing to treat cancer.

Acknowledgements

The authors are thankful to Department of Pharmaceutics Sant Gajanan Maharaj College of Pharmacy Mahagaon and Trustees of Sant Gajanan Maharaj College of Pharmacy Mahagaon for providing required guidance and support for completion of this work.

Conflict of interest

The authors declare no conflict of interest.

Notes/thanks/other declarations

Special thanks to **Supriya S. Galatage** and **Shivtej S. Galatage** for their continuous support throughout the work.

Abbreviations

API	active pharmaceutical ingredient
HA	hyaluronic acid
LP	liposomes
PCB	poly carboxybetaine
PEG	poly ethylene glycol
NDDS	nanoparticulate drug delivery
WHO	World Health Organization
EPR	enhanced permeability and retention effect

Author details

Sunil T. Galatage[1*], Arehalli S. Manjappa[2,3], Raghwendra R. Waghmode[4], Swapnil S. Harale[1], Rushikesh B. Katkar[5], Sujit A. Desai[6], Swapnil S. Chopade[2], Kranti S. Bille[1], Rubina U. Watangi[1], Shweta N. Kalebere[7], Aditya S. Hebalkar[8], Shradhey V. Dhobale[9], Harshada N. Gunjate[1], Poonam R. Dhenge[1], Purva S. Ikke[1], Saheblal A. Shaikh[1], Rutuja J. Patil[1], Sakshi B. Shinde[1], Rutuja V. Khatavakar[1], Anuja B. Patil[1], Prajakta N. Khatavakar[1], Sourabh S. Hegaje[2] and Suresh G. Killedar[1]

1 Sant Gajanan Maharaj College of Pharmacy Mahagaon, Maharashtra, India

2 Tatyasaheb Kore College of Pharmacy, Kolhapur, Maharashtra, India

3 Vasantidevi Patil Institute of Pharmacy, Kolhapur, Maharashtra, India

4 Krishna Institute of Pharmacy, Krishna Vishwa Vidyapeeth, Karad, Maharashtra, India

5 Vijayrao Naik College of Pharmacy, Shirval Kankavali, Maharashtra, India

6 Annasaheb Dange College of D Pharmacy, Ashta, Walawa, Maharashtra, India

7 Genesis Institute of Pharmacy, Radhanagari, Maharashtra, India

8 IQVIA Biotech, Thane, Maharashtra, India

9 National Institute of Pharmaceutical Education and Research (NIPER), Ahmadabad, India

*Address all correspondence to: gsunil201288@gmail.com

References

[1] Reza Mozafari M, Johnson C, Hatziantoniou S, Demetzos C. Nanoliposomes and their applications in food nanotechnology. Journal of Liposome Research. 2008;**18**(4):309-327

[2] Laliani G, Sorboni SG, Lari R, Yaghoubi A, Soleimanpour S, Khazaei M, et al. Bacteria and cancer: Different sides of the same coin. Life Sciences. 2020;**246**:117398

[3] Sawant S, Shegokar R. Cancer research and therapy: Where are we today. International Journal of Cancer Therapy and Oncology. 2014;**2**(4):02048

[4] Weilbaecher KN, Guise TA, McCauley LK. Cancer to bone: A fatal attraction. Nature Reviews Cancer. 2011;**11**(6):411-425

[5] Misra R, Acharya S, Sahoo SK. Cancer nanotechnology: Application of nanotechnology in cancer therapy. Drug Discovery Today. 2010;**15**(19-20):842-850

[6] Bayda S, Adeel M, Tuccinardi T, Cordani M, Rizzolio F. The history of nanoscience and nanotechnology: From chemical–physical applications to nanomedicine. Molecules. 2019;**25**(1):112

[7] Loomans-Kropp HA, Umar A. Cancer prevention and screening: The next step in the era of precision medicine. NPJ Precision Oncology. 2019;**3**(1):1-8

[8] Greene RJ, Harris ND. Pathology and Therapeutics for Pharmacists. London: Pharmaceutical Press; 2020

[9] Schirrmacher V. From chemotherapy to biological therapy: A review of novel concepts to reduce the side effects of systemic cancer treatment. International Journal of Oncology. 2019;**54**(2):407-419

[10] Masuda T, Tsuruda Y, Matsumoto Y, Uchida H, Nakayama KI, Mimori K. Drug repositioning in cancer: The current situation in Japan. Cancer Science. 2020;**111**(4):1039-1046

[11] Shim JS, Liu JO. Recent advances in drug repositioning for the discovery of new anticancer drugs. International Journal of Biological Sciences. 2014;**10**(7):654

[12] Pandita V, Parihar A, Parihar DS, Panda S, Shanmugarajan D, Kumari L, et al. System and network biology-based computational approaches for drug repositioning. In: Computational Approaches for Novel Therapeutic and Diagnostic Designing to Mitigate SARS-CoV-2 Infection. 2022. pp. 267-290. DOI: 10.1016/B978-0-323-91172-6.00003-0. Epub 2022 Jul 15. PMCID: PMC9300680

[13] Pantziarka P, Verbaanderd C, Sukhatme V, Capistrano IR, Crispino S, Gyawali B, et al. ReDO_DB: The repurposing drugs in oncology database. Ecancermedicalscience. 2018;**2**:1-12

[14] Abbruzzese C, Matteoni S, Signore M, Cardone L, Nath K, Glickson JD, et al. Drug repurposing for the treatment of glioblastoma multiforme. Journal of Experimental & Clinical Cancer Research. 2017;**36**(1):1-11

[15] Nishimura Y, Tagawa M, Ito H, Tsuruma K, Hara H. Overcoming obstacles to drug repositioning in Japan. Frontiers in Pharmacology. 2017;**8**:729

[16] Ahmed K, Shaw HV, Koval A, Katanaev VL. A second WNT for old drugs: Drug repositioning against

WNT-dependent cancers. Cancers. 2016;**8**(7):66

[17] Pawar HR, Bhosale SS, Derle ND. Use of liposomes in cancer therapy: A review. International Journal of Pharmaceutical Sciences and Research. 2012;**3**(10):3585

[18] Dalton LR, Press CRC, editors. EPR and Advanced EPR Studies of Biological Systems. Vol. 1. Boca Raton: CRC Press; 1985. pp. 1-10

[19] Finean JB, Rumsby MG. Negatively stained lipoprotein membranes. Nature. 1963;**200**(4913):1340-1340

[20] Bangham AD, Horne RW. Action of saponin on biological cell membranes. Nature. 1962;**196**(4858):952-953

[21] Bangham AD, Horne RW. Negative staining of phospholipids and their structural modification by surface-active agents as observed in the electron microscope. Journal of Molecular Biology. 1964;**8**(5):660-IN10

[22] Gomez-Hens A, Fernandez-Romero JM. Analytical methods for the control of liposomal delivery systems. TrAC Trends in Analytical Chemistry. 2006;**25**(2):167-178

[23] Barani H, Montazer M. A review on applications of liposomes in textile processing. Journal of Liposome Research. 2008;**18**(3):249-262

[24] Meure LA, Knott R, Foster NR, Dehghani F. The depressurization of an expanded solution into aqueous media for the bulk production of liposomes. Langmuir. 2009;**25**(1):326-337

[25] Zhang L, Gu FX, Chan JM, Wang AZ, Langer RS, Farokhzad OC. Nanoparticles in medicine: Therapeutic applications and developments. Clinical Pharmacology & Therapeutics. 2008;**83**(5):761-769

[26] Patra JK, Das G, Fraceto LF, Campos EVR, Rodriguez-Torres MDP, Acosta-Torres LS, et al. Nano based drug delivery systems: Recent developments and future prospects. Journal of Nanobiotechnology. 2018;**16**(1):1-33

[27] Shoji Y, Nakashima H. Nutraceutics and delivery systems. Journal of Drug Targeting. 2004;**12**(6):385-391

[28] Weaver CM, Dwyer J, Fulgoni VL III, King JC, Leveille GA, MacDonald RS, et al. Processed foods: Contributions to nutrition. The American Journal of Clinical Nutrition. 2014;**99**(6):1525-1542

[29] Mbah CC, Builders PF, Attama AA. Nanovesicular carriers as alternative drug delivery systems: Ethosomes in focus. Expert Opinion on Drug Delivery. 2014;**11**(1):45-59

[30] Imaizumi K. Digestive absorption and physiological activity of phospholipids in clinical nutrition. The American Journal of Clinical Nutrition. 1999;**1**:127-134

[31] Kryou C, Leva V, Chatzipetrou M, Zergioti I. Bioprinting for liver transplantation. Bioengineering. 2019;**6**(4):95

[32] Saraf S, Jain A, Tiwari A, Verma A, Panda PK, Jain SK. Advances in liposomal drug delivery to cancer: An overview. Journal of Drug Delivery Science and Technology. 2020;**56**:101549

[33] Shelke O, Kulkarni A. Formulation, development and evaluation of nano ethosomal gel of tramadol hydrochloride. Journal of Nanomedicine & Nanotechnology. 2018;**9**:514

[34] Verma P, Pathak K. Therapeutic and cosmeceutical potential of ethosomes:

An overview. Journal of Advanced Pharmaceutical Technology & Research. 2010;**1**(3):274

[35] Kumar N, Dubey A, Mishra A, Tiwari P. Ethosomes: A novel approach in transdermal drug delivery system. International Journal of Pharmacy & Life Sciences. 2020;**11**(5):1-7

[36] Jain NK. Controlled and Novel Drug Delivery. Daria Gang, New Delhi: CBS publishers & distributors; 1997. pp. 101-127

[37] Vyas SP, Khar RK. Controlled drug delivery concepts and advances. vallabh prakashan. 2002;**1**:411-447

Chapter 2

A Computational Approach for Identifying Experimental or Approved Drugs That Can Be Repurposed for the Treatment of Type-2 Diabetes

Gemma Topaz, Dongjun Yoo, Richard Anderson and Kimberly Stieglitz

Abstract

Approved and experimental drugs can be utilized for new indications as illustrated in the case study presented herein. In this case study, allopurinol (trade name Zyloprim and Aloprim) which is currently utilized for gout, was retrieved from the Drug Bank and evaluated for a new indication. Utilizing a catechin derivative as a scaffold, a derivative was designed incorporating allopurinol. This novel molecule was predicted to act as an allosteric inhibitor of fructose 1,6-bisphosphatase (FBPase), a control point for entry into the biochemical pathway gluconeogenesis. The predicted inhibition was validated with a colorimetric assay. Potential toxicity was assessed using a HepG2 MTT assay. As an inhibitor of this enzyme, the novel molecule proved to be both potent and non-toxic in cell-based assays. Once optimized and tested *in vivo*, the novel molecule may be potentially used as a therapeutic agent for type-2 diabetes mellitus inhibiting FBPase. This action prevents the *de novo* synthesis of glucose and potentially contributes to lowering blood glucose levels for patient populations that are genetically prone to chronic high blood glucose leading to insulin resistance. The computational approach to the design of the novel potential lead compound is discussed in detail and validation data presented.

Keywords: allosteric regulation, enzyme inhibition, structure-based drug discovery, geometric docking, molecular dynamics

1. Introduction

Type-2 diabetes mellitus is recognized as a global epidemic by the World Health Organization with an estimated 500 million affected worldwide. The Center for Disease Control (CDC) estimates that 30 million in the US are affected. Most of this is caused by lifestyle and improper diet, a direct result of the mismanagement of agricultural and food distribution systems. Certain populations, such as Native Americans and Polynesians, appear to be predisposed to type-2 diabetes. This might be a result of genetic adaptations brought on by chronic food scarcity [1]. In both cases, type-2 diabetes is characterized by impaired insulin sensitivity or availability and increased endogenous glucose production (EGP). The primary source of EGP is gluconeogenesis in the liver, which is typically three-fold greater in type-2 diabetics. It is widely recognized that when gluconeogenesis is curtailed, this provides a valuable therapy for type-2 diabetes [2]. Analysis of the gluconeogenesis pathway has suggested that the best target for inhibition is the fructose 1,6-bisphosphatase (FBPase) enzyme. Yet after many years of work, there is no FBPase inhibitor that has reached the market. The FBPase molecule is a homotetramer, each monomer with an active site and two allosteric binding sites. The active site contains highly conserved amino acids and so is not a suitable drug target. The AMP binding site is an allosteric site, which has been known and targeted for many years for drug development [1–4]. A novel allosteric site was discovered at the tetramer interface by Pfizer [5]. Although a potent inhibitory site, the volume of the pocket is made up of contributions from the four monomers and is highly mobile, so there is difficulty in predicting the actual binding modes of selected molecules. In addition, a 2:1 molar ratio of drug to protein is often required for effective inhibition, which makes drug studies challenging. This study focuses on the FBPase protein target AMP binding site relying heavily on similarity searches with the natural inhibitor AMP.

Herein is a case study focused on the early stages of the development of an FBPase inhibitor (lead compound) that targets the adenosine monophosphate (AMP) allosteric binding site is presented. This has led to the computational identification and assay verification of several effective compounds in the Drug Bank database. The compounds are currently approved drugs. If any of these drugs can be fully verified to be effective for a new application, this could lead to a breakthrough treatment for type-2 diabetes mellitus.

2. Strategies and methods

As shown in **Figure 1**, the repurposing workflow is a linear process. The process begins with literature searches then similarity searches of known inhibitors with searches of the Drug Bank database [6]. Once compounds are identified, molecular docking is done using AutoDock Vina for both fixed and flexible (side chain) docking protocols [7]. Molecular dynamics follows for accurate physiological check on the binding score of the ligand/protein complex [8] followed by laboratory validation [9]. In the hit-to-lead optimization stage, there was a reiterative process of modifying the hit repurposed compound (treated as a scaffolding compound) with substituted functional groups. This process refines the molecule eliminating derivatives issues such as low solubility, cellular toxicity, and PAINS (pan assay interference screening) before proceeding to optimize the lead compound for *in vivo* animal studies and finally clinical trials.

Key research performed already published that supports this strategy includes:

1. The ZINC15 database of 3D structures of small molecules [10].

2. The Drug Bank database of approved and experimental drugs [6].

3. The 3D structures of human and pig liver fructose 1,6-bisphosphatase (FBPase), PDB code 1FTA [11], and 1KZ8 [5] for FBPase in complex with AMP.

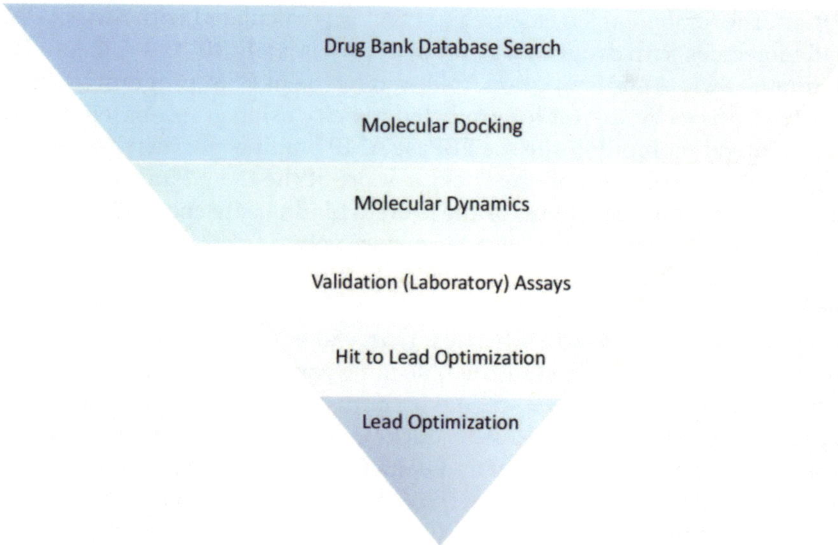

Figure 1.
A virtual drug development platform (VDDP): a schematic representation of repurposing workflow.

4. Colorimetric assays able to confirm inhibition of FBPase [12, 13].

5. Site-directed mutagenesis studies on FBPase used to validate binding site residues and significant residues for allosteric mechanism [11, 13, 14].

6. The recognition of the AMP binding site on fructose 1,6-biphosphatase as an important allosteric drug target for type-2 diabetes [2–4, 11–14].

7. A 2- stage process of docking and molecular dynamics to screen millions of compounds [15].

Research conducted by symmetric computing supports this case study includes the development of the virtual drug discovery platform (VDDP), which performs high throughput virtual screening by combining molecular docking with molecular dynamics. Screening of millions of small molecules from the ZINC15 database was done using VDDP, in order to identify high-scoring binders to the AMP binding site on fructose 1,6-biphosphatase. Identification of high-scoring binders that are Phase I approved deployed or experimental drugs that were also included in the Drug Bank database were cross-referenced.

3. Flexible docking and MD protocols

3.1 Preparation of small molecules and protein target for MD and geometric docking

Once repurposing molecules for the target were identified through literature searches to be the appropriate for alternative medicinal activities, the PubChem and Drug Bank database was searched these compounds and derivatives. Following identification, the total polar surface area (TPSA) was calculated with SwissADME [16]. Small molecules with druggable TPSA of approximately 90–120 A^2 [16–18] were fed into the SwissADME program, followed by the pkCSM program to screen for central ADMET properties to test for predicted toxicity using graph-based patterns [17]. The protein target binding site the FBPase AMP binding site was then selected based on geometric attributes and the docking score of the Drug Bank scaffolds. More specifically, the geometric attributes of the protein binding site coordinates were selected according to the ratio of molecular surface volume of the cavity over the total molecular surface volume of the protein. Ratios below 0.15 A^3 were not considered druggable target binding sites [19]. In addition, the docking score of the ligand to the protein was considered reasonable when less than ~50 micromolar. Once the protein target binding site was correctly identified, docking was performed with all of the selected drugs for repurposing (n = ~525) with both flexible and rigid residues. After initial docking (rigid) followed by flexible docking, a molecular dynamics protocol in NAMD was executed to check contacts and delta G of binding scores. Since convergence with flexible docking scores and MD scores occurred, flexible docking was used for drugs that were then altered with specific functional groups for further protein/drug docking studies.

The initial workflow for ligand and FBPase protein target preparation is shown in **Figure 2**. Two protein target PDBs that were chosen of FBPase were 1KZ8 [5] and 1FTA [2] to capture the AMP binding site and the dimer and tetramer interfaces in different starting conformations.

A guide of the initial identification of potentially druggable binding sites for a given target and previously approved drugs appropriate for drug repurposing studies.

Initially, the RCSB was searched for human and pig kidney structures of FBPase as these species have >85% identity and ~95% homology of amino acid sequences. Although the location of the AMP binding site of FBPase is known, the conformation of the amino acid side chains that make up the "gateway" and interior of the binding site change position when substrate or product is bound in the active site. The enzyme has two canonical states the T state known as inactive state and the R state the active state. The enzyme rotates around the dimer interface of the tetramer. Since the AMP binding site is on exterior side of the homotetramer on each monomer individual amino acid side chains shift position during this rotation.

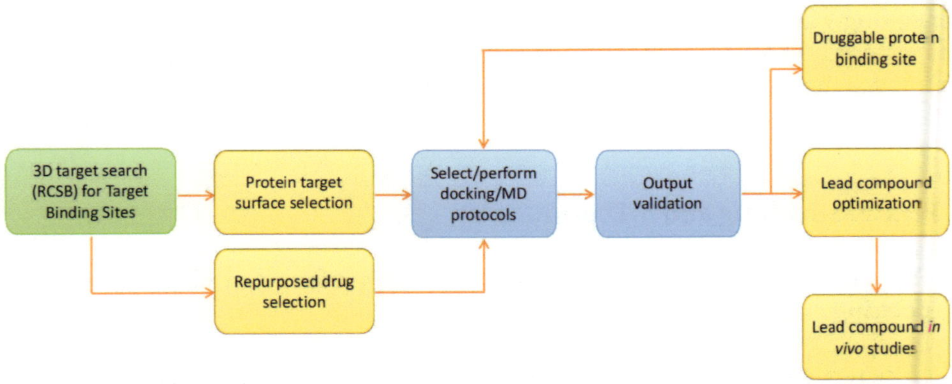

Figure 2.
Ligand/protein target computational platform workflow chart.

DOI: http://dx.doi.org/10.5772/intechopen.110812

The repurposed drugs were selected based on similarity searches to natural allosteric inhibitor in both PubChem and Drug Bank databases. Once the protein target center of position coordinates are selected and the repurposed drugs identified, static docking followed by flexible docking was done with the FBPase-repurposed drug complex. After molecular docking, the coordinates were run in MD protocols to check overall energy of the system and calculate the binding energy of the protein-drug complex. From the output from the VDDP, repurposed drugs from the Drug Bank were chosen for laboratory validation, derivatized as needed to enhance binding and the process of optimization towards lead compounds was done. In addition, the processed target protein can be "recycled" in its altered conformation out of MD to be tested with other repurposed drugs. In a reiterative process tailored to each small molecule, different amino acids can be made flexible prior to computationally expensive MD, simulating an induced fit model of protein-ligand binding using the platform. The reiterative process of flexible docking coupled with MD protocols decreases the computational time to generate new protein conformers significantly.

4. Molecular dynamics

4.1 MD simulations

Preparations for MD simulations were done using SwissDock parameter files for the catechin derivatives for MD [20]. The protein structure files were generated with docked ligands in VMD [21]. Molecular dynamics simulations were performed with the NAMD Program [8] using CHARMM37 parameters along with complementary CHARMM General Force Field optimized for ligand parameter files for each protein target/catechin derivative complex [22]. Periodic boundary conditions were imposed and explicit solvent/implicit solvent boundaries defined using a truncated rectangular box, ensuring a solvent shell of at least 10 A around the solute surrounding the protein-ligand complex. The solute was neutralized with potassium ions (K^+/Cl^- ion pairs) to a concentration of 150 mM. The ions were initially placed at random, but at least 5 A from ligands and 3.5 A from one another. The resulting systems contained between 10,500 and 15,250 water molecules, corresponding to a total of 30–45,000 atoms.

Simulations employed periodic boundary conditions and electrostatic interactions were treated using the particle-mesh Ewald algorithm [23, 24] with a real space cutoff of pair list was built with a buffer region, and a list update was triggered whenever a particle moved by more than 0.5 A with respect to the previous update. Each system was initially subjected to energy minimization with harmonic restraints of 2 kcal mol^{-1} $A^{\circ -2}$ on the solute atoms. The system was then heated to 310 K at constant volume during 100 ps. Constraints were then relaxed from 5 to 1 kcal mol^{-1} $A^{\circ\ -2}$ during a series of 1000 steps of energy minimization (500 steps of steepest descent and 500 steps of conjugate gradient) followed by 50 ps of equilibration with restraints of 0.5 mol^{-1} $A^{\circ -2}$ and 50 ps without solute restraints. The 50 ns production simulations were carried out at constant temperature (300 K) and pressure (1 bar) with a 2 fs time step. This was reiterated 10×. During these simulations, pressure and temperature were maintained using the Berendsen algorithm [25] with a coupling constant of 5 ps, and SHAKE constraints were applied to all bonds involving hydrogens [26]. Conformational snapshots were saved for further analysis every 10 ps.

For comparison purposes, the isolated catechin complexes from each complex were also simulated alone using an identical protocol, creating a second set of ten 50 ns trajectories.

4.2 Potential energy of binding and free energy of binding calculations for MD output

The overall potential energy of protein-ligand system was evaluated by adding the final potential energy of the small molecule alone, and the final potential energy of the protein alone run through the same MD protocol. These values were compared with the protein/ligand complex. An expected, drop in the potential energy of the complex was confirmed. Absolute binding free energy (ABFE) calculation, with total annihilation of the ligand in the binding pocket followed by its reappearance at bulk state where the target protein was absent, was part of this process. As free energy is a state function, the alchemical FEP route to getting binding free energy of these derivates was as follows: (1) 'locking the ligand', restraining conformational, translational, and rotational degrees of freedom at bound state, (2) 'disappearing the locked ligand', turning off the interaction between ligand and its surroundings, (3) 'translocating ligand' of which corresponding free energy is zero, (4) 'reappearance of the locked ligand', turning on the interaction between ligand and its surroundings at bulk state, and (5) 'unlocking the ligand', releasing of the three restraints from [1]. Lenselink et al. tested binding free energies of congeneric ligands to four different using FEP+ from Schrödinger and obtained results in great agreement with our experimental results [27].

5. Laboratory validation

In order to validate the binding of the Drug Bank compounds, colorimetric kinetic assays were conducted. To perform these tests recombinant FBPase protein was over-expressed and purified. The construct was transformed into competent cells, and the purified construct used to over-express protein, which was harvested and purified prior to use.

5.1 Transformation(s) and purification of FBPase plasmid

Plasmids containing FBPase sequence underwent transformation with XL Blue super-competent cells [13]. Cells were plated on Luria Bertani (LB) agar plates and colonies selected for 5 mL overnights for plasmid purification using various kits [28]. Following purification, FBPase plasmids were screened for integrity and run on an agarose gel and sequenced. A transformation protocol for over-expression was then performed as previously described [13]. The contents of the tubes were transferred to LB ampicillin plates using a sterile technique. Plates were incubated for 18 h at 37°C and stored for 2.5 weeks at 4°C.

5.2 Protein over-expression, isolation, and purification

To prepare the recombinant human or closely related pig kidney FBPase enzymes for kinetic and binding assays, the recombinant proteins were over-expressed, isolated, and purified as previously described using ampicillin resistance for selection of cells containing the construct [13]. Briefly, the host cell translation was inhibited with 34 mg/mL chloramphenicol (in isopropanol). The solution was shaken again for 2–3 h at 37°C to ensure optimal growth of the host cells. Cells were isolated by pelleting in 250 mL flasks in a centrifuge at 4000 rpm. After the cells were frozen, each cell pellet was resuspended in 20 mL of 50 mM Tris pH 7.5. The supernatant was lysed *via* sonication to release cell contents. Each protein solution was sonicated as previously described. Sonication settings were at 10% duty cycle for 5 min, pulsing 10 s on, and 10 s off ×3. Each supernatant cell lysate was centrifuged for 30 min at 13,500 rpm at 4°C and transferred to dialysis tubing for dialysis in 50 mM Tris pH 8.0. Protein was then purified *via* NTA nickel affinity column as previously described [13]. In addition, gel filtration was run on a G250 column in Tris buffer pH 7.5 in 0.150 M NaCl as eluent buffer to investigate the oligomeric status of inhibitor-bound protein compared to FBPase enzyme alone.

5.3 Characterization of purified recombinant enzymes and preparation for enzyme kinetic assays

The purity of the recombinant FBPase was assessed *via* SDS-PAGE, and the oligomeric state was identified with native gel electrophoresis. An SDS-PAGE gel electrophoresis was used to separate and identify proteins with the correct molecular weight [9]. For the kinetic assay, a standard curve was obtained from an ammonium molybdate malachite green inorganic phosphate assay (OD660 nm) [5, 6]. The purified FBPase protein was dialyzed ×3 in 50 mM Tris buffer at pH 7.5 at 4°C. For enzyme concentration, absorbency values were recorded using spectrophotometer readings at OD280 nm. To quantify enzyme concentration, the enzyme concentration was calculated based on the quantity of micrograms per microliter (μg/μL) present. Final concentration FBPase enzyme was between 2.5 and 5.0 μg/μL. Using a colorimetric assay as described below, specific activity (SA) was determined in the absence and presence of Drug Bank inhibitors.

5.4 Kinetic assays on FBPase/ligand complexes

A colorimetric malachite green kinetic assay was utilized for FBpase activity levels to validate inhibition of the enzyme predicted with selected Drug Bank molecules. FBPase cleaves fructose 1,6-bisphosphate to fructose 6 phosphate and inorganic phosphate. The malachite green colorimetric assay is based on the change in color from brown to blue, observed when a complex is formed between malachite green, ammonium molybdate, and the product inorganic phosphate. For calculating Ki values, data was collected with varying substrate FBP concentrations (100–500 μM at pH 7.5). Malachite green dye was prepared under acidic conditions to activate the color change and quench the FBPase activity at fixed time points [13]. Absorbance readings were recorded at OD660 nm. Data collected was input to the inorganic phosphate standard curve equation to calculate product formed. Micromoles of product inorganic phosphate were calculated to determine the specific activity (SA) of FBPase enzyme +/− inhibitor. The IC50 assay was designed with fixed high concentration of substrate varying the inhibitor concentration to calculate IC50 values. For each Drug Bank ligand, the kinetic assay was performed in duplicates of triplicates. All kinetic data were fit using origin software based on methods previously described [13]. More specifically, for kinetic parameters established to fin Ki's *via* curve fitting the equation $y = d + (a - d) / 1 + (x / c)b$ was used where "x" is represented by apparent Ki when y = Vmax. IC50s were also determined with origin curve-fitting software [29].

To avoid high background due to malachite green dye interaction with some Drug Bank ligands cleavage assays utilizing phosphoglucose isomerase and glucose-6-phosphate dehydrogenase were used as coupling enzymes in validation assays for FBPase [18]. For specific activity measurements, reduction of NADP to NADPH was monitored by absorbance at 340 nm. Other assays used the same coupling enzymes but monitored the formation of NADPH by its fluorescence emission at 470 nm using an excitation wavelength of 340 nm. Assays were performed at 22°C in 50 mM Hepes, pH 7.5. Data for inhibitor (inhibition) were fit to several models using origin or sigma plot software with a Hill equation model [6]. These assays are robust and unbiased as they follow the ASBMB standard for rigor and reproducibility [30]. In addition, these assays have been published in many peer reviewed research articles [1–5, 14].

6. Case study analysis and discussion

6.1 Case study: allopurinol as a scaffolding molecule for drug design

The approved Drug Bank compound allopurinol is already on the market to relieve symptoms of gout. Also known as Zyloprim and Aloprim, allopurinol is composed of a dihydroxy substituted pyrimidine ring that is fused to a pyrazole ring. Allopurinol is shown below in green in **Figure 3A**. Allopurinol alone is not large enough to bind to the entire allosteric binding site, and more than one allopurinol molecule may bind at a time resulting in a 1:2 binding ratio. For every target allosteric binding site, 2 allopurinol compounds can fit in the allosteric binding pocket. In this study, allopurinol molecules docked in the FBPase AMP binding site were used as scaffolding molecules upon which functional groups were added to enhance their binding affinity for the FBPase. As shown below in **Figure 3A**, allopurinol top scoring position (Ki ~300 micomolar) overlays with the crystallographic AMP molecule adenine ring. Interestingly, with another allopurinol docked, the predicted Ki dropped to ~150 micromolar. The residues shown here Phe184, Leu173, Glu20, Val160, Arg140, Tyr113, Lys112, Glu 29, and Thr27 were all separately made flexible during reiterative runs of docking followed by full-scale MD runs for scoring predicted Ki's. In **Figure 3B**, the Zinc38643891 (pink) literally straddles the AMP binding site. The predicted Ki is ~50 nM for this catechin derivative discovered in the PubChem database after similarity searches for catechin EGCG as previously described (ref). Note when compared to the crystallographic position of the AMP co-crystallized with FBPase in PDB 1FTA, the predicted position of the phenyl ring aligns in the position where the adenine ring is located. Leu174, Phe184, and Val60 alternate to interact with the zinc molecule and stabilize its position during simulations. During simulations the helix behind these three residues shifts slightly out of position causing a "domino effect" and the zinc molecule moves deeper into the AMP binding site cleft.

Figure 3C shows the best docking pose predicted for Zinc38643891 and allopurinol. This figure illustrates how allopurinol may be modified to bind tighter by derivatizing the heterocyclic ring. Details of the synthesis are preserved for a future manuscript.

Figure 3A shows the 1FTA protein coordinates with a close-up of the AMP binding site with the crystallographic ligand AMP in dark gray. The best score for the docked allopurinol is in green. **Figure 3B** shows the same coordinates docked with a catechin derivative (pink) from the PubChem database cross-referenced to the zinc database

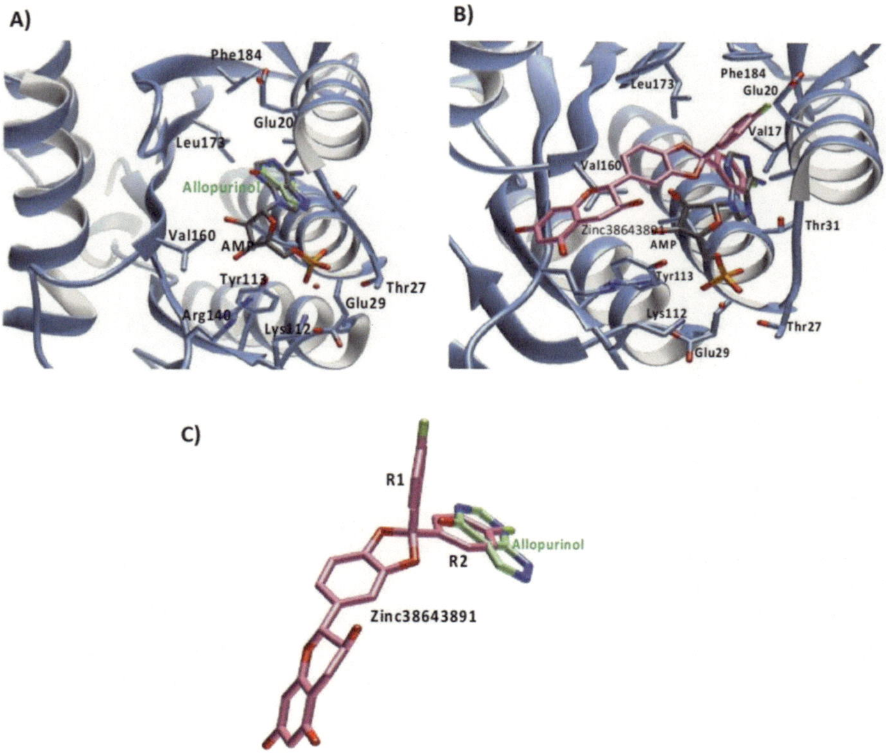

Figure 3.
Docking of allopurinol and Zinc38643891 into the AMP allosteric binding site of FBPase.

as Zinc38643891. **Figure 3C** shows the best docking results of the two compounds Zinc38643891 (pink) and allopurinol (green).

Figure 4A shows allopurinol derivative (orange) and Zinc38643891 (blue) in an FBPase activity assay showing relative activity as a function of compound concentration. The average specific activity of each concentration (triplicates) was normalized against FBPase with no inhibitor. **Figure 4B** shows the relative viability of HepG2 cells as a function of inhibitor concentration. The raw data from the MTT assay was normalized with HepG2 cells with no inhibitor present.

As shown in **Figure 4A**, both the allopurinol derivative and Zinc inhibit the activity of the isolated recombinant FBPase activity with ~50% inhibition in the low nanomolar range. The allopurinol derivative reaches the 50% inhibition mark at exactly 100 nM whereas the Zinc compound reaches 50% inhibition at ~25 nM, nearly 4-fold more potent than the allopurinol derivative in this cell-free activity assay. This is considered a promising hit for moving forward in the drug development pipeline to a lead compound.

However, it was surprising in **Figure 4B** that within the same concentration range, the Zinc38643891 was at 50% viability in the MTT viability assay with the HepG2 cells. Whereas the allopurinol derivative remained 90% viable in this range and beyond. In fact, allopurinol did not show significant drop in viability until the mid-high micromolar range. Initially, the expectation was that a derivative of a natural product catechin, the Zinc compound would have a better toxicological profile. The allopurinol derivative of Zinc38643891 was able to overcome the toxicological barrier of the original zinc molecule by substituting out the fluorophenyl rings for allopurinol in a novel synthesis

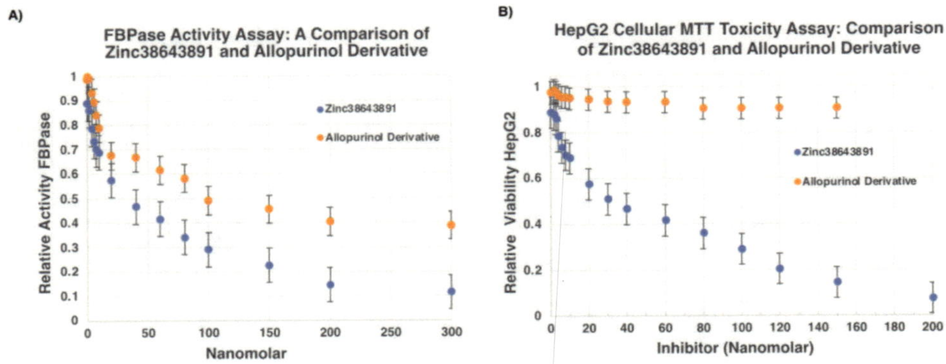

Figure 4.
Inhibition and toxicity assays comparing Zinc38643891 and sllopurinol derivative.

protocol (manuscript under preparation). Insights from this case study that have led to the synthesis of the novel allopurinol derivative were discovered by visual analysis of the output frames of the MD runs of the allopurinol and Zinc38643891 protein-ligand complexes. During this visual inspection process (which was laborious), it became apparent that the allopurinol molecule(s) in the allosteric binding site were localizing in the same area as Zinc38643891 fluorophenyl rings. The VDDP was an integral part of the drug discovery process for this project. Currently, the lead compound(s) from this case study are being evaluated for *in vivo* studies.

7. Conclusions

Using our virtual drug discovery platform, symmetric computing has identified potential therapeutic small molecules used as scaffolding molecules that are approved drugs. The repurposed compounds were selected based on theoretical binding score (Ki) of the FBPase protein-compound complex. Initial validation in a colorimetric enzymatic inhibitory assay and a toxicity assay led the way to derivatives of these repurposed drugs from validated hits to lead optimization. The next steps to validate the predicted activity of each of these compounds would be an animal model (*in vivo* studies targeting the liver) utilizing a rat animal model. In the future, a decision will be made on which Drug Bank derivative will be advanced to human clinical studies.

Acknowledgements

We thank Jason Gao of Northeastern University for the use of the NMR facility to track synthesis of the Drug Bank derivatives. Also thank you to Jeffrey Turner and the symmetric computing support staff for this project, and Professor Nurit Haspel for valuable insight and discussions on the molecular dynamics protocols. As well as the Biotechnology Division at Roxbury Community College. Thank you to Northeastern Professional Studies College Department of Biotechnology for assistance with HepG2 toxicity assays.

Conflict of interest

None.

Author details

Gemma Topaz[1], Dongjun Yoo[2], Richard Anderson[1] and Kimberly Stieglitz[1*]

1 Venture Development Center, Symmetric Computing Inc., University of Massachusetts Boston, Boston, USA

2 University of Massachusetts Boston Psychology Department, Boston, USA

*Address all correspondence to: kstieglitz@rcc.mass.edu

References

[1] Kelley-Loughnane N, Kantrowitz ER. AMP inhibition of pig kidneyfructose-1,6-bisphosphatase. Biochimica et Biophysica Acta. 2001;**1548**(1): 66-71

[2] Hines JK, Kruesel CE, Fromm HJ, Honzatko RB. Structure of inhibited fructose-1,6-bisphosphatase from *Escherichia coli*: Distinct allosteric inhibition sites for AMP and glucose 6-phosphate and the characterization of a gluconeogenic switch. Journal of Biological Chemistry. 2007;**282**(34):24697-24706

[3] Heng S, Gryncel KR, Kantrowitz ER. A library of novel allosteric inhibitors against fructose 1,6-bisphosphatase. Bioorganic & Medicinal Chemistry. 2009;**17**(11):3916-3922. DOI: 10.1016/j.bmc.2009.04.030

[4] Heng S, Harris KM, Kantrowitz ER. Designing inhibitors against fructose 1,6-bisphosphatase: Exploring natural products for novel inhibitor scaffolds. European Journal of Medicinal Chemistry. 2009;**45**(4):1478-1484. DOI: 10.1016/j.ejmech.2009.12.055

[5] Wright SW, Carlo AA, Carty MD, Danley DE, Hageman DL, Karam GA, et al. Anilinoquinazoline inhibitors of fructose 1,6-bisphosphatase bind at a novelallosteric site: Synthesis, in vitro characterization, and X-ray crystallography. Journal of Medicinal Chemistry. 2002;**45**(18):3865-3877

[6] Wishart DS, Knox C, Guo AC, Cheng D, Shrivastava S, Tzur D, et al. DrugBank: A knowledgebase for drugs, drug actions and drug targets. Nucleic Acids Research. 2008;**36**(Database issue):D901-D906. DOI: 10.1093/nar/gkm958

[7] Trott O, Olson AJ. AutoDockVina: Improving the speed and accuracy of docking with a new scoring function, efficient optimization and multithreading. Journal of Computational Chemistry. 2010;**31**:455-461

[8] Phillips JC, Braun R, Wang W, Gumbart J, Tajkhorshid E, Villa E, et al. Scalable molecular dynamics with NAMD. Journal of Computational Chemistry. 2005;**26**:1781-1802

[9] Ninfa AJ, Ballou DP, Benore M, Hoboken NJ. Fundamental Laboratory Approaches for Biochemistry and Biotechnology. Wiley: University of Michigan; 2009. p. 161

[10] Sterling T, Irwin JJ. ZINC 15—Ligand discovery for everyone. Journal of Chemical Information and Modeling. 2015;**55**(11):2324-2337. DOI: 10.1021/acs.jcim.5b00559

[11] Gidh-Jain M, Zhang Y, van Poelje PD, Liang JY, Huang S, Kim J, et al. The allosteric site of human liver fructose-1,6-bisphosphatase. Analysis of six AMP site mutants based on the crystal structure. The Journal of Biological Chemistry. 1994;**269**(44):27732-27738

[12] Stieglitz KA, Johnson KA, Yang H, Roberts MF, Seaton BA, Head JF, et al. Crystal structure of a dual activity IMPase/FBPase (AF2372) from Archaeoglobusfulgidus. The story of a mobile loop. The Journal of Biological Chemistry. 2002;**277**(25):22863-22874

[13] Topaz G, Epiter-Smith V, Robalo C, Emad M, Ford V, Daley J, et al. Characterization of recombinant fructose-1,6-bisphosphatase gene mutations: Evidence of inhibition/activation of FBPase protein by

gene mutation. Bioscience Reports. 2019;**39**(2):BSR20180960. DOI: 10.1042/BSR20180960

[14] Kelley-Loughnane N, Kantrowitz ER. Binding of AMP to two of the four subunits of pig kidney fructose-1,6-bisphosphatase induces the allosteric transition. Proteins. 2001;**44**(3):255-261

[15] Shukla R, Shukla H, Sonkar A, Pandey T, Tripathi T. Structure-based screening and molecular dynamics simulations offer novel natural compounds as potential inhibitors of *Mycobacterium tuberculosis* isocitrate lyase. Journal of Biomolecular Structure & Dynamics. 2018;**36**(8):2045-2057. DOI: 10.1080/07391102.2017.1341337

[16] Daina A, Michielin O, Zoete V. SwissADME: A free web tool to evaluate pharmacokinetics, drug-likeness and medicinal chemistry friendliness of small molecules. Scientific Reports. 2017;**3**(7):42717. DOI: 10.1038/srep42717

[17] Pires DEV, Blundell TL, Ascher DB. pkCSM: Predicting small-molecule pharmacokinetic and toxicity properties using graph-based signatures. Journal of Medicinal Chemistry. 2015;**58**(9):4066-4072. DOI: 10.1021/acs.jmedchem.5b00104

[18] Mannhold R. Molecular Drug Properties: Measurement and Prediction. 2007. Print ISBN: 9783527317554 OnlineISBN:9783527621286. DOI: 10.1002/9783527621286

[19] Renee MK, Ervin P, Kazuo K, Ken H, Aleksandra R, Boguslaw S, et al. Shape matters: Improving docking results by prior analysis of geometric attributes of binding sites. JSM Chemistry. 2016;**4**:1020

[20] Grosdidier A, Zoete V, Michielin O. SwissDock, a protein-small molecule docking web service based on EADock DSS. Nucleic Acids Research. 2011;**39**:W270-W277. DOI: 10.1093/nar/gkr366

[21] Humphrey W, Dalke A, Schulten K. VMD—Visual molecular dynamics. Journal of Molecular Graphics. 1996;**14**:33-38

[22] CHARMM36m and the complementary CHARMM General Force Field (CGenFF) have extensively optimized and validated parameters for proteins, lipids, and drug-like ligands (Huang et al., 2017; Klauda et al., 2010; Vanommeslaeghe and MacKerell Jr, 2012)

[23] Available from: https://www.ks.uiuc.edu/Research/namd/2.9/ug/node33.html

[24] Di Pierro M, Elber R, Leimkuhler B. A stochastic algorithm for the isobaric-isothermal ensemble with Ewald summations for all long range forces. Journal of Chemical Theory. 2015;**11**(12):5624-5637. DOI: 10.1021/acs.jctc.5b00648

[25] Berendsen HJC, Postma JPM, van Gunsteren WF, DiNola A, Haak JR. Molecular dynamics with coupling to an external bath. The Journal of Chemical Physics. 1984;**81**:3684-3690

[26] Ryckaert JP, Ciccotti G, Berendsen HJC. Numerical-integration of cartesian equations of motion of a system with constraints—Molecular-dynamics of N-alkanes. Journal of Computational Physics. 1977;**23**:327-341

[27] Lenselink EB, Louvel J, Forti AF, Van Veldhoven JPD, Vries HD, Mulder-Krieger T, et al. Predicting binding affinities for GPCR ligands using free-energy perturbation. ACS Omega. 2016;**1**(2):293-304. DOI: 10.1021/acsomega.6b00086

[28] Zhang S, Cahalan MD. Purifying plasmid DNA from bacterial colonies using the Qiagen Mini prep kit. Journal of Visualized Experiments. 2007;**6**:e247. DOI: 10.3791/247

[29] Di Veroli GY, Fornari C, Goldlust I, Mills G, Boon Koh SB, Bramhall JL, et al. An automated fitting procedure and software for dose-response curves for multiphasic features. Nature Scientific Reports. 2015;**2015**:14701

[30] Fosang AJ, Colbran RJ. Transparency is the key to quality. JBC. 2015;**290**(5):29692-29694

Chapter 3

Targeted Modification of Physical-Chemical Properties of Drugs as a Universal Way to Transform "Old" Drugs into "New" Drugs

Aleksandr Urakov, Natalya Urakova, Yulia Sorokina, Aleksandr Samorodov and Evgeny Fisher

Abstract

Historically, the bulk of known drugs was created for resorptive action. Therefore, the mechanism of action of drugs was attributed to the specific action of the main ingredients once they were absorbed into the bloodstream. In recent years, it has been found that the mechanism of local action of drugs is determined not only by the specific activity of their main ingredients but also by the nonspecific activity of the excipients and formulation ingredients included in the ready-to-use drug: tablet, injectable solution, aerosol, etc. In this regard, there is an opportunity to repurpose drugs by purposefully changing their quality by changing the physical, chemical, and physical-chemical properties of the finished products. As an example, two new groups of drugs intended for local application to dissolve dense pus and discolor blood stains, namely, piolytics and drugs that bleach bruises, have been created. It is shown that the advantage and at the same time the limitation of the upgraded preparations is their local application, as their peculiarity is the realization of the physical-chemical principle of the drug action in local interaction with the selected part of the patient's organism.

Keywords: new drugs, repurposing, physical-chemical features, financial cost, search, development, screening

1. Introduction

Traditional ways of searching for and developing new drugs require large financial, time, and human costs. It is reported that with traditional research design, it would take more than 12 years and $800 million to create a new drug and conduct the entire set of preclinical studies [1, 2]. However, even these costs do not guarantee success, since all traditional drugs have toxicity. Therefore, all drug candidates are traditionally tested for general (resorptive) toxicity. However, no amount of testing can completely eliminate drug toxicity. Therefore, it is no coincidence that most of today's projects aimed at finding and developing new drugs designed for resorptive action are doomed to fail, as they have in the past. In particular, specialists know that under the traditional scheme of search and development of new drugs out of several thousand substances that participated in trials at the beginning of the complex of these trials, only 1–2 substances can survive all trials more or less successfully and obtain the status of a drug [3]. All other substances will be rejected and forgotten.

That is why it is very important to choose the right design for the search and development of new drugs at the very beginning of this journey in order to reduce the risk of a pharmacological project, the financial and human costs, and to win in time. One very profitable decision these days may be the decision to develop a new drug intended not for general (resorptive) but for local application [4, 5]. The essence of this innovation lies in the fact that in order to reduce financial, human, and time costs when searching for and developing new drugs, it is proposed to abandon the idea of discovering absolutely new chemical compounds intended for resorptive action and to aim at modernizing the formulation of "old" (known) drugs by turning them from resorptive drugs into drugs of local action when applied locally. In other words, it is proposed to create new drugs by purposeful changes in the formulation of known drugs providing them with a new mechanism of local action when applied locally. It has been shown that the transformation of drugs known for their general action into drugs with a new mechanism of local action provides a change in their quality indicators and especially in their physicochemical properties [6, 7].

The author's experience in using this design for the search and development of new drugs showed the high promise and competitive benefit of the proposed research design compared to the conventional design. It was also confirmed that artificial imparting of quite certain physicochemical properties to ready-made drugs and/or artificial provision of certain physicochemical factors of their local interaction during local application can provide the required mechanism of local drug action and become an alternative to traditional performers of this role in pharmacology, namely, original chemical compounds (substances) with specific pharmacological activity inherent in each of them.

2. Methods

The study is based on Russian research, as there are no similar studies in other countries. The contents of the following materials were included in the analysis:

1. "Development of a remedy for bleaching the skin of the face with black eyes"—report on the implementation of the State Innovation Support Fund grant N 24398 (under the application N C1-19369) (Moscow, Russia).

2. Financial support of research work on the implementation of grant N 24398 from 2016 to 2018. Proceedings of the Institute of Thermology (Izhevsk, Russia).

3. Annual Reports on scientific and inventive work of the Institute of Thermology (Izhevsk, Russia) and the Department of General and Clinical Pharmacology of Izhevsk State Medical Academy in the period from 2016 to 2022 (Izhevsk, Russia);

4. Descriptions of inventions created with the participation of Alexander Urakov and devoted to the development of new drugs from "old" drugs in the period from 2012 to 2022 (Federal Institute of Industrial Property, Moscow, Russia).

5. Official website of the Federal Institute of Industrial Property www1.fips.ru, section "Patent fees" (Moscow, Russia).

3. Results

The first announcement that new materials can be created from old materials by changing their physical and chemical properties was made at the 3rd International Conference on Competitive Materials and Technology Processes (IC-CMTP3) (6–10 October 2014, Miskolc-Lillafüred, Hungary) [4]. Several examples of creating new drugs created from "old", that is, known drugs by purposeful modification of their physical and chemical properties were shown as evidence of the real possibility of this direction. Thus, there was an example of creating a "floating tablet" due to the fact that the well-known tablet, which is an artificial stone, is made porous, consisting of individual isolated cavities filled with air, and the specific gravity of the tablet is less than 1 g/cm^3 (RU 2254121). It has been clearly demonstrated that the specific gravity and strength values of conventional drug tablets are similar to pieces of chalk, natural stone, river pebbles, and even concrete since the tablets are produced from dry powders by pressing them without maintaining isolated cavities filled with air. Therefore, when taken orally, regular pills sink in gastric juice, sink quickly to the very bottom of the stomach and remain at the bottom, no matter how much water the patient drank before, during, or after taking the pills. Moreover, "sinking" pills are very salty and acidic, so they have a local irritating effect on the mucous membrane of the stomach in the area of their contact with it. That is why all the pills cause erosive damage to the mucous membrane of the stomach and gastric ulcers precisely in the pyloric region. At the same time, a floating tablet is lighter and floats on the surface of the gastric juice, not in contact with the pyloric mucosa. Moreover, it has been shown that taking water and raising the liquid level in the stomach cavity causes the floating tablet to move along with the liquid level. Therefore, the floating tablet cannot have a local irritant and ulcerogenic effect on the mucous membrane of the pyloric region of the stomach. The higher the level of liquid in the stomach cavity rises, the higher the floating pill rises.

In addition, it has been convincingly shown that increasing the temperature, alkaline activity, and gas content of conventional drugs can turn them into new drugs, for example—into solvent drugs for thick and dry biological masses (pus, blood clots, blood stains, mucus, sputum, sulfur plugs, etc.). It has been reported that almost any drug can be turned into a solvent for thick pus and blood stains if sodium bicarbonate, hydrogen peroxide, and/or carbon dioxide under increased pressure are additionally introduced into the drug formulation and the drug is heated to a temperature of 37–45°C. In particular, it has been reported that such drug solutions acquire the physicochemical properties of alkaline carbonated drinking beverages.

However, drugs differ from the known carbonated drinking beverages in that they have hydrogen peroxide in their composition. The fact is that the addition of hydrogen peroxide to such solutions further changes their physicochemical properties, especially during local interaction with biological tissues containing the enzyme catalase, which decomposes hydrogen peroxide into oxygen gas and water very quickly. Therefore, warm alkaline solutions of hydrogen peroxide in local interaction with thick pus, mucus, sputum, blood, feces, meconium, sulfur plugs, and other biological objects containing catalase enzyme immediately "explode" them due to cold boiling process. As a result, the above biological objects turn into a soft oxygen foam of white color, because at the same time, oxygen decolorization of hemoglobin and its colored metabolites occurs.

On this basis, it was concluded that by giving drugs physical and chemical properties such as hyperthermia, alkalinity, increased gas content under increased pressure, and the ability to release molecular oxygen under the influence of catalase can provide drugs with the ability to bleach blood spots, bruises, and hematomas, as well as dissolve thick pus and thick sulfur plugs.

Finally, based on the results obtained, it was concluded that a new direction in pharmacology and materials science was discovered, namely, physicochemical pharmacology and physicochemical materials science.

A few years after the first official communication, the assumption was realized in Russia with the help of the State Fund for Innovation Support. This fund provided a grant for the development of the first drug to bleach the skin in the area of the black eye. The first drug, a skin-bleaching agent in the area of a black eye, was successfully developed by the team of the Institute of Thermology (Izhevsk, Russia) in the period from 2016 to 2018. Analysis of the reports of the Institute of Thermology showed that it took 2 years to find and develop a new drug, a skin-bleaching agent for the bruise area, at a cost of $27,132. It is important to emphasize that 10 qualified physicians participated in the development. One of them was a doctor of medicine, a professor in the field of pharmacology, and four doctors had Ph.D. degrees. In addition, five students helped the team to carry out the research on their own initiative, that is, free of charge.

At the same time, in Russia, a group of specialists and students conducted laboratory screening of several dozens of known drugs and some physical, chemical, and physicochemical factors of local interaction between 2015 and 2022. The results obtained made it possible to establish that such "old" drugs as hydrogen peroxide and sodium bicarbonate have weak dissolving and bleaching activity, and such physical–chemical factors of local interaction such as hyperthermia, alkalinity and hypergazing, and increase and accelerate their bleaching and pyolytic action several times.

In addition, this research team conducted several series of experiments on the non-specific pharmacological activity of warm alkaline hydrogen peroxide solutions when injected into the skin in the area of bruises in awake piglets, by cutaneous and intradermal injection in the area of artificial bruises created in isolated pig skin segments and in models of blood spots on dressing materials. In parallel, laboratory studies were conducted on the transformation of thick pus, mucus, sputum, and meconium into fluffy oxygenated foam under laboratory conditions with the corresponding isolated biological objects of patients, as well as in experiments on rabbits and isolated rabbit lungs. The results confirmed the correctness of the assumption that it is possible to create new drugs from old drugs by artificially and purposefully changing their physical and chemical properties such as temperature, acidity (alkalinity), osmotic explosive, and oxygen-releasing activity. Examples are new drugs-bleaching stains, traces of blood, bruises, and hematomas, as well as new medical technologies of skin whitening in the area of bruises, developed in Russia on the basis of physical–chemical pharmacology (RU 2539380, RU2589682, RU 2573382, RU 2653465, RU 264737[illegible], RU 2639485, RU 2586278, RU 2582215, RU 2577510, RU 2600504, RU 2634268, RU 2631593, RU 2631592, RU 2641386, RU 2639283, RU 2679334) [5, 7].

Another example of the successful use of the basics of physicochemical pharmacology to transform "old" drugs into new drugs is the development of new aerosols for inhalations and new solutions for intrapulmonary injections based on the original warm alkaline hydrogen peroxide solutions, which provide urgent recanalization of the airways and oxygen saturation of blood through the lungs due to oxygen foaming of thick mucus, sputum, and pus inside the airways during respiratory obstruction caused by COVID-19 (RU Patent No. 2742505, RU Patent No. 2735502, RU Application No. 2021102618, RU Application No. 2021114105) [8].

4. Discussion

In the period from 2012 to 2022, the foundations of physical-chemical pharmacology, pharmacy, and materials science were laid [5, 8]. The essence of the new direction is that new drugs, or rather drugs with a new mechanism of local action, can be created from well-known and proven drugs (that is, old drugs) by purposefully changing their physical-chemical properties. It is reported that a targeted change in the physical-chemical properties of finished drugs (tablets, solutions, aerosols, etc.) allows you to radically change the local mechanism of action of traditional drugs (chemical compounds) with local interaction inside the stomach (with enteral administration), inside blood vessels (with intravenous injections), inside the skin (with intradermal injections), on the surface of the skin and mucous membranes (with applications), as well as inside sulfur plugs, purulent masses, blood clots, thick masses of mucus, sputum, meconium, and other biological masses. It has been convincingly shown that the mechanism of local action of drugs with local application is determined not only by the specific activity of their main ingredients but also by the nonspecific activity of auxiliary and formative ingredients included in the composition of drugs, as well as the physical-chemical properties of finished drugs. That is why for the development of new drugs intended for topical use, "old" drugs can be used, but with artificially altered physical-chemical properties. The new mechanism of local action of "old" drugs can be adjusted by changing the mechanical, physical, chemical, and physical–chemical properties of drugs in specific dosage forms, that is, by changing the quality of tablets, solutions, ointments, creams, aerosols, etc.

It is paradoxical, but the results obtained convince us of the prospects of searching for drugs with new mechanisms of local action among the "old" drugs by purposefully changing their quality (from the standpoint of traditional ideas about the quality of drugs).

Indeed, using the example of ordinary tablets, it was shown that they sink to the bottom of the stomach and move inside its cavity under the influence of gravity in the same way as river sand, pieces of chalk, clay, gravel, and pebbles [9]. It turned out that the specific gravity of all modern tablets exceeds 1 g/cm^3, and, therefore, all tablets sink in gastric juice, water, and milk. It has been shown that in the vertical position of the patient's torso, all tablets fall into the pyloric part of the stomach despite the added liquid. At the same time, it was found that all tablets have an aggressive effect on the gastric mucosa since they corrode the stomach wall and can lead to the formation of ulcers. At the same time, a decrease in the specific gravity of tablets of less than 1 g/cm^3 due to the creation of isolated cavities in them by the type of solid or thick foam makes it possible to radically change the intra-stomach pharmacokinetics and pharmacodynamics of tablet drugs.

Further studies have shown that tablets, which are considered high-quality today, cannot be considered such in comparison with natural food lumps that a person swallows with high-quality chewing of food [9]. It is reported that not only the specific gravity of the tablets but also the shape of the tablets distinguish them from natural food lumps. This approach is recommended for the future adjustment of modern standards of quality control of tablets. It was reported that the manufacturing of tablets by pressing dry powders up to their transformation into artificial stones in the form of a round disk is a pharmaceutical mistake since the disc-shaped shape of tablets with the properties of stones is incompatible with the specifics of the human digestive system. In addition, it was reported that the sizes of modern tablets, which are considered high-quality, do not correspond to the sizes of natural food lumps. It has been shown that high–quality tablets from different manufacturers can differ in height by 3 times, and in volume by 10 times. It was also reported that the natural food lump has the shape of an olive with the largest diameter of up to 1 cm and a maximum length of 2 cm. At the same time, food lumps have an average elasticity, a hardness value of about zero, food lumps are porous and have a specific gravity of less than 1 g/cm^3, and are also devoid of aggressive osmotic action on the mucous membranes of the mouth and stomach. At the same time, modern tablets considered to be of high quality may differ from each other in terms of their hardness by 500 times, since the hardness of the tablets is not controlled [9].

Therefore, it was not by chance that it was stated that the human stomach is not adapted to the introduction of such pills into it (and in fact—artificial stones), since a person is not a bird. Based on these data, it was proposed to modernize the quality standard of tablets, since to increase their safety there is no alternative to their similarity to natural human food lumps in shape, size, and physical-chemical properties. In particular, tablets–analogs of natural food lumps were developed (RU 2533840).

In parallel with the studies of the physical-chemical properties of tablets, the physical-chemical properties of solutions of drugs intended for injection and considered to be of high quality (from the standpoint of drug quality standards) were carried out. It was reported that most of the modern high-quality drug solutions have acidic activity, that is, a pH value of less than 7.0. At the same time, blood and most human tissues have alkaline activity with a pH value of 7.4 [4, 5]. Therefore, some solutions of drugs, which are considered to be of high quality today, can have a local irritating effect and even post-injection necrosis and abscesses at the sites of intramuscular and intravenous injections [10].

In this regard, it was proposed to modernize the pharmacopeia requirements for drug solutions intended for injection. In particular, it was proposed to replace the traditional division of medicinal solutions by the magnitude of their acid (alkaline) activity from pH 7.0 (that is, acidic and alkaline drugs) with a more physiological division of drugs into groups compared to pH 7.4, namely, acidifying and alkalizing drugs (RU 2219958, RU 2221248). The fact is that the acidic activity of drug solutions coagulates proteins and protein-lipid complexes, and also has a local irritant effect on tissues, causing local aseptic inflammation in the injection and/or application sites (for example, when injecting drug solutions into the conjunctival cavity). On the other hand, the alkaline activity of drug solutions liquefies colloidal tissues and can saponify protein and protein-lipid complexes. Therefore, drug's alkaline activity optimizes the rheological properties of blood after local interaction of drug solutions with blood inside veins and vascular catheters, preventing clogging. Additionally, it is reported that alkaline activity of drug solutions promotes liquefaction and dissolution of thick mucus, sputum, pus, and blood clots, especially when local temperature increases, namely, when heating solutions to +37 – +45°C [5, 8].

In addition to this, the great importance of the temperature of drug solutions has been shown. The fact is that temperature according to the Arrhenius and Van Goff law is of great importance for the intensity of all metabolic and vital processes at all levels of organization of living systems, including protein molecules. At the same time, there are reports that modern standards of treatment do not take into account the temperature of drugs when they are administered to patients. Because of this, drugs are not heated to human body temperature and most often the drugs are at room temperature, that is, about +24°C [5, 8]. Therefore, during local interactions, cold drugs cool the tissues in the area of local interactions. Thus, the drugs cause formation of a zone of local hypothermia. In its turn, local hypothermia compacts biological tissues and slows down the rate of biochemical processes in them. In particular, it was reported that temperature decrease from +37 to +24°C significantly slows down the process of blood clotting inside the vascular catheters and blood vessels, which reduces the risk of vein and vascular catheter thrombosis formation, especially during infusion of infusion fluids. In addition, during intravenous injections, cold drug solutions cool the veins, the localization of which can be detected using a thermal imaging device by appropriate zones of local hypothermia in the area of vein projection. This role of cold solutions during intravenous injections was the basis of a new method of infrared imaging of subcutaneous veins (RU 2389429).

On the other hand, it is reported that another very important physicochemical property of drug solutions is their osmotic activity. For a long time, ready-to-inject drug solutions were thought to be of impeccable quality and to be isotonic. However, studies conducted in recent years have shown that the drug quality standard includes control of the concentration value of drug ingredients, but does not include control of osmotic activity and local irritant effect of drug solutions on tissues at injection sites [11]. In this regard, any drug in a particular series (or batch) with a particular manufacturer may sooner or later have excessive hypertonic and/or acidic activity.

Using the example of nonsteroidal anti-inflammatory drugs (NSAIDs), it was shown that some of these drugs have a local irritant effect due to the high concentration of ingredients and hypertonic activity [11]. In laboratory conditions, using an osmometer, it was found that a solution of 50% sodium metamizole has an osmotic activity of 4638 ± 12.5 mosmol/l of water, that is, it is a hypertonic solution. In experimental and clinical conditions, it was shown that intramuscular and subcutaneous injections of a solution of 50% metamizole sodium caused aseptic inflammation, necrosis, and abscess. However, preliminary dilution of a 50% metamizole sodium solution with water by 10 times completely prevented the development of postinjection necrosis and abscess during subcutaneous and intramuscular injections. At the same time, the effectiveness of the protective action of water was explained by its physicochemical role in reducing the concentration of ingredients and the hypertonic activity of the diluted sodium metamizole solution.

These reports convince us that one of the causes of acute post-injection local complication, which is manifested by aseptic inflammation, necrosis, and abscess of tissues at the injection sites of drugs, may be an excessively strong dehydrating effect of drugs on tissue cells due to their hypertensive activity. The dehydrating effect is exerted by an excessively large hyperosmotic activity (hypertonic activity) of drugs, which is created by a large concentration of dissolved ingredients. It has been shown that medicinal solutions containing ingredients in the range of 1–10% are isotonic, either weak hypotonic or weak hypertonic solutions. Such solutions have moderate postinjection safety. Drug solutions containing ingredients in the range of 10–76% are strong hypertonic solutions and have an excessively strong dehydrating effect on cells with local interaction. In this regard, solutions with a total concentration of ingredients of more than 10% are excessively hypertensive and have excessively low postinjection safety, since their injections cause excessive dehydration of cells, necrosis, and abscess [12].

Based on the results, it was concluded that traditional drug quality control requirements are responsible for the fact that some drug solutions, now considered to be of high quality, may have excessive hypertonic activity. In turn, hypertonic drug activity may cause local irritation, aseptic postinjection necrosis, and injection site abscesses. In this regard, ignoring the actual values of osmotic and acidic activity of drugs in the drug form "solution for injection" during injection reduces postinjection drug safety. Therefore, in order to improve postinjection drug safety, it is proposed to monitor the osmotic and acidic activity and the local irritant effect of drugs on the tissues at the injection sites. At the same time, it is reported that postinjection necrosis and abscess in the place of subcutaneous injection of hypertonic solution of almost any drug can be prevented by immediate injection of water for injection (not later than 5–6 minutes after the injection) under control of the dynamics of local skin temperature in the injection site using a thermal imager (RU 2326662, RU 2304769, RU 2396562).

Consequently, convincing evidence has been obtained that eliminating the hypertonic activity of highly concentrated drug solutions by diluting them 2–10 times with water increases the safety of drug injections. Therefore, there are grounds for including this recommendation in the instructions for medical use of highly concentrated drug solutions.

5. Conclusion

Thus, in 2014, an affordable way was proposed to transform "old" quality drugs into new drugs by purposefully changing their quality by artificially changing the physical, chemical, and physicochemical properties of finished drugs: tablets, injectable solutions, aerosols, etc. From the point of view of traditional ideas, the newly created drugs in this way may seem to be spoiled or defective. However, this is not the case. Simply known (old) drugs were traditionally developed mainly for the general (resorptive) mechanism of action. Therefore, the "old" drugs have outdated requirements for their quality. Pharmaceutical and pharmacological progress is impossible without revising the pharmacopeia and traditional drug quality control standards, because "old" drug quality standards preclude their qualitative modernization. It is shown that the advantage and at the same time the limitation of modernized drugs is their local application since their peculiarity is the implementation of the physicochemical principle of drug action in local interaction with a selected part of the patient's (or animal's) body.

Acknowledgements

We express gratitude to Professor László A Gömze for his constant support and assistance in the formation of physicochemical materials science.

Conflict of interest

The authors declare no conflict of interest.

Author details

Aleksandr Urakov[1*], Natalya Urakova[1], Yulia Sorokina[2], Aleksandr Samorodov[3] and Evgeny Fisher[1]

1 Izhevsk State Medical University, Izhevsk, Russia

2 Volga Medical Research University, Nizhny Novgorod, Russia

3 Bashkir State Medical University, Ufa, Russia

*Address all correspondence to: urakoval@live.ru

References

[1] Wyatt PG, Gilbert IH, Read KD, Fairlamb AH. Target validation: Linking target and chemical properties to desired product profil. Current Topics in Medicinal Chemistry. 2011;**11**:1275-1283. DOI: 10.2174/156802611795429185

[2] Frearson JA, Wyatt PG, Gilbert IH, Fairlamb AH. Target assessment for antiparasitic drug discovery. Trends in Parasitology. 2007;**23**(12):589-595. DOI: 10.1016/j.pt.2007.08.019

[3] Brown M, Bennett P, Sharma P. Discovery and Development of Drugs. 11th ed. Edinburgh: Churchill Livingstone; 2012. p. 680

[4] Urakov AL. Development of new materials and structures based on managed physical-chemical factors of local interaction. IOP Conference Series Materials Science and Engineering. 2016;**123**:012008. DOI: 10.1088/1757-899X/123/1/012008

[5] Urakov AL, Urakova NA, Stolyarenko AP. How to turn an old medicine into a new medicine. Journal of Bio Innovation. 2020;**9**(5):774-777. DOI: 10.46344/JBINO

[6] Urakov AL. The change of physical-chemical factors of the local interaction with the human body as the basis for the creation of materials with new properties. Epitőanyag – Journal of Silicate Based and Composite Materials. 2015;**67**(1):2-6. DOI: 10.14382/epitoanyag-jsbcm.2015.1

[7] Urakov A, Urakova N, Nikolenko V, Belkharoeva R, Achkasov E, et al. Current and emerging methods for treatment of hemoglobin related cutaneous discoloration: A literature review. Heliyon. 2021;**7**(1):e059542. DOI: 10.1016/j.heliyon.2021.e05954

[8] Fisher E, Urakov A, Svetova M, Suntsova D, Yagudin I. COVID-19: Intrapulmonary alkaline hydrogen peroxide can immediately increase blood oxygenation. Medicinski Casopis. 2021;**55**(4):135-138. DOI: 10.5937/mskg55-3524

[9] Urakov A, Urakova N, Reshetnikov A, Kasatkin A, Kopylov M, Baimurzin D. About what is happening in the stomach after swallowing human river pebbles, gravel, chalk, clay and tablets drugs. Epitőanyag – Journal of Silicate Based and Composite Materials. 2016;**68**(4):110-113. DOI: 10.14382/epitoanyag-jsbcm.2016.19

[10] Urakov AL. Nikolau syndrome: Necrotic activity of drugs and ways to prevent post-injection abscesses (In memory of Professor László A Gömze). Creative Surgery and Oncology. 2022;**12**(2):159-163. (In Russ.). DOI: 10.24060/2076-3093-2022-12-2-159-163

[11] Kasatkin AA, Urakov AL, Lukoyanov IA. Nonsteroidal antiinflammatory drugs causing local inflammation of tissue at the site of injection. Journal of Pharmacology and Pharmacotherapeutics. 2016;**7**(1):26-28. DOI: 10.4103/0976-500x.179359

[12] Urakov A, Urakova N. Osmotic activity of drugs is an important factor of their local action at their injection site: What we don't use to prevent post-injection abscesses. Journal of Pharmaceutical Research International. 2021;**33**(59B):647-650. DOI: 10.9734/jpri/2021/v33i59B34428

Chapter 4

Recent Advancements in Phyto Component Based Nanocarriers for Improved Treatment of Brain Disorders

Bhabani Sankar Satapathy, Snigdha Pattnaik, Sangram Keshari Biswal, Biswabhusan Biswal, Pralaya Kumar Sahoo, Himansu Bhusan Samal and Binapani Barik

Abstract

Effective treatment of brain disorders remains a tough task in medical science. Age-old brain disorders like Parkinson's (PD) and Alzheimer's (AD) are yet to be managed effectively in spite of fabulous scientific progress over the last decades. Presently available treatment strategies have been found insufficient to tackle the out bursting cases of AD and PD. Indeed, presence of blood-brain barrier (BBB) highly hijacks success of conventional drug therapy. In this regard, phyto bioactive components delivered through nanocarrier (NCs) systems hold ray of hope in improving treatment benefits in brain disorders. Several NCs including polymeric nanoparticles, nanoliposomes, micelles, dendrimers have now being heavily researched to effectively deliver the phyto active components to brain tissue. NCs owing to their structural and physiological uniqueness have now been evolved with great potential for the treatment of brain disorders. Functionalization of brain specific ligands on the surface of NCs further makes them target specific, which might significantly improve bioavailability or reduce the off-target adverse effects. This chapter primarily focuses on recent advancements in phyto component loaded NCs employed for the treatment of brain disorders. The chapter especially covers existing impediments of phyto component based NCs for Parkinson and Alzheimer's disease.

Keywords: phyto component, nanocarriers, blood-brain barrier, brain disorder, treatment strategies, recent advances

1. Introduction

Brain disorders refer to non-transmittable but widely inherited disease problems caused by disruptions in normal body structure and functioning caused by birth abnormalities or genetic malfunctions [1]. There are many different types of brain problems and diseases that impact the brain, such as infections, tumors, traumas, and neurological abnormalities [2]. Present time demands rapid development of diagnostic, therapeutic, and effective preventive agents to tackle the rising prevalence of cerebral illnesses brought on by the aging global population. The BBB, a unique brain capillary control mechanism that prevents the majority of blood molecules from accessing the central nervous system, has severely hampered brain drug development [3]. As a result, unlike other organs, over than 98% of micro therapeutic compounds and about 100% of bigger therapeutic molecules are unable to reach the brain via the circulatory system. Researchers have found that because of their small size, nanocarriers (NCs) can enter most cells through endocytosis and transcytosis. NCs are sub micrometer objects that act as a unified entity in terms of transport and characteristics. NCs have been extensively researched in recent times for brain medication delivery [4]. Previously, various co-solvents/surfactants like dimethyl sulfoxide, polysorbate 80, ethyl alcohol etc. were used with medications to promote BBB penetration. However, such substances pose high risk for integrity of BBB and might disrupt its protective features. NCs-based therapeutics have recently emerged as a prospective therapeutic for brain diseases and disorders due to their easy transportability across the BBB and distinctive qualities like low toxicity, specificity, biocompatible, tiny size, and solubility [5]. However, conventional drugs used for brain disorders possess lots of severe healthy tissue toxic effects along with low bioavailability at brain tissue, which limits their effective clinical application. In view of this, the secondary metabolites of plants known as phytochemicals or phytonutrients such as alkaloids, saponins, indoles, phytosterols, phenolic acids, isothiocyanates, and phytoprostanes/furanes etc. are being largely investigated in recent days [6]. Phyto bioactive constituents have a long history of use in the management of illnesses and brain disorders in people. Nanocarriers are intended to more effectively carry phytochemicals to the target region (brain). Depending on the carrier material, both hydrophilic and hydrophobic molecules can be loaded inside them. For instance, polar and non-polar molecules are both transported by lipid-based nanocarriers (in the aqueous core and the membrane, respectively) [7]. Owing to their nanosize, tunable surface nature, several nanocarriers like polymeric nanoparticles, nanoliposomes, niosomes, magnetic nano-carriers, dendrimers etc. have been investigated largely over the past years to improve treatment outcomes in brain disorsders. Many phytochemicals delivered through polymeric/lipid based nanocarriers have already shown effective potential in increasing the therapeutic efficacy of phytochemicals. In the present chapter, we want to highlight the major phytocomponents those have been delivered through nanocarriers for improved therapeutic effect in brain disorders. We have mostly covered two important brain disorders, *Viz*. Parkinson's (PD) and Alzheimer's disease (AD) with their recent reports on the use of phtonanocarriers. We summarized potential targets, phytoconstituents, brain medication delivery methods, and nanocarrier systems used in the disease management and therapy in this chapter.

1.1 Blood brain barrier (BBB)

BBB is essential for allowing biomolecules to enter and exit the brain's neuronal system. Therefore, comprehension of the functional structure and characteristics of BBB is required to increase medication transport to the brain. This protective unit component helps to stop the shuttling of chemicals between the blood and the brain [8]. It consists of layers of vascular endothelial cells that are restrained by tight junctions and other supporting structures. The astrocyte end-feet of the basement membrane surround the endothelial cells discontinuously scanned by microglial cells. Endothelial cells cohesive regions give persistence for the deliberate movement of tiny substances across the BBB. Transcytosis is a type of regulated intracellular transport that occurs to meet the protein and peptide needs of the brain [9]. Depending on the type of molecules, endothelial cells may be able to promote transfer with the help of numerous unique transporting proteins (hydrophilic or hydrophobic) [10]. In recent times, many NCs based novel formulations have been investigated at pre-clinical stage to treat brain disorders like AD and PD. The NCs can encapsulate anti-AD/anti-PD drugs and can efficiently transport them across the BBB.

1.2 Role of P-gp in brain disorders

The most difficult challenges have been passing the BBB and the blood-cerebrospinal fluid (CSF) barrier in treating brain diseases and disorders. As P-gp carefully mediates material efflux across the BBB, its down-regulation has been linked to the advancement of neurodegenerative disorders and tumors [11]. P-gp inhibition improves medication penetration and subsequent effects across the BBB. Poly(butylcyanoacrylate) NCs have been shown to reduce with P-gp-mediated phenytoin tolerance in rats [12]. Furthermore, when compared to free drug, the incorporation of andrographolide (a neuroprotective agent) into solid lipid NCs increases their permeation to the BBB. In summary, the data suggest that by controlling p-gp, NCs can improve predicted drug penetration and targetability [13].

1.3 Types of nanodrug carriers for brain targeting

1.3.1 Solid lipid nanoparticles (SLNs)

SLNs are nanoscale dispersal made of fatty acids, biocompatible triglycerides, or waxes that have been steady by emulsifiers with HLB values less than 12 [14]. SLNs are unique lipid-based biocompatible nanocarrier systems mainly constituting lipid or modified lipid (triglycerides, fatty acids, or waxes) nanostructures (10–1000 nm diameter size range). SLNs have a solid hydrophobic lipid core, in which both hydrophilic and lipophilic drugs can be dispersed. In vitro, SLNs containing stearic acid and pluronic®F68 were added to demonstrate the ability of Atazanavir to successfully penetrate human brain vascular endothelium. In vivo testing on rats revealed that Riluzole-loaded SLNs were more effective at transporting the medication into the brain [15]. Docetaxel-loaded SLNs composed of soya lecithin, monostearin, vitamin E, and stearyl amine-betreliesoxybutyric acid (HBA, a ketone body and substrate for the monocarboxylic acid carrier conveyed on the BBB) conjugation showed effective permeation across the intact BBB. Despite the fact that SLNs are easily cleared by the reticuloendothelial system due to their hydrophobicity, they have demonstrated the benefits, biocompatibility, good degradability, and the ability to be surface-covalently for brain targeting [16].

1.3.2 Nanoemulsions

Nanoemulsions are biphasic dispersion of two immiscible liquids: either water in oil (W/O) or oil in water (O/W) droplets stabilized by an amphiphilic surfactant. These are the thermodynamically stable isotropic system in which two immiscible liquids are mixed to form a single phase by means of an emulsifying agent, i.e., surfactant and co-surfactant [17]. Nano emulsions are promising drug delivery vehicles across the BBB, because they can solubilize either hydrophilic (W/O nanoemulsions) or hydrophobic (O/W nanoemulsions) drugs. The typical mean droplet diameter of nanoemulsions obtained is around 500 nm or smaller [18]. They have a transparent or hazy look due to their small droplet size, as opposed to the milky white due to attachment with coarse emulsion (whose micron sized droplets partake in multiple light scattering). Additionally, surface functionalization for targeting may make it easier for cells to take up nanoemulsions and the drugs they contain through receptor-mediated endocytosis [19].

1.3.3 Gold NPs

Gold nanoparticles (AuNPs) provide non-toxic carriers for drug and gene delivery applications. AuNPs have been widely studied for their neuroprotective and BBB penetration characteristics in the diagnosis of AD [20]. AuNPs use their special chemical and physical characteristics to load and unload medicines. The gold core is basically inert and non-toxic, which is the first advantage. Another benefit is their simple steps of production. A study reported the production of Au-NPs in the range of 150 nm and the experimental Au-NPs conjugated with glutathione were examined for potential anti-AD effect and it was found that these nanoparticles prevented amyloid aggregation and had a strong anti-AD effect [21].

1.3.4 Nanoliposomes (NLs)

NLs are lipid based nanoparticles with one or more layers of phospholipid bilayers [22]. Natural sphingomyelin, phosphatidylcholine, and glycerophospholipids are common elements of the phospholipid bilayer. NLs have received a lot of attention because of their good biocompatibility and potential for uploading pharmaceuticals in the aqueous core for systemic therapeutic medication delivery [23]. Another strategy to increase the penetration rate of NLs crossing the BBB is cationization of the conjugated ligands. Other challenges affecting NLs brain delivery include poor stability and low drug loading capacity. Due to the limited number of accessible surface groups, binding ligands to the surface is problematic, and steric hindrance exists [16].

1.3.5 Polymeric nanoparticles (PNPs)

PNPs have attracted considerable interest over the last few years due to their unique properties and behaviors resulting from their small size. PNPs have the potential for a variety of uses including medication delivery and diagnostics. PNPs are formed of natural or synthetic polymers and have a diameter of 1 to 1000 nm [24]. Depending on the drug-loading techniques, PNPs can either form thermodynamically stable nanocapsules (drugs are encircled by a polymeric shell) or nanospheres (drugs are embedded into polymeric matrix) [25]. PNPs possess certain qualities such as controlled and/or sustained medication release profiles, better half-life, along with easy surface manipulation for site-specific targeting [26].

One of the best-studied biodegradable copolymers is poly (lactic-co-glycolic acid) (PLGA), which breaks down into non-toxic chemicals that the body excretes (H2O and CO2). Through hydrolysis of the ester linkages to its monomeric anions, the polymer degrades in vivo (lactate and glycolate). PEG-PLGA/PLA-PEG NPs were only used in one Phase II clinical trial for metastatic castration-resistant cancer (BIND-014) [27]. There is no PLGA NPs available for the clinical trial in the market for treatment of brain disorders right now. In reality, a variety of pre-clinical studies based on drug-loaded NCs are being done. Drugs like curcumin, levodopa, cholesterol, rapamycin etc. have already been investigated for the treatment of AD, PD, high blood pressure, and multiple sclerosis [28]. As a result of the lack of drug-specific transport systems at BBB, many neuroprotective medications are unable to reach the brain. PLGA NPs in such cases have the capacity to carry the loaded drugs across BBB to elicit improved brain delivery [29].

1.3.6 Dendrimers

The symmetric monodispersed macromolecules known as dendrimers are built from a collection of branching units that are clustered around in an inner core [30]. When there are numerous responsive groups on the surface, the number of arms and

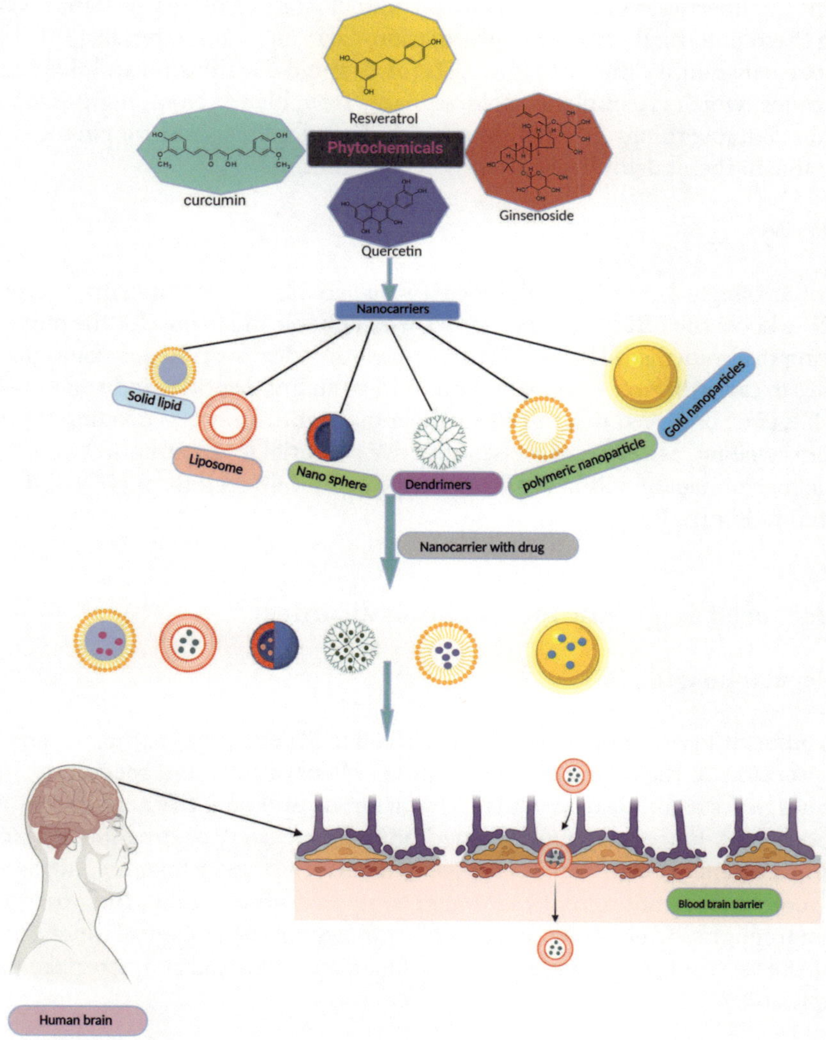

Figure 1.
Selected phyto chemicals and their delivery mechanism through various nanocarrier platforms for improved brain permeation.

surface groups increases dramatically with each generation [31]. They can be used to determine receptor-ligand affinities, administer targeted drugs, or to conduct imaging studies. In case of insoluble and hydrophobic drugs, it is considered as a useful nanocarrier. The interaction of dendrimers with cells is dependent on the hydrophobic contact between the dendrimer arms and the lipid chains of the cell membrane's phospholipid bilayer. Drug distribution to the target site is enabled by the functional groups on the dendrimer's exterior because they act as attachment sites for ligands [32]. Drug is released from dendrimers either through enzymatic dendrimer-drug bond degradation or as a result of environmental changes like temperature and pH [33].

1.3.7 Carbon dots (CDs)

The performance of CDs, a new type of zero-dimensional carbonaceous nanomaterials, is superior to that of novel metal nanoclusters or inorganic nanocrystals, making them potentially effective information-carrying nanomaterials [34]. The ability to easily modify the surface of CDs for targeted distribution and their tunable fluorescence, which is completely color-tunable from blue to close, regions are two of its most notable things [35]. These novel carriers could be used for chemo- or bio sensing due to their customizable luminous capabilities.

1.3.8 Micelles

These are single-layered amphiphilic NCs that enable for regulated drug release. These NCs boost the BBB's ability to absorb hydrophobic medicines for the purpose of treating the brain disorders [36]. Micelles have also demonstrated encouraging outcomes to carry different potent compounds, including peptides and small molecules [37]. It has been observed that micelles deliver magnetic resonance imaging for strokes and brain swelling, as well as possesses effective potential for treating AD [38].

Basic mechanism of action of phyto components delivered through NCs has been presented in **Figure 1**.

2. Widely used diagnostic tools in brain disorders

2.1 Molecular imaging (MI)

An important area of biomedical science called MI examines pathogenesis or bodily processes at the molecular level. With great sensitivity and specificity, imaging techniques make it simple to visualize, characterize, and quantify activities of interest in the body [39]. It uses cutting-edge methods with a variety of capabilities, including as bioluminescence imaging, microscopy, magnetic resonance imaging, ultrasound, single-photon, x-ray radiography emission computed tomography, and positron emission tomography etc. Infections, brain tumors, and neurological illnesses are just a few of the several brain diseases that have been analyzed and characterized using MI techniques [40].

2.2 Biomarker detection

Basically, a biomarker is a distinguishable molecule that is linked to a specific disease or protein. A biomarker's ability to distinguish between healthy and ill persons, as well as its precision in determining illnesses stage is the critical component in disease management [41]. Many biomarkers for illnesses and abnormalities of the brain have been identified. However, the lack of suitable methodologies makes its clinical application difficult. Ubiquitin-C-terminal hydrolase-L1 (UCH-L1) plasma limits have been found to be significantly higher in TBI patients than in healthy people, implying that UCH-L1 could be a viable diagnostic marker for the situation [42]. An innovative technique based on the surface plasmon resonance of Au NPs has recently been shown to successfully and swiftly identify the biomarker UCH-L1 in TBI patients with 100% sensitivity and specificity [43].

3. Some important brain disorders, their etiology and treatment strategies

3.1 Alzheimer's disease (AD)

AD is caused by a mix of genetically determined and environmental risk factors. Age is the most major risk factor [44]. At the age 65, the chance of developing this disease is about 3 percentages and increasing in to more than 30 percentages by the age of 85. Although the frequency of AD among persons under the age of 65 is unclear, it is estimated that this age group accounts for around 3 percentages of all AD patients [45]. While overall numbers of AD continue to rise with the aging population, age-specific incidence too appears to be declining in a number of countries [46]. The accumulation of amyloid-β protein on neuronal cells after exposure to iron, copper, aluminum, cadmium, and zinc chloride salts suggests that heavy metals might be associated with the development or progression of AD [47]. Researchers have also interlinked the AD pathogenesis with presence of toxic metals such as vanadium, nickel, lead etc. Along with that, certain gases like SO2, NOx, and CO found in polluted air may cause chronic neuroinflammation, cerebrovascular damage, oxidative stress reactive oxygen species (ROS) production, neuron damage/loss and peptide accumulation [48]. Also exposure to high amount of pesticides and insecticides in the environment has also been assigned as other major contributing factors for the progression of AD [49]. The etiology of AD has been summarized in **Figure 2**.

Current therapeutic approaches give symptomatic relief of AD, but do not ensure complete recovery. Phytochemical components in this regard are getting more importance owing to their neuroprotective properties, less toxicity and potential to target various pathogenic pathways implicated in AD. Given the limits of currently available AD medications, the different types of phytocompounds have been suggested as therapeutic agents for the disease management. However, phyto components in their native form show poor bioavailability, low solubility and insufficient BBB permeability, which restrict their effective application. Nanotechnology in this regard has been accepted as an innovative technique to overcome these brain medication delivery restrictions [50]. Phyto constituents loaded NCs have the potential to overcome these challenges while also improving neuroprotective effects in BBB. A numbers of pre-clinical studies on phyto component loaded NCs nanocarriers to treat AD have been reported [28, 50]. However, development of NCs for delivery of phyto componets in AD is still limited due to challenging formulation procedures at industrial prospects [51]. Though, several in-vitro and in-vivo studies have been carried out; however, detailed studies by using small laboratory animals to human testing is still very necessary. When administering medicines for the treatment of AD, precise analysis of important parameters like physicochemical

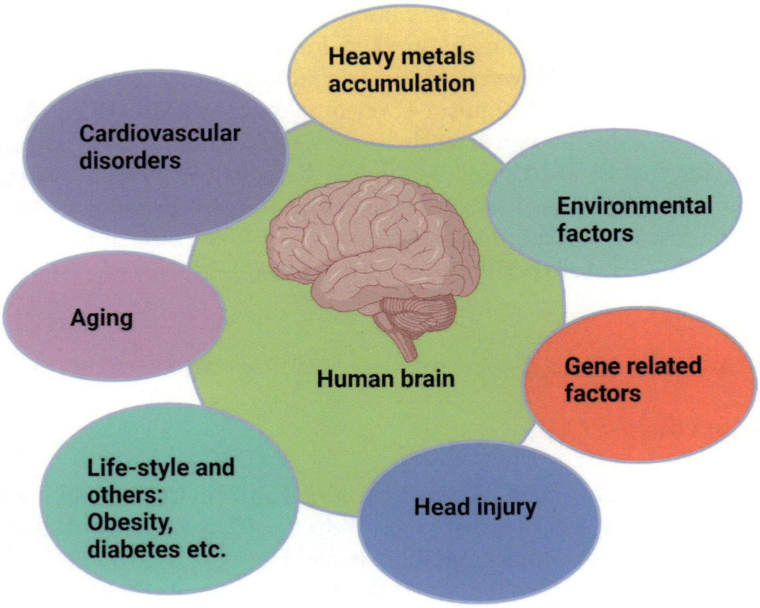

Figure 2.
Probable causes/risk factors involved in the progression of Alzheimer's disease.

properties, particle size, biodistribution, and bioavailability of loaded drug(s) is extremely necessary [52]. Furthermore, the stability of NCs is another striking factor in decreasing the toxic metabolites agglomeration in the BBB. While the conventional formulation of compounds remains difficult to show their action at brain tissue, NCs could be alternative strategy for effective permeation across the BBB with utmost specificity. Problems of instability, limited solubility, low bioavailability issue associated with phytocomponents could be sufficiently addressed by suitable NCs. Clinical studies have also demonstrated efficacy of phyto component loaded NCs in various brain disorders [53].

Further, concerns of safety and brain absorption of NCs must be addressed in AD patients. At present, creating nano phytopharmaceuticals for large-scale production in line with good laboratory practice standards is required to maintain the quality of end product, while retaining patient compliance.

3.1.1 Recent research findings on phyto component based NCs for AD

Over the past years, many active phyto components have been delivered through NCs and have been shown to elicit better pharmacological effect than the free phyto components. Multi-functional liposomal NPs were prepared and coated with an amyloid-binding curcumin-lipid ligand to target amyloid. Along with that two other ligands were also conjugated with the liposomal NPs to target transferrin and LDL receptors present over BBB. The study indicated excellent brain targeting and amyloid peptide aggregation of experimental NCs [54].

The functionalization of NPs with plant phytochemicals has been investigated by Zhang J. et al., 2014. Polyphenols were used to functionalize selenium NPs. The nanosized selenium in the study was coated with epigallocatechin gallate (EGCG), a polyphenol found in green tea. EGCG is well-known for its neuroprotective properties, specifically its ability to limit the formation of many amyloid-forming proteins engaged in the course of Alzheimer's disease. The EGCG-stabilized selenium prevented atrial fibrillation while also dissolved the developed fibrils. Furthermore, at very low concentrations, the specified NCs was observed to decrease DNA fragmentation and ROS generation [55].

In another research, A. Mathew, et al., 2012 investigated the potential of curcumin loaded NCs in in neuronal targeting in vitro. Curcumin is one of the widely investigated phytocomponent over the past decade for the treatment of several brain disorders. In the study, Tet-1 targeted PLGA loaded curcumin nanoparticles with anti-amyloid and anti-oxidant capabilities was found effective in the diagnosis of AD. The incorporation of Tet-1 neuropeptide into the PLGA-curcumin nanoparticle increased its neuronal targeting efficacy in vitro. Although additional conclusions can only be formed after extensive in vivo research, the findings of this exploratory investigation suggested that curcumin could be a promising drug in the treatment of AD [56]. Resveratrol is another important phytocomponent, which is now heavily investigated for its neuroprotective properties. Grape seed and grape skin extracts containing resveratrol were shown to be more efficient at suppressing aggregation. However, after the intravenous injection, resveratrol is quickly metabolized (in less than 2 hours) in the liver and intestinal epithelial cells into glucuronic acid and sulphate conjugations of phenolic groups, which are subsequently excreted. According to a recent study, anti-transferrin receptor monoclonal antibody (OX26 mAb) functionalized SLNs was found as an efficient carrier system for transporting the extract into the target encephalon [57]. In vitro studies on human brain like endothelial cells showed that OX26 SLNs were significantly more effective at cellular absorption than conventional SLNs and SLNs functionalized with an unspecific antibody. Experimental SLNs functionalized with OX-26 showed higher transcytosis capacity [57].

3.2 Parkinson's disease (PD)

PD is a complicated condition with biological as well as environmental origins. The common major risk factor for PD is age, with a median onset age of 60 years. The prevalence of the condition rises with age, peaking at 93.1 (per 100,000 person-years) in people aged 70 to 79 [58]. Though, the exact etiology of PD is yet to be understood. But several risk factors like accumulation of heavy metals, cigarette smoking, pesticides, herbicides, genetic factors, high amount caffeine consumption etc. have been identified for the development and progression of PD. The basic etiology of PD has been summarized in **Figure 3**.

Nanosizing the formulation is an option for increased PD protection to improve the efficiency and bioavailability of crude extracts. Furthermore, adding one or two phytonanocarrier of nano-sized range bioactive chemicals delivers considerable health advantages for specific conditions, thus reducing the need for several drugs. Example like Curcumin and resveratrol NLs exhibited anticancer activity against prostate cancer. According to research curcumin loaded NCs improved the therapeutic and bioavailability efficacy during PD [59]. Experimental NCs significantly lowered oxidative stress and apoptotic cell death in fly model of PD. Similarly, an alginate curcumin nanocomposite also showed a lowering in brain oxidative stress and cell death in a transgenic Drosophila PD model [60]. Curcumin loaded NCs improved bioavailability of curcumin in the blood circulation and also the brain pharmacokinetic [61, 62]. The methods of administration utilized were more significant in increasing nanocurcumin bioavailability in the circulatory system and penetrating to the BBB. Ginsenoside also

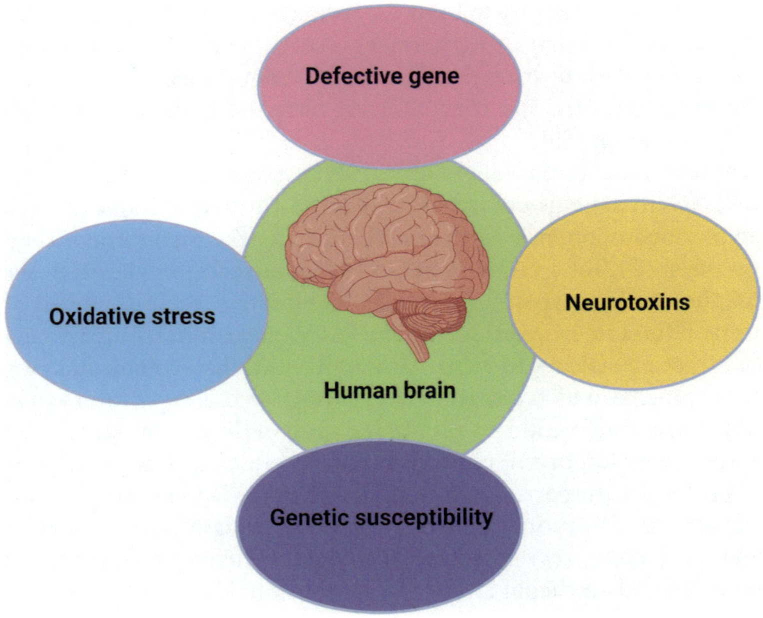

Figure 3.
Probable causes/risk factors involved in the progression of Parkinson's disease.

protects neurons against 6-hydroxydopamine- and iron-induced neurotoxicity. These compounds have an important role in lowering oxidative stress as reported in the recent experiment [63]. Various studies have also indicated that nanoresveratrol can aid in the prevention of PD and enhance neuronal survival in the face of oxidative stress [64].

3.2.1 Recent research findings on phyto component based NCs for PD

Aggregation of amyloid protein in the brain as a result of oxidative stress causes the formation of Lewy bodies and the selective death of dopamine neurons [65]. Polyphenolic substances have poor oral bioavailability, higher metabolic turnover, and decreased BBB permeability. The effect of a produced alginate-curcumin nanocomposite on the climbing capacity of PD model flies, apoptosis, and lipid peroxidation in the brain of PD model flies was investigated in a recent work [65]. The chow was supplied at the known concentrations of 105, 103, and 101 g/mL of alginate-curcumin nanocomposite, and the flies were allowed to consume for 24 days. In the Drosophila model of PD, there was a substantial dose-dependent delay in the reduction in climbing ability, as well as a lowering in apoptosis and oxidative stress.

Another recent work highlighted the neuro protective effect of *Bacopa monnieri* loaded SLNs in vivo. The work involved incorporation of *Bacopa monnieri* extract into SLNs to develop dissolvable microneedle arrays and evaluate its neuroprotective activity. Quality by design approach was employed for optimizing the SLNs formulations based on several in vivo and in vitro properties. Mechanical strength, in vitro release studies, permeation studies, skin irritation test, histopathological analysis, biochemical studies, and behavioral tests of SLNs loaded microneedle arrays were performed. The experimental phyto constituent loaded microneedle patches were shown to be mechanically robust, nonirritant. The optimized formulation was also found to produce decreased degree of bradykinesia along with high motor coordination, and balance ability [66].

In another study, neuronal protective effect of photoactive component of Ginsen delivered in nanoparticle formulation was investigated. The principal active component of the plant, ginsenoside (Rg1) has been reported to protect the neurons against 6-hydroxydopamine-induced death and neuronal toxicity [67]. Although the photoactive components of Ginsen play a critical role in reducing oxidative stress, but the poor bioavailability problem has always been an issue In the work, Rg1 loaded nanoparticles were found to enhance the in vivo activity and bioavailability of these compound than the crude extracts. Nanosizing the formulation showed an enhanced protective effect against PD. The nano ginsenosides were developed using a nanoemulsion technique with average particle diameter of 19.9 nm. Bioavailability of the selected Rg1 loaded nanoparticles showed significantly higher bioavailability than the crude extract in the rat brain tissue [63].

Numerous studies have reported that different nanoparticle-loaded phytochemicals (e.g., vitamin E, resveratrol, curcumin, and hyaluronic acid) with an average particle size of 100 nm resulted in higher ROS scavenging efficiency and lower lipid peroxidation in patients with PD. A work by Pangeni R et al., evidenced antioxidant and neuroprotective effect of nanoencapsulated thymoquinone (TQ) in PD induced rat model. The experimental TQ-loaded mesoporous silica NPs (90 nm in size) were able to cross the BBB. Results showed that the experimental silica NPs enhanced drug delivery to all major brain areas including cortex, thalamus, midbrain, and hypothalamus and significantly reduced oxidative stress biomarkers [64]. Few significant recent research outcomes on phyto component based NCs on AD and PD has been summarized in **Table 1**.

Name of the plant	Major active biocomponent	Nano carrier formulation	Model	Outcome	Reference
Turmeric	Curcumin	Alginate–curcumin nanocomposite	In-vivo	In Parkinson's disease, improve bioavailability while decreasing oxidative stress and apoptosis.	[65]
		Caprylic and capric triglycerides, sorbitan monostearate	In-vitro	Curcumin-NPs protect against A42-induced behavioral and neurochemical alterations in AD mice model.	[68]
		PLGA nanoparticles	In-vitro	Reduced the protection of neurons protected against oxidative damage in AD.	[69]
		curcumin-loaded NP	In-vivo	synergistic delivery of Levodopa curcumin that would be able to pass the blood–brain barrier	[70]

Name of the plant	Major active biocomponent	Nano carrier formulation	Model	Outcome	Reference
Panax ginseng	Ginsenosides	Nanoliposome	In-vitro	Improved the survival of H2 O2-damaged cells	[71]
		PGL-1 nanoparticles	In-vivo	protective effect on apoptosis SH-SY5Y induced by Aβ25–35	[72]
		glipopolysaccharide	In-vivo	ginsenoside Rg3 effective for slowing the development of neurological disorders	[73]
Grapes (*Vitis vinifera*), Cranberry (*Vaccinium macrocarpon*), and Peanut (*Arachis hypogaea*)	Resveratrol	Nanocapsule	In-vivo	Bioavailability enhancement in AD sickness	[74]
		PCL–PEG polymeric micelles	In-vitro	Bioavailability improvement in AD dementia	[75]
		RSV loaded lipid nanocarrier	In-vivo	Induced AD rat model Restoration of the deteriorative effects of Aβ1–42 in animals	[76]
Tea, red wine, apples, parsley, citrus fruits, sage and onions	Quercetin	Solid lipid nanoparticles	In-vivo	Increased the antioxidant capacity of the brain.	[77]
		Nanoliposome	In-vitro	Improved bioavailability	[78]
		(QC- and RA-loaded liposome with conjugated phosphatidic acid and grafted apolipoprotein E	In-vivo	Neurotoxicity was recovered and drug was able to penetrate BBB in AD induced rat model	[79]
		Epigallocatechin-3-gallateloaded nanoparticles	In-vivo	Reduced atherosclerosis	[80]

Table 1.
List of some important phyto components delivered through nanocarrier systems for the treatment of Parkinson (PD) and Alzheimer's disease (AD) [63].

4. Conclusion

Technological advancements in the scientific tools along with exploration of novel formulation strategies have made a substantial impact on diagnosis and treatment of major brain disorders like AD/PD. Undoubtedly, delivery of phyto components through nanocarrier based platforms will bring significant impact on the management and treatment outcome of AD and PD in future days. Most phyto active components show poor BBB penetration capacity, yet possess effective brain therapy potential, which can be overcome by loading the phyto active components suitable nanocarriers. Further, the nanocarriers could be functionalized with brain-specific ligands for effective BBB permeation. However, despite of huge progress in disease diagnosis, health infrastructure, and newer treatment strategies, the clinical use of phyto nanotherapeutics has yet to gain commercial acceptance. There still exists long gap between in vivo data and effective clinical use. Poor yield percentage, low encapsulation efficiency, lack of efficient purification techniques, high production cost, stability issues are some of the crucial problems, which need to be addressed cautiously. Some of the key factors that need urgent attention include: Optimization and standardization of laboratory techniques for effective isolation of phyto active components, optimization of formulation steps of nanocarriers to achieve reasonable loading capacity and stability, in vitro- in vivo correlation, establishment effective process for technology transfer etc. Seeing the diversifying area of brain diseases, interdisciplinary research should be the need of the hour. Neurosurgeons/neuroscientists, formulation scientists, industrial experts and drug researchers should come together for continuous research collaboration to utilize the power of nanotechnology and phyto pharmaceuticals for effective treatment of brain diseases. Only a well-organized, planned interdisciplinary research outlook could offer promising avenue for phyto active chemicals to get clinical approval.

Acknowledgements

The authors are very much grateful to Prof. Manoj Ranjan Nayak, President, Siksha 'O' Anusandhan (Deemed to be University) for providing necessary facilities and encouragement.

Disclosure statement

The authors of the article have no conflict of interest to declare.

Author details

Bhabani Sankar Satapathy[1*], Snigdha Pattnaik[1], Sangram Keshari Biswal[1], Biswabhusan Biswal[1], Pralaya Kumar Sahoo[1], Himansu Bhusan Samal[2] and Binapani Barik[2]

1 School of Pharmaceutical Sciences, Siksha 'O' Anusandhan University, Bhubaneswar, Odisha, India

2 Centurion University of Technology and Management, Bhubaneswar, Odisha, India

*Address all correspondence to: bbhabanisatapathy@yahoo.com; bhabanisatapathy@soa.ac.in

References

[1] Ngowi EE, Wang YZ, Qian L, Helmy YA, Anyomi B, Li T, et al. The application of nanotechnology for the diagnosis and treatment of brain diseases and disorders. Frontiers in Bioengineering and Biotechnology. 2021;**9**:629832. DOI: 10.3389/fbioe.2021.629832

[2] Herman ST. Epilepsy after brain insult: Targeting epileptogenesis. Neurology. 2002;**59**(Suppl 5):S21-S26. DOI: 10.1212/WNL.59.9_suppl_5.S21

[3] Zhou Y, Peng Z, Seven ES, Leblanc RM. Crossing the blood-brain barrier with nanoparticles. Journal of Controlled Release. 2018;**270**:290-303. DOI: 10.1016/j.jconrel.2017.12.015

[4] Borm PJ, Robbins D, Haubold S, Kuhlbusch T, Fissan H, Donaldson K, et al. The potential risks of nanomaterials: A review carried out for ECETOC. Particle and Fibre Toxicology. 2006;**3**:1-35

[5] Kaushik A, Jayant RD, Sagar V, Nair M. The potential of magneto-electric nanocarriers for drug delivery. Expert Opinion on Drug Delivery. 2014;**11**(10):1635-1646. DOI: 10.1517/17425247.2014.933803

[6] Ahmad R, Srivastava S, Ghosh S, Khare SK. Phytochemical delivery through nanocarriers: A review. Colloids and Surfaces. B, Biointerfaces. 2021;**197**:111389. DOI: 10.1016/j.colsurfb.2020.111389

[7] Gordillo-Galeano A, Mora-Huertas CE. Solid lipid nanoparticles and nanostructured lipid carriers: A review emphasizing on particle structure and drug release. European Journal of Pharmaceutics and Biopharmaceutics. 2018;**133**:285-308. DOI: 10.1016/j.ejpb.2018.10.017

[8] Xie J, Shen Z, Anraku Y, Kataoka K, Chen X. Nanomaterial-based blood-brain-barrier (BBB) crossing strategies. Biomaterials. 2019;**224**:119491. DOI: 10.1016/j.biomaterials.2019. 119491

[9] Maher S, Geoghegan C, Brayden DJ. Intestinal permeation enhancers to improve oral bioavailability of macromolecules: Reasons for low efficacy in humans. Expert Opinion on Drug Delivery. 2021;**18**(2):273-300. DOI: 10.1080/17425247.2021.1825375

[10] Tuma PL, Hubbard AL. Transcytosis: Crossing cellular barriers. Physiological Reviews. 2003;**83**(3):871-932. DOI: 10.1152/physrev.00001.2003

[11] Furtado D, Björnmalm M, Ayton S, Bush AI, Kempe K, Caruso F. Overcoming the blood–brain barrier: The role of nanomaterials in treating neurological diseases. Advanced Materials. 2018;**30**(46):1801362. DOI: 10.1002/adma.201801362

[12] Joshi SA, Chavhan SS, Sawant KK. Rivastigmine-loaded PLGA and PBCA nanoparticles: Preparation, optimization, characterization, in vitro and pharmacodynamic studies. European Journal of Pharmaceutics and Biopharmaceutics. 2010;**76**(2):189-199. DOI: 10.1016/j.ejpb.2010.07.007

[13] Gomes MJ, Kennedy PJ, Martins S, Sarmento B. Delivery of siRNA silencing P-gp in peptide-functionalized nanoparticles causes efflux modulation at the blood–brain barrier. Nanomedicine. 2017;**12**(12):1385-1399. DOI: 10.2217/nnm-2017-0023

[14] Khater D, Nsairat H, Odeh F, Saleh M, Jaber A, Alshaer W, et al. Design, preparation, and characterization of effective dermal and transdermal lipid nanoparticles: A review. Cosmetics. 2021;**8**(2):39. DOI: 10.3390/cosmetics8020039

[15] Bondì ML, Craparo EF, Giammona G, Drago F. Brain-targeted solid lipid nanoparticles containing riluzole: Preparation, characterization and biodistribution. Nanomedicine. 2010;**5**(1):25-32. DOI: 10.2217/nnm.09.67

[16] Ahlawat J, Guillama Barroso G, Masoudi Asil S, Alvarado M, Armendariz I, Bernal J, et al. Nanocarriers as potential drug delivery candidates for overcoming the blood–brain barrier: Challenges and possibilities. ACS Omega. 2020;**5**(22):12583-12595. DOI: 10.1021/acsomega.0c01592

[17] Nikam TH, Patil MP, Patil SS, Vadnere GP, Lodhi S. Nanoemulsion: A brief review on development and application in parenteral drug delivery. Advanced Pharmaceutical Journal. 2018;**3**(2):43-54. DOI: 10.31024/apj.2018.3.2.2

[18] Kedzior SA, Gabriel VA, Dubé MA, Cranston ED. Nanocellulose in emulsions and heterogeneous0020water-based polymer systems: A review. Advanced Materials. 2021;**33**(28):2002404. DOI: 10.1002/adma.202002404

[19] Patel MM, Patel BM. Crossing the blood–brain barrier: Recent advances in drug delivery to the brain. CNS Drugs. 2017;**31**:109-133. DOI: 10.1007/s40263-016-0405-9

[20] Zhao J, Xu N, Yang X, Ling G, Zhang P. The roles of gold nanoparticles in the detection of amyloid-β peptide for Alzheimer's disease. Colloid and Interface Science Communications. 2022;**46**:100579. DOI: 10.1016/j.colcom.2021.100579

[21] Singh M, Arseneault M, Sanderson T, Murthy V, Ramassamy C. Challenges for research on polyphenols from foods in Alzheimer's disease: Bioavailability, metabolism, and cellular and molecular mechanisms. Journal of Agricultural and Food Chemistry. 2008;**56**(13):4855-4873. DOI: 10.1021/jf0735073

[22] Sheikholeslami B, Lam NW, Dua K, Haghi M. Exploring the impact of physicochemical properties of liposomal formulations on their in vivo fate. Life Sciences. 2022;**2022**:120574. DOI: 10.1016/j.lfs.2022.120574

[23] Abdel-Mageed HM, AbuelEzz NZ, Radwan RA, Mohamed SA. Nanoparticles in nanomedicine: A comprehensive updated review on current status, challenges and emerging opportunities. Journal of Microencapsulation. 2021;**38**(6):414-436. DOI: 10.1080/02652048.2021.1942275

[24] Calzoni E, Cesaretti A, Polchi A, Di Michele A, Tancini B, Emiliani C. Biocompatible polymer nanoparticles for drug delivery applications in cancer and neurodegenerative disorder therapies. Journal of Functional Biomaterials. 2019;**10**(1):4. DOI: 10.3390/jfb10010004

[25] Vrignaud S, Benoit JP, Saulnier P. Strategies for the nanoencapsulation of hydrophilic molecules in polymer-based nanoparticles. Biomaterials. 2011;**32**(33):8593-8604. DOI: 10.1016/j.biomaterials.2011.07.057

[26] Nahar M, Dutta T, Murugesan S, Asthana A, Mishra D, Rajkumar V, et al. Functional polymeric nanoparticles: An efficient and promising tool for active delivery of bioactives. Critical Reviews™ in Therapeutic Drug Carrier

Systems. 2006;**23**(4):1615. DOI: 10.1615/CritRevTherDrugCarrierSyst.v23.i4.10

[27] Tomalia DA, Naylor AM, Goddard WA III. Starburst dendrimers: Molecular-level control of size, shape, surface chemistry, topology, and flexibility from atoms to macroscopic matter. Angewandte Chemie International Edition in English. 1990;**29**(2):138-175. DOI: 10.1002/anie.199001381

[28] Rahman MM, Islam MR, Akash S, Harun-Or-Rashid M, Ray TK, Rahaman MS, et al. Recent advancements of nanoparticles application in cancer and neurodegenerative disorders: At a glance. Biomedicine & Pharmacotherapy. 2022;**153**:113305. DOI: 10.1016/j.biopha.2022.113305

[29] Mishra I. Dendrimer: A novel drug delivery system. Journal of Drug Delivery and Therapeutics. 2011;**1**(2):22270. DOI: 10.22270/jddt.v1i2.46

[30] Crespo L, Sanclimens G, Pons M, Giralt E, Royo M, Albericio F. Peptide and amide bond-containing dendrimers. Chemical Reviews. 2005;**105**(5):1663-1682. DOI: 10.1021/cr030449l

[31] Cunha A, Gaubert A, Latxague L, Dehay B. PLGA-based nanoparticles for neuroprotective drug delivery in neurodegenerative diseases. Pharmaceutics. 2021;**13**(7):1042. DOI: 10.3390/pharmaceutics13071042

[32] Mukherjee S, Mukherjee S, Abourehab MA, Sahebkar A, Kesharwani P. Exploring dendrimer-based drug delivery systems and their potential applications in cancer immunotherapy. European Polymer Journal. 2022;**2022**:111471. DOI: 10.1016/j.eurpolymj.2022.111471

[33] Asil SM, Ahlawat J, Barroso GG, Narayan M. Nanomaterial based drug delivery systems for the treatment of neurodegenerative diseases. Biomaterials Science. 2020;**8**(15):4109-4128. DOI: 10.1039/D0BM00809E

[34] Farzin L, Sheibani S, Moassesi ME, Shamsipur M. An overview of nanoscale radionuclides and radiolabeled nanomaterials commonly used for nuclear molecular imaging and therapeutic functions. Journal of Biomedical Materials Research Part A. 2019;**107**(1):251-285. DOI: 10.1002/jbm.a.36550

[35] Liu ML, Chen BB, Li CM, Huang CZ. Carbon dots: Synthesis, formation mechanism, fluorescence origin and sensing applications. Green Chemistry. 2019;**21**(3):449-471

[36] Desai HR, Shinde UA. Hybrid nanoparticles to cross the blood–brain barrier. In: Nanocarriers for Drug-targeting Brain Tumors. Netherlands: Elsevier; 2022. pp. 565-586. DOI: 10.1016/B978-0-323-90773-6.00002

[37] Lu CT, Zhao YZ, Wong HL, Cai J, Peng L, Tian XQ. Current approaches to enhance CNS delivery of drugs across the brain barriers. International Journal of Nanomedicine. 2014;**9**:2241. DOI: 10.2147%2FIJN.S61288

[38] Mi P, Cabral H, Kataoka K. Ligand-installed nanocarriers toward precision therapy. Advanced Materials. 2020;**32**(13):1902604. DOI: 10.1002/adma.201902604

[39] Villemagne VL, Doré V, Burnham SC, Masters CL, Rowe CC. Imaging tau and amyloid-β proteinopathies in Alzheimer disease and other conditions. Nature Reviews. Neurology. 2018;**14**(4):225-236. DOI: 10.1038/nrneurol.2018.9

[40] Hu Z, Chen WH, Tian J, Cheng Z. NIRF nanoprobes for cancer molecular

imaging: Approaching clinic. Trends in Molecular Medicine. 2020;**26**(5):469-482. DOI: 10.1016/j.molmed.2020.02.003

[41] Orru G, Pettersson-Yeo W, Marquand AF, Sartori G, Mechelli A. Using support vector machine to identify imaging biomarkers of neurological and psychiatric disease: A critical review. Neuroscience and Biobehavioral Reviews. 2012;**36**(4):1140-1152. DOI: 10.1016/j.neubiorev.2012.01.004

[42] Bazarian JJ, Biberthaler P, Welch RD, Lewis LM, Barzo P, Bogner-Flatz V, et al. Serum GFAP and UCH-L1 for prediction of absence of intracranial injuries on head CT (ALERT-TBI): A multicentre observational study. The Lancet Neurology. 2018;**17**(9):782-789. DOI: 10.1016/S1474-4422(18)30231-X

[43] Peng F, Jeong S, Ho A, Evans CL. Recent progress in plasmonic nanoparticle-based biomarker detection and cytometry for the study of central nervous system disorders. Cytometry Part A. 2021;**99**(11):1067-1078. DOI: 10.1002/cyto.a.24489

[44] Nutten S. Atopic dermatitis: Global epidemiology and risk factors. Annals of Nutrition & Metabolism. 2015;**66**(Suppl. 1):8-16. DOI: 10.1159/000370220

[45] Arvanitakis Z, Shah RC, Bennett DA. Diagnosis and management of dementia. Journal of the American Medical Association. 2019;**322**(16):1589-1599. DOI: 10.1001/jama.2019.4782

[46] Matthews FE, Stephan BC, Robinson L, Jagger C, Barnes LE, Arthur A, et al. A two-decade dementia incidence comparison from the Cognitive Function and Ageing Studies I and II. Nature Communications. 2016;**7**(1):11398. DOI: 10.1038/ncomms11398

[47] Kawahara M, Kato-Negishi M. Link between aluminum and the pathogenesis of Alzheimer's disease: The integration of the aluminum and amyloid cascade hypotheses. International Journal of Alzheimer's Disease. 2011;**2011**:1-17. DOI: 10.4061/2011/276393

[48] Moulton PV, Yang W. Air pollution, oxidative stress, and Alzheimer's disease. Journal of Environmental and Public Health. 2012;**2012**:1-9. DOI: 10.1155/2012/472751

[49] Ascherio A, Chen H, Weisskopf MG, O'Reilly E, McCullough ML, Calle EE, et al. Pesticide exposure and risk for Parkinson's disease. Annals of Neurology: Official Journal of the American Neurological Association and the Child Neurology Society. 2006;**60**(2):197-203. DOI: 10.1002/ana.20904

[50] Paramanick D, Singh VD, Singh VK. Neuroprotective effect of phytoconstituents via nanotechnology for treatment of Alzheimer diseases. Journal of Controlled Release. 2022;**351**:638-655. DOI: 10.1016/j.jconrel.2022.09.058

[51] Wen MM, El-Salamouni NS, El-Refaie WM, Hazzah HA, Ali MM, Tosi G, et al. Nanotechnology-based drug delivery systems for Alzheimer's disease management: Technical, industrial, and clinical challenges. Journal of Controlled Release. 2017;**245**:95-107. DOI: 10.1016/j.jconrel.2016.11.025

[52] Kassem LM, Ibrahim NA, Farhana AS. Nanoparticle therapy is a promising approach in the management and prevention of many diseases: Does it help in curing Alzheimer disease? Journal of Nanotechnology. 2020;**2020**:1-8. DOI: 10.1155/2020/8147080

[53] Patra JK, Das G, Fraceto LF, Campos EV, Rodriguez-Torres MD,

Acosta-Torres LS, et al. Nano based drug delivery systems: Recent developments and future prospects. Journal of Nanobiotechnology. 2018;**16**(1):1-33. DOI: 10.1186/s12951-018-0392-8

[54] Papadia K, Giannou AD, Markoutsa E, Bigot C, Vanhoute G, Mourtas S, et al. Multifunctional LUV liposomes decorated for BBB and amyloid targeting-B. In vivo brain targeting potential in wild-type and APP/PS1 mice. European Journal of Pharmaceutical Sciences. 2017;**102**:180-187. DOI: 10.1016/j.ejps.2017.03.010

[55] Zhang J, Zhou X, Yu Q, Yang L, Sun D, Zhou Y, et al. Epigallocatechin-3-gallate (EGCG)-stabilized selenium nanoparticles coated with Tet-1 peptide to reduce amyloid-β aggregation and cytotoxicity. ACS Applied Materials & Interfaces. 2014;**6**(11):8475-8487. DOI: 10.1021/am501341u

[56] Mathew A, Fukuda T, Nagaoka Y, Hasumura T, Morimoto H, Yoshida Y, et al. Curcumin loaded-PLGA nanoparticles conjugated with Tet-1 peptide for potential use in Alzheimer's disease. PLoS One. 2012;7(3):e32616. DOI: 10.1371/journal.pone.0032616

[57] Loureiro JA, Andrade S, Duarte A, Neves AR, Queiroz JF, Nunes C, et al. Resveratrol and grape extract-loaded solid lipid nanoparticles for the treatment of Alzheimer's disease. Molecules. 2017;**22**(2):277. DOI: 10.3390/molecules22020277

[58] Bower JH, Maraganore DM, McDonnell SK, Rocca WA. Incidence and distribution of parkinsonism in Olmsted County, Minnesota, 1976-1990. Neurology. 1999;**52**(6):1214. DOI: 10.1212/WNL.52.6.1214

[59] Cheng KK, Yeung CF, Ho SW, Chow SF, Chow AH, Baum L. Highly stabilized curcumin nanoparticles tested in an in vitro blood–brain barrier model and in Alzheimer's disease Tg2576 mice. The AAPS Journal. 2013;**15**:324-336. DOI: 10.1208/s12248-012-9444-4

[60] Siddique YH, Naz F, Jyoti S. Effect of curcumin on lifespan, activity pattern, oxidative stress, and apoptosis in the brains of transgenic Drosophila model of Parkinson's disease. Biomed Research International. 2014;**2014**:1-6. DOI: 10.1155/2014/606928

[61] Anand P, Nair HB, Sung B, Kunnumakkara AB, Yadav VR, Tekmal RR, Aggarwal BB. RETRACTED: Design of curcumin-loaded PLGA nanoparticles formulation with enhanced cellular uptake, and increased bioactivity in vitro and superior bioavailability in vivo. 10.1016/j.bcp.2009.09.003

[62] Liu Q, Kou JP, Yu BY. Ginsenoside Rg1 protects against hydrogen peroxide-induced cell death in PC12 cells via inhibiting NF-κB activation. Neurochemistry International. 2011;**58**(1):119-125. DOI: 10.1016/j.neuint.2010.11.004

[63] Ryu JS, Lee HJ, Bae SH, Kim SY, Park Y, Suh HJ, et al. The bioavailability of red ginseng extract fermented by Phellinus linteus. Journal of Ginseng Research. 2013;**37**(1):108. DOI: 10.5142/jgr.2013.37.108

[64] Pangeni R, Sharma S, Mustafa G, Ali J, Baboota S. Vitamin E loaded resveratrol nanoemulsion for brain targeting for the treatment of Parkinson's disease by reducing oxidative stress. Nanotechnology. 2014;**25**(48):485102. DOI: 10.1088/0957-4484/25/48/485102

[65] Siddique YH, Khan W, Singh BR, Naqvi AH. Synthesis of alginate-curcumin nanocomposite and its protective role in transgenic Drosophila

model of Parkinson's disease. International Scholarly Research Notices. 2013;**2013**:1-8. DOI: 10.1155/2013/794582

[66] Joy D, Jose J, Bibi S, Bandiwadekar A, Gopan G, et al. Development of Microneedle Patch Loaded with Bacopa monnieri Solid Lipid Nanoparticles for the Effective Management of Parkinson's Disease. Bioinorganic Chemistry and Applications. 2022;**2022**:1-17. DOI: 10.1155/2022/9150205

[67] Xu H, Jiang H, Wang J, Xie J. Rg1 protects iron-induced neurotoxicity through antioxidant and iron regulatory proteins in 6-OHDA-treated MES23. 5 cells. Journal of Cellular Biochemistry. 2010;**111**(6):1537-1545. DOI: 10.1002/jcb.22885

[68] Bhattacharya T, Soares GA, Chopra H, Rahman MM, Hasan Z, Swain SS, et al. Applications of phyto-nanotechnology for the treatment of neurodegenerative disorders. Materials. 2022;**15**(3):804. DOI: 10.3390/ma15030804

[69] Pocernich C, Lange M, Sultana R, Butterfield D. Nutritional approaches to modulate oxidative stress in Alzheimer's disease. Current Alzheimer Research. 2011;**8**(5):452-469. DOI: 10.2174/156720511796391908

[70] Mogharbel BF, Cardoso MA, Irioda AC, Stricker PE, Slompo RC, Appel JM, et al. Biodegradable nanoparticles loaded with levodopa and curcumin for treatment of Parkinson's disease. Molecules. 2022;**27**(9):2811. DOI: 10.3390/molecules27092811

[71] Tsai WC, Li WC, Yin HY, Yu MC, Wen HW. Constructing liposomal nanovesicles of ginseng extract against hydrogen peroxide-induced oxidative damage to L929 cells. Food Chemistry. 2012;**132**(2):744-751. DOI: 10.1016/j.foodchem.2011.11.026

[72] Liu M, Bai X, Yu S, Zhao W, Qiao J, Liu Y, et al. Ginsenoside re inhibits ROS/ASK-1 dependent mitochondrial apoptosis pathway and activation of Nrf2-antioxidant response in beta-amyloid-challenged SH-SY5Y cells. Molecules. 2019;**24**(15):2687

[73] Lee B, Sur B, Park J, Kim SH, Kwon S, Yeom M, et al. Ginsenoside rg3 alleviates lipopolysaccharide-induced learning and memory impairments by anti-inflammatory activity in rats. Biomolecules & Therapeutics. 2013;**21**(5):381. DOI: 10.4062/biomolther.2013.053

[74] Frozza RL, Bernardi A, Paese K, Hoppe JB, Silva TD, Battastini AM, et al. Characterization of trans-resveratrol-loaded lipid-core nanocapsules and tissue distribution studies in rats. Journal of Biomedical Nanotechnology. 2010;**6**(6):694-703. DOI: 10.1166/jbn.2010.1161

[75] Lu X, Ji C, Xu H, Li X, Ding H, Ye M, et al. Resveratrol-loaded polymeric micelles protect cells from Aβ-induced oxidative stress. International Journal of Pharmaceutics. 2009;**375**(1-2):89-96. DOI: 10.1016/j.ijpharm.2009.03.021

[76] Kanojia N, Thapa K, Kaur G, Sharma A, Puri V, Verma N. Update on Therapeutic potential of emerging nanoformulations of phytocompounds in Alzheimer's and Parkinson's disease. Journal of Drug Delivery Science and Technology. 2022;**2022**:104074. DOI: 10.1016/j.jddst.2022.104074

[77] Dhawan S, Kapil R, Singh B. Formulation development and systematic optimization of solid lipid nanoparticles of quercetin for improved brain delivery. The Journal of Pharmacy and Pharmacology. 2011;**63**(3):342-351. DOI: 10.1111/j.2042-7158.2010.01225.x

[78] Zou LQ, Peng SF, Liu W, Gan L, Liu WL, Liang RH, et al. Improved in vitro digestion stability of (−)-epigallocatechin gallate through nanoliposome encapsulation. Foodservice Research International. 2014;**64**:492-499. DOI: 10.1016/j.foodres.2014.07.042

[79] Shahbaz SK, Koushki K, Sathyapalan T, Majeed M, Sahebkar A. PLGA-based curcumin delivery system: An interesting therapeutic approach in the treatment of Alzheimer's disease. Current Neuropharmacology. 2022;**20**(2):309-323. DOI: 10.2174/1570159X19666210823103020

[80] Hong Z, Xu Y, Yin JF, Jin J, Jiang Y, Du Q. Improving the effectiveness of (−)-epigallocatechin gallate (EGCG) against rabbit atherosclerosis by EGCG-loaded nanoparticles prepared from chitosan and polyaspartic acid. Journal of Agricultural and Food Chemistry. 2014;**62**(52):12603-12609. DOI: 10.1021/jf504603n

Chapter 5

Utilizing 505(b)(2) Regulatory Pathway for New Drug Applications: An Overview on the Advanced Formulation Approach and Challenges

Jiayi Chen, Zhifeng Zhao, Xinyu Wang and Jingjun Huang

Abstract

More than 50% of approved drugs on the market contain poorly water-soluble APIs, which typically are associated with poor bioavailability, suboptimal drug delivery, ineffective drug efficacy, and side effects. This creates a huge opportunity in generating 505(b)(2) products, which address unmet medical needs by applying formulation technologies to overcome those difficulties. A key feature of the 505(b)(2) pathway is the 505(b)(2) sponsor can rely upon clinical data or literature produced by other companies. The 505(b)(2) pathway allows manufacturers to acquire FDA approval without performing all the work required with a traditional NDA. The 505(b)(2) strategy can be an option to improve existing drug products with a new indication, dosage form, dosing regimen, strength, combination with other products, new route of administration, elimination of food effect, switching from a prescription drugs (Rx) to an over-the-counter (OTC), non-prescription product that differs from the OTC monograph, and orphan drug indications. Both generic and brand companies are turning to more complex 505(b)(2) products to avoid the commoditized generic competition. Revitalization of older marketed drug products using innovative drug delivery technologies or platforms can provide new marketing exclusivity and new patent protection, and thus offer an effective tool for product life cycle management.

Keywords: NDA, 505(b)(2), liposome, nanoemulsion, long-acting injectable, suspension, polymer microsphere

1. Introduction

The United States Food and Drug Administration (FDA) published the Draft Guidance for Industry Applications Covered by Section 505(b)(2) in 1999 which for the first time introduced this section of the Federal Food, Drug, and Cosmetic Act (FFDC). By definition, the 505(b)(2) application is "a new drug application (NDA) that contains full reports of investigations of safety and effectiveness but where at least some of the information required for approval comes from studies not conducted by or for the applicant and for which the applicant has not obtained a right of reference" [1]. It is submitted under Section 505(b)(1) of the Act and approved under Section 505(c) of the Act. Compared to the other two types of application described under Section 505, i.e., Section 505(b)(1), an application that contains full reports of investigations of safety and effectiveness; and Section 505(j), sometimes referred to as abbreviated new drug application (ANDA), an application that contains information to show that the proposed product is identical in active ingredient, dosage form, strength, route of administration, labeling, quality, performance characteristics, and intended use, among other things, to a previously approved product, 505(b)(2) pathway offers unique benefits for drug developers and sponsors: (i) Low risk, time and cost effectiveness. 505(b)(2) allows the sponsor to rely on the FDA's previous findings of approved drug's safety and effectiveness, and publicly available literature without the right of reference. The substantially reduced studies and required resources result in a 2–5 years program prior to the FDA approval as compared to 8–15 years for a full NDA, and meanwhile cut the cost from 0.5–2 billion to 3–7 million dollars [2]. (ii) Flexibility. Contrary to 505(j) pathway which only permits certain degree of flexibility in terms of additional physicochemical characterization to demonstrate therapeutically equivalence (TE), 505(b)(2) encourages additional clinical studies to assess drug safety and efficacy profiles, which renders a scientifically more robust alternative for approving complex generics with unnecessarily a TE rating. (iii) Market exclusivity. The 505(b)(2) approved drug product may be warranted by FDA a 3 to 5 years market exclusivity depending upon the extent of changes to the reference product and the type of clinical data included, new intellectual property rights and/or an "AB" substitution rating in the Orange Book (AB: actual or potential bioequivalence problems have been resolved through adequate *in vivo* and/or *in vitro* testing) [3].

In short, 505(b)(2) provides a midway between 505(b)(1) and 505(j) in terms of the volume of new evidence required to be generated and submitted to the FDA. For sponsors and investors, 505(b)(2) pathway presents as a lower risk, time and cost option, and meantime a great market potential especially as many of the "blockbuster drugs" patents and other protected drugs are expiring. **Figure 1** is a schematic representation of the three FDA approval pathways [4]. **Table 1** lists some major differences and similarities in the registration process among the three pathways [2].

The aforementioned features of 505(b)(2) have driven industry's growing interest to utilize this pathway. It was barely used following the first a few years after it was codified by the Hatch-Waxman Act. However, the number of 505(b)(2) approvals slowly increased in the beginning of the 1990s and sharply increased around 2003–2004, when the number of approved drugs through 505(b)(2) superseded new molecular entities (NMEs) approved through 505(b)(1). Nowadays, 505(b)(2) accounts for more than 60% of the total approved new drug applications. **Figure 2** shows the number of drugs approved through 505(b)(2) compared with 505(b)(1) [5].

By nature, 505(b)(2) is an NDA which can be an option to improve existing drug products with new indication, route of administration, dosage form, formulation, strength, multiple drugs combination, dosing regimen, over-the-counter (OTC) switch from prescription drug (Rx), and orphan drug indications, etc. [6], which means that there are numerous approaches to fully take advantage of the 505(b)(2) pathway. A retrospective analysis revealed that out of 224,505(b)(2) NDAs approved by FDA between January 2012 and December 2016, the most prevalent type of FDA submission class fell in type 5 (new formulation or new manufacturer; 43.3%),

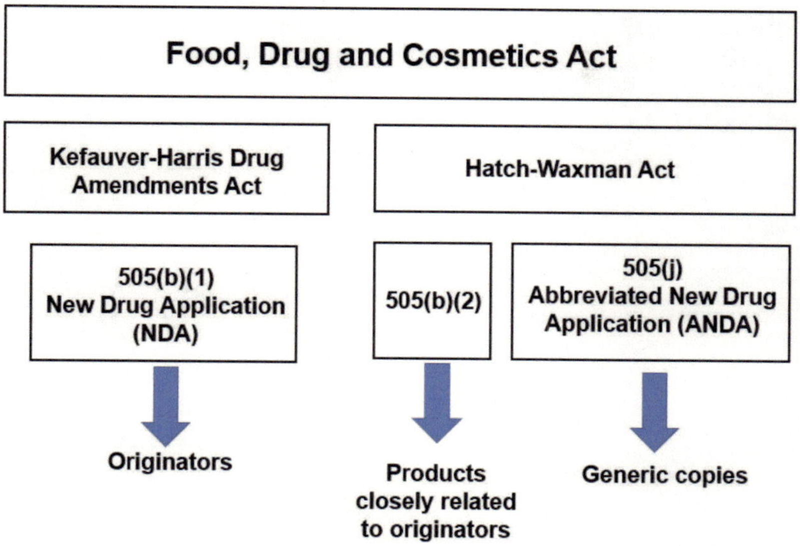

Figure 1.
Schematic representation of the three FDA drug approval pathways [4].

Component	505(b)(1)	505(b)(2)	505(j)
Studies	Full	Partial	BA/BE
New ingredients	Yes	Yes	No
New Formulations	Yes	Yes	No
Patented	Yes	Yes	No
Market exclusivity	5 years	3–5 years	6 months
Agency meetings	Yes	Yes	No
Review classification	9 months	9 months	6–12 months
Timing	8–15 years	2–5 years	1–2 years
Costs	\$500 m – 2b	\$3 m – 7 m	\$50 k – 750 k
Clinical trials	Yes	Maybe	No
Non-clinical / Toxicology data	Yes	Maybe	No
PK/BA/BE studies with RLD	N/A	Yes	Yes
New dosage form/strength	Yes	Yes	No
Combination product	Yes	Yes	Maybe

Table 1.
Differences and similarities in the registration process as per NDA (505(b)(1)), 505(b)(2), and ANDA (505(j)) [2].

followed by type 3 (new dosage form; 28.6%) and type 4 (new drug-drug combination; 12.9%) [7]. It is clear that both generic and brand companies are turning to more complex 505(b)(2) products to avoid the commoditized generic competition [4]. In addition, reformulation of a conventional drug product by newly emerged technologies is an effective way to improve the drug efficacy, safety and patient compliance, and to grant new marketing exclusivity and patent protection.

Year	Number of 505(b)(1) approvals (NMEs only)	Number of 505(b)(2) approvals
2003	15	19
2004	31	44
2005	18	29
2006	18	35
2007	16	27
2008	21	33
2009	20	38
2010	15	29
2011	24	43
2012	33	37
2013	25	39
2014	30	43
2015	33	45
2016	15	45
2017	34	63
2018	42	75
2019	38	64
2020	40	68

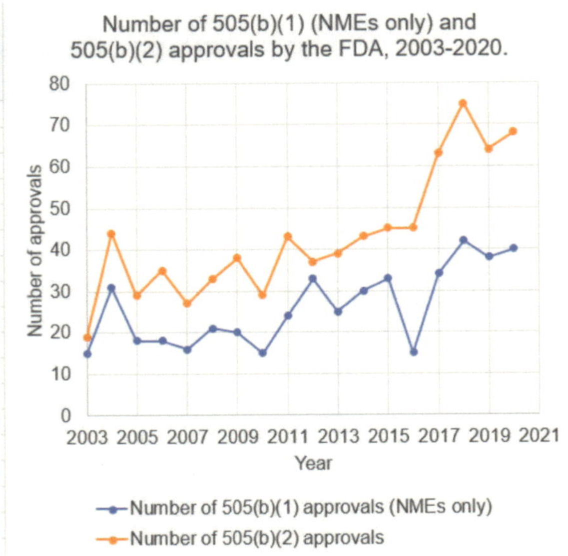

Figure 2.
FDA approvals of 505(b)(1) (NMEs only) and 505(b)(2) applications, 2003–2020.

This chapter, hence, aims to provide an overview on selected advanced formulation technologies including liposome, nanoemulsion, long-acting suspension, polymeric microsphere and their respective 505(b)(2) approved products. The features of each formulation approach are elaborated. Typical case is illustrated. The challenges within the analytical characterizations and testing of these complex 505(b)(2) products, and the potential obstacles with regards to the manufacturing and regulatory perspectives are also highlighted.

2. Liposome

Tracing back to as early as 1960's, liposomes – the microscopic phospholipid bubbles with single or several concentric lipid bilayered structure, have drawn tremendous research interest as potential pharmaceutical carriers due to attractive biological properties. They are biocompatible; they have capability of entrapping hydrophilic pharmaceutical moiety in the inner aqueous compartment as well hydrophobic pharmaceutical agent into the lipid membrane; liposomes are highly tunable in size (from less than 100 nm to several micron), charge and surface properties (PEGylated or ligand modified) by formulation and/or preparation methods to achieve favorable physicochemical and biological features; they also offer unique opportunity to protect the encapsulated cargo from undesired environment and to deliver pharmaceutical agents to target cells, or even sub-cellular compartments. These advantages and highly tunability have made liposome an ideal drug delivery system (DDS) for various pharmaceutical agents including water-soluble/insoluble small molecules, peptides, proteins, DNAs, imaging agents, etc., in therapeutical and diagnostic applications. The research and development effort, and clinical investigation led to the breakthrough as Doxil® (liposomal doxorubicin) was approved by the FDA as the first nanodrug. Thereafter, numerous liposomal drugs have been successfully developed and marketed (**Table 2**).

Product name	Indication	Route of administration	Active substance/ Strength	Excipient formulation
Abelcet	Invasive fungal infection	i.v. infusion	Amphotericin B / 5 mg/mL	l-α-dimyristoylphosphatidylcholine (DMPC) 3.4 mg/mL, l-α-dimyristoylphosphatidylglycerol (DMPG) 1.5 mg/mL, NaCl 9.0 mg/mL, WFI q.s. 1 mL
Ambisome	Severe fungal infection	i.v. infusion after reconstitution	Amphotericin B / 50 mg/vial	Alpha tocopherol 0.64 mg, cholesterol 52 mg, distearoylphosphatidylglycerol 84 mg, hydrogenated soy phosphatidylcholine 213 mg, disodium succinate hexahydrate 27 mg, sucrose 900 mg, and HCl and/or NaOH
Arikayce[1]	*Mycobacterium avium* complex (MAC) lung disease	Oral inhalation	Amikacin sulfate / 590 mg/8.4 mL base	Cholesterol, dipalmitoylphosphatidylcholine (DPPC), NaCl[2], NaOH and WFI
Daunoxome[2]	HIV related Kaposi's sarcoma	i.v. infusion	Daunorubicin citrate 2 mg/mL base	Distearoylphosphatidylcholine 28.2 mg/mL, cholesterol 6.7 mg/mL, sucrose 85.0 mg/mL, glycine 3.8 mg/mL, calcium chloride dihydrate 0.3 mg/mL
Depocyt[2]	Lymphomatous meningitis	Intrathecal	Cytarabine / 10 mg/mL	Cholesterol 4.1 mg/mL, triolein 1.2 mg/mL, dioleoylphosphatidylcholine (DOPC) 5.7 mg/mL, dipalmitoylphosphatidylglycerol (DPPG) 1.0 mg/mL, NaCl 9.0 mg/mL
Depodur[1,2]	Surgery pain	Epidural administration	Morphine sulfate pentahydrate/ 10 mg/mL	1,2-dioleoyl-sn-glycero3-phosphocholine (DOPC) 4.2 mg/mL, cholesterol 3.3 mg/mL, 1,2-dipalmitoyl-sn-glycero3-phospho-rac-(1-glycerol) (DPPG) 0.9 mg/mL, tricaprylin 0.3 mg/mL, triolein 0.1 mg/mL, NaCl 9 mg/mL
Doxil	Kaposi's sarcoma, ovarian/breast cancer, multiple myeloma	i.v. infusion	Doxorubicin hydrochloride / 2 mg/mL base	N-(carbonyl-methoxypolyethylene glycol 2000)-1,2-distearoyl-sn-glycero-3-phosphoethanolamine sodium salt (MPEG-DSPE) 3.19 mg/mL, fully hydrogenated soy phosphatidylcholine (HSPC) 9.58 mg/mL, cholesterol 3.19 mg/mL, ammonium sulfate, approximately 2 mg, histidine, sucrose, HCl or NaOH
Exparel[1]	Postsurgical analgesia	Local infiltration	Bupivacaine / 13.3 mg/mL	Cholesterol 4.7 mg/mL, 1, 2-dipalmitoyl-sn-glycero-3 phospho-rac-(1-glycerol) (DPPG) 0.9 mg/mL, tricaprylin 2.0 mg/mL, 1, 2-dierucoylphosphatidylcholine (DEPC) 8.2 mg/mL, NaCl 9.0 mg/mL
Marqibo[1,2]	Acute lymphoblastic leukemia	i.v. infusion	Vincristine sulfate / 0.16 mg/mL after preparation	Kit contains vincristine sulfate injection, USP (5 mg/5 mL), sphingomyelin/cholesterol liposome injection (103 mg/mL), sodium phosphate injection (355 mg/25 mL)

Product name	Indication	Route of administration	Active substance/ Strength	Excipient formulation
Onivyde[1]	Metastatic pancreas adenocarcinoma	i.v. infusion	Irinotecan hydrochloride trihydrate / 4.3 mg/ mL base	1,2-distearoyl-sn-glycero-3-phosphocholine (DSPC) 6.81 mg/mL, cholesterol 2.22 mg/mL, methoxy-terminated polyethylene glycol (MW 2000)-distearoylphosphatidyl ethanolamine (MPEG-2000-DSPE) 0.12 mg/mL, 2-[4-(2-hydroxyethyl) piperazin-1-yl] ethanesulfonic acid (HEPES) 4.05 mg/mL, NaCl 8.42 mg/mL
Visudyne	Macular degeneration	i.v. injection	Verteporfin / 15 mg for reconstitution	Lactose, egg phosphatidylglycerol, dimyristoyl phosphatidylcholine, ascorbyl palmitate and butylated hydroxytoluene
Vyxeos[1]	Acute myeloid leukemia	i.v. infusion	Daunorubicin and cytarabine / 44 and 100 mg	Distearoylphosphatidylcholine 454 mg, distearoylphosphatidylglycerol 132 mg, cholesterol HP 32 mg, copper gluconate 100 mg, triethanolamine 4 mg, and sucrose 2054 mg

Information acquired from FDA Orange Book as of January 2023.
Abbreviation: i.v.: intravenous; NaCl: sodium chloride; NaOH: sodium hydroxide; HCl: hydrochloric acid; WFI: sterile water for injection.[1]*Product approved via 505(b)(2) pathway.*
[2]*Product with marketing status "discontinued."*

Table 2.
FDA approved liposomal drug products via 505(b) pathway.

Year	Event
1979	Fundamental research on liposomal doxorubicin initiated by Gabizon and Barenholz
1984	"First in man" (FIM) trial with "first generation" of liposomal doxorubicin (OLV-DOX) initiated
1987	OLV-DOX clinical trial failed
1988	"Remote loading" of doxorubicin was patented
1989	Doxil development initiated
1991	FIM trial on Doxil initiated in Jerusalem, Israel
1994	Major publication on Doxil clinical trials (Cancer Research 1994)
1995	FDA approval of Doxil
2010	US patent expired

Table 3.
Historical timeline of Doxil development and regulatory affairs [8].

The development of Doxil® is enlightening as a showcase of an NDA using advanced formulation approach. A brief historical perspective (**Table 3**) is elaborated herein but readers are highly encouraged to dig through the publication by Barenholz [8] for more details. The selection of the model drug Doxorubicin (DOX), an anthracycline chemotherapeutic agent, was deliberated. DOX is effective against a broad spectra of cancer types than any other class of chemotherapy agents, thus it has remained the "first line" anticancer drug from discovery till today [9]. Nevertheless, the use of free drug solution (Adriamycin) was limited by toxicities, especially dose-dependent cardiotoxicity which causes irreversible congestive heart failure, among other side effects [10]. The drug's physicochemical properties were well established, as were its stability [11] and ADME (Absorption, Distribution, Metabolism and Excretion) knowledge [12]. The distinct spectral properties of DOX (high molar extinction at 486 nm, long wavelength > 550 nm and high quantum yield fluorescence emission) makes the quantification sensitive and accurate [13]. Its state of aggregation, hygroscopicity, chemical degradation, pH change in its local environment, etc. are all well-known at the time of the development. Taking advantage of the aforementioned drug properties, the "first generation" liposomal DOX was developed using negatively charged, medium sized oligolamellar liposomes (OLV-DOX) composed of two low chain melting - phospholipids (egg phosphatidylcholine and egg phosphatidylglycerol) and cholesterol. DOX was passively loaded during the lipid hydration and hence membrane associated. Unfortunately, OLV-DOX did not survive in the First in Man (FIM) trial due to multiple folds of reasons: (i) rapid release of DOX in plasma, likely due to the drug location in the liposome bilayer as opposed to encapsulation in the aqueous interior [14]; (ii) high mole fraction of phosphatidylcholine in the bilayer accelerates uptake by reticular-epithelial system (RES) [15] and (iii) size is too large to allow for extravasation in extra-hepatic tissues [16] and to fully utilize the enhanced permeability and retention (EPR) effect [17, 18].

Though not successful, the failure of OLV-DOX served as the main driving force towards two unrelated technologies to address the shortcomings in OLV-DOX, both of which ultimately became the foundation of Doxil. Notably, Doxil does not have direct patent on itself. Rather, it is based on the two families of patents which will be further elaborated, and indeed Doxil enjoyed 14 years of patent protection in the US thanks to the underlying cornerstones. The first technology, namely "remote (active) loading", was to achieve a viable formulation with desired intra-liposome drug concentration, usually defined as drug to lipid molar ratio [19], by pH gradient for many amphipathic weak bases [20], or in the case of Doxil, based on a transmembrane gradient of ammonium sulfate to load drug into preformed liposomes [19, 21]. The second technology was to formulate long circulating liposome with extend plasma half-life ($t_{1/2}$), reduced RES uptake and increased intra-tumor accumulation. Several approaches to alter the lipid composition thus to create a steric stabilized lipid bilayer were studied to achieve the goal, which includes the addition of GM_1 ganglioside [22], the use of hydrogenated phosphatidylinositol (HPI) [15] and synthetic pegylated phospholipids (PEG-DSPE) with different PEG chain length ranging from 350 to 15,000 Da [23, 24]. Small unilamellar liposomes with narrow unimodal size distribution having a mean size of ~100 nm was prepared by medium pressure extrusion using polycarbonate filters with defined pore size [25]. Considering the availability and cost, etc. factors, GM_1 ganglioside-based formulation was excluded in the race [24]. Subsequently after a critical comparative PK study in Beagle dogs [26], 2000 Da PEG-DSPE was demonstrated superior over HPI as the steric stabilizer for the similar nano-liposomes, which was ultimately determined to be the integral component of Doxil.

3. Nanoemulsion

Emulsion, a heterogeneous mixture of two or more immiscible liquids stabilized by a third component (emulsifier), can be generally categorized into two types: oil in water (o/w) and water in oil (w/o), whereas the former liquid is dispersed and stabilized in the latter liquid. Lipid emulsion of the o/w type was firstly evolved in the World War II to serve as an intravenous source of calories and essential fatty acids. The development is based on the rationale that such emulsion is very similar in structure as chylomicrons produced by human body, which is comprised of triglycerides, proteins, free cholesterol and phospholipids. After about 14 years of safe clinical use in European countries, Intralipid® was approved and launched in the US in 1975 for parenteral nutrition indication [27]. However, it was not until late 1980's that lipid emulsion has started to draw researchers' interest as a carrier system for drug delivery. Indeed, the generally non-toxic components of the lipid emulsion alleviate the safety concerns. Besides, lipid emulsion offers some important advantages such as:

i. reduction in pain, irritation, and thrombophlebitis when administered by injection,

ii. reduced systemic toxicity from the free drug or the solvent/surfactant used,

iii. improved lipophilic drug solubility, as well as stability especially in the case of susceptibility to oxidation or hydrolysis, and

iv. potential targeted delivery [28].

To fully utilize emulsion as an effective DDS, a major formulation concern is the physical stability of the formulation, besides other considerations such as drug compatibility, etc. Hence, a subtype of emulsion, the nanoemulsion, has evolved and become a viable approach to deliver drug systematically or locally (**Table 4**). These nanoemulsions are named after their submicron droplet size ranging from 10

Product name	Indication	Route of administration	Active substance / Strength	Excipient formulation
Aponvie[2]	Postoperative nausea and vomiting	Short i.v. infusion over 30 s	Aprepitant / 32 mg/4.4 mL	In 4.4 mL: dehydrated alcohol 0.13 g, egg lecithin 0.64 g, sodium oleate 0.02 g, soybean oil 0.42 g, sucrose 0.24 g, and WFI 2.97 g
Camcevi[2]	Advanced prostate cancer	s.c. injection	Leuprolide mesylate / 42 mg/pre-filled syringe	Each pre-filled syringe contains: poly(D, L-lactide) 184 mg and N-methyl-2-pyrrolidone 136 mg
Cinvanti[2]	Emetogenic chemotherapy associated nausea and vomiting	i.v. infusion	Aprepitant / 130 mg/18 mL	In 18 mL: egg lecithin 2.6 g, ethanol 0.5 g, sodium oleate 0.1 g, soybean oil 1.7 g, sucrose 1 g, and WFI 12 g
Cleviprex	Blood pressure reduction	i.v. infusion	Clevidipine butyrate / 0.5 mg/mL	Soybean oil 200 mg/mL, glycerin 22.5 mg/mL, purified egg yolk phospholipids 12 mg/mL, NaOH, WFI q.s.
Clinolipid 20%	Parenteral nutrition	i.v. infusion	Refined olive oil / 160 mg/mL; Refined soybean oil / 40 mg/mL	Egg phospholipids NF 12 mg/mL, glycerin 22.5 mg/mL, sodium oleate 0.3 mg/mL, NaOH, and WFI q.s.
Durezol	Inflammation and pain associated with ocular surgery	Topical, ophthalmic	Difluprednate / 0.5 mg/mL	Boric acid, castor oil, glycerin, polysorbate 80, purified water, sodium acetate, sodium EDTA, NaOH and sorbic acid 1 mg/mL
Estrasorb[3]	Menopause associated vasomotor symptoms	Topical	Estradiol hemihydrate / 2.5 mg/g	Soybean oil, water, polysorbate 80 and ethanol
Kabiven[2]	Total parenteral nutrition	i.v. infusion, central vein only	Dextrose, amino acids, electrolytes, Intralipid® 20%	Soybean oil 200 mg/mL, glycerin 22.5 mg/mL, purified egg yolk phospholipids 12 mg/mL, NaOH and WFI
Omegaven	Parenteral nutrition-associated cholestasis in pediatric	i.v. infusion, central or peripheral vein	Fish oil / 100 mg/mL	Glycerin 25 mg/mL, egg phospholipids 12 mg/mL, D,L-α-tocopherol 0.15 to 0.3 mg/mL, sodium oleate 0.3 mg/mL, NaOH and WFI
Perikabiven[2]	Total parenteral nutrition	i.v. infusion, central or peripheral vein	Dextrose, amino acids, electrolytes, Intralipid® 20%	Soybean oil 200 mg/mL, glycerin 22.5 mg/mL, purified egg yolk phospholipids 12 mg/mL, NaOH and WFI

Product name	Indication	Route of administration	Active substance / Strength	Excipient formulation
Restasis	Promotion of tear production	Topical, ophthalmic	Cyclosporine / 0.5 mg/mL	Glycerin, castor oil, polysorbate 80, carbomer 1342, NaOH and WFI
Smoflipid	Parenteral nutrition	i.v. infusion	Soybean oil / 60 mg/mL; MCTs / 60 mg/mL; olive oil / 50 mg/mL; fish oil / 30 mg/mL	Glycerin 25 mg/mL, egg phospholipids 12 mg/mL, all-rac-α-tocopherol 0.163 to 0.225 mg/mL, sodium oleate 3 mg/mL, NaOH and WFI
Varubi[3]	Emetogenic chemotherapy associated nausea and vomiting	i.v. infusion	Rolapitant / 1.8 mg/mL	Dibasic sodium phosphate, anhydrous 2.8 mg/mL, MCTs 11 mg/mL, polyoxyl 15 hydroxystearate 44 mg/mL, sodium chloride 6.2 mg/mL, soybean oil 6.5 mg/mL, NaOH or HCl, and WFI
Verkazia[2]	Vernal keratoconjunctivitis	Topical, ophthalmic	Cyclosporine / 1 mg/mL	Cetalkonium chloride, glycerol, MCT, Poloxamer 188, tyloxapol, NaOH and WFI
Xelpros[2]	Reduction of intraocular pressure	Topical, ophthalmic	Latanoprost / 0.05 mg/mL	Castor oil, sodium borate, boric acid, propylene glycol, edetate disodium, polyoxyl 15 hydroxystearate, potassium sorbate 4.7 mg/mL, NaOH or HCl, and WFI

Information acquired from FDA Orange Book as of January 2023.
Abbreviation: i.v.: intravenous; s.c.: subcutaneous; NaOH: sodium hydroxide; MCT: medium chain triglycerides; WFI: sterile water for injection; HCl: hydrochloric acid.[1]*Some discontinued products including: Hexa-Germ, Lipo Gantrisin, Phisohex, Soy-dome, Turgex are not listed due to limited information.*
[2]*Product approved via 505(b)(2) pathway.*
[3]*Product with marketing status "discontinued."*

Table 4.
FDA approved emulsion drug products[1] *via 505(b) pathway.*

to 1000 nm. Unlike solution, they are thermodynamically unstable systems that trend towards separation into two discrete phases over time. However, by deliberate selection of the type of oil and surfactant type and composition ratio, the stability time frame of the formed nanoemulsion can be substantially extended to a sufficient shelf life for months or even years, given the system is kinetically stable. In addition to the improved stability, suitable droplet size (as characterized by particle size distribution (PSD)) and surface properties of nanoemulsion also dictate their in vivo performances after systemic administration, usually governed by the biodistribution, cellular uptake, etc. Studies have revealed larger sized droplets

(>250 nm compared to <100 nm) were cleared faster from the body, indicating a great role of mononuclear phagocyte system (MPS) in the clearance of these nanoemulsion [29]. Moreover, droplet size has also been demonstrated to determine the intratumor distribution versus the peripheral tissues [30]. Therefore, it is in common agreement that nanoemulsions with mean droplet size of less than 150 nm and a narrow, unimodal distribution is highly favored. Besides, a slightly negative charged surface of the nanoemulsion can efficiently prevent the interaction with cells due to electrostatic repulsion thus are not readily taken up by liver and macrophage cells [31]. Therefore, egg derived phospholipids are generally formulated into the nanoemulsion to provide this negative charge besides its overall profound emulsifying and stabilizing properties. Neutral droplet surface or stealth coating can be alternative ways to provide similar "inert" effect, fulfilled by using non-ionic surfactants and/or PEG [32].

Although nanoemulsion presents numerous advantages, not quite many have been successfully launched to the market. Some of the major formulation challenges preventing a broader application of nanoemulsion as DDS are: (i) The disperse phase comprised of long chain triglycerides (LCT) and/or medium chain triglycerides (MCT) are not necessarily good solvents for lipophilic drugs; (ii) Drug loading. As generally the lipid phase cannot exceed 30% in the formulation, many - time it is challenging to load therapeutic-relevant dose of drug in the lipid; (iii) The incorporated drugs may render instability of the nanoemulsion, physically and/or chemically. The hydrolysis of the lipids, usually free fatty acids, could also be detrimental to the drug. (iv) There is a very limited number of approved oils and surfactants, and strict regulatory restrictions on their total content in the product that can be used to formulate, especially injectable emulsions [28].

4. Suspensions

Long-acting injectables (LAIs) are parenteral drug formulations that provide a slow and sustained release of the Active Pharmaceutical Ingredient (API) following administration. Compared to conventional oral formulations, LAIs have many advantages, including sustained exposure of API, reduced administration frequency, enhanced therapy adherence and patient compliance, and potentially lower level of adverse effects [33]. Major classes of LAI formulation technologies are suspensions, polymer microspheres, multi-vesicular liposomes (MVLs), oily solutions, and in situ forming implants.

Aqueous suspensions are solid drug particles produced in micro- or nanometer ranges in water and often have a stabilizer or surfactant to stabilize the particle size distribution and particle morphology during storage. Suspensions are most likely applied for APIs with low water solubility and relatively high lipophilicity, and drug molecule dissolution occurs slowly *in vivo*. Suspensions can be maintained as liquid suspensions ready for injection or further lyophilized into dry powders to be reconstituted before administration [34, 35]. For APIs chemically stable in aqueous solutions, the suspension can be made as a ready-to-use product for direct injection. For APIs with poor chemical stability in aqueous solutions, the suspension is preferred to be formulated as a lyophilized powder and reconstituted prior to administration. In liquid suspension products, particles may sediment at the bottom of the container during storage, and hence the suspension would need to be resuspended prior to administration.

The physical stability of suspensions relies on whether the suspended solids remain dispersed or flocculate upon sedimentation [36]. If all the particles remain discrete, the suspension is considered to be physically stable. Flocculation should be carefully controlled, especially during long-term storage. The viscosity of suspensions should not be too high to make redispersion difficult [37]. To formulate a physical stable suspension, several approaches can be employed, including controlled particle size, the use of structured vehicles, and the use of flocculating agents [38]. The particle size of suspensions is crucial and must be reduced within certain range during development stage. Large particles (> 5 μm diameter) will impart a gritty texture to the product and might cause irritation upon injection or instillation into eyes. Typical structured vehicles are aqueous solutions of polymeric materials, which are usually charged to maintain the suspension [39]. Flocculating agents are added in the suspension to form loosely bound aggregates that settle rapidly but resuspend easily upon agitation. Common flocculating agents include electrolytes, surfactants, and polymers [40]. Suspensions may also be formulated with other excipients, such as solvents, wetting agents, anti-oxidants, preservatives, chelating agents, buffering agents [41]. To develop a successful suspension, the compatibility of excipients with API, the container closure system, and the manufacturing process should be investigated.

Upon administration, the API release from suspended solids is controlled by the API solubility in the surrounding fluids and the accessible surface area of the API particles [42]. API solubility is determined by the physicochemical properties of the API, in which APIs with greater lipophilicity tend to show slower release. In most long-acting suspensions, the API is designed as a prodrug with lower solubility to achieve extended release at the injection site. Accessible surface area is usually controlled by the particle size of the API. Smaller particle size means larger surface area to volume ratio, resulting in faster release. Accessible surface area can also be controlled by the microfractures or surface roughness of the API. In addition, injection volume and injection site could also affect the *in vivo* release of the API [43].

In the manufacturing of suspensions, critical steps include API introduction, vehicle formulation, particle size reduction, sterilization, and filling. To introduce API, it can be done in sterile or non-sterile, micronized or un-micronized manner. Aqueous vehicles are prepared by the dissolution and filtration of surfactants, flocculating agents, and other excipients. High-shear mixing is normally needed to fully wet the API in the suspension vehicle. Particle size reduction of the crystallized API is required when the API is introduced in an un-micronized manner. Microfluidics, wet milling, and high-shear homogenization are options to achieve this purpose [44–46]. Selection of the proper particle size reduction strategy depends on the final target particle size and size distribution, as well as the physicochemical property of the API.

So far, numerous suspensions have been approved by the U.S. FDA via 505(b)(2) pathway. Some of the approved long-acting suspensions and their drug product information are summarized in **Table 5**. One example is Aristada, which is an injectable suspension for intramuscular use. Aristada delivers aripiprazole lauroxil, an atypical antipsychotic, for the treatment of schizophrenia in adults. In clinic, Aristada Initio (675 mg dose) is used as initial regimen in Aristada-based therapy in combination with oral aripiprazole (30 mg dose). Aripiprazole lauroxil is a prodrug of aripiprazole, and it has a lower aqueous solubility than aripiprazole, which allows the preparation of a crystal suspension [47]. After intramuscular injection, the aripiprazole lauroxil crystal suspension forms a local depot, resulting in a sustained release of aripiprazole lauroxil more than 4 weeks [47]. The clinical efficacy and safety of

Product name	Indication	Route of administration	Active substance / Strength	Formulation
Aristada	Schizophrenia	Intramuscular injection	Aripiprazole lauroxil / 441 mg, 662 mg, and 882 mg	Sorbitan monolaurate (3.8 mg/mL), polysorbate 20 (1.5 mg/mL), sodium chloride (6.1 mg/mL), sodium phosphate dibasic anhydrous, sodium phosphate monobasic and WFI
Depo-Medrol	Anti-inflammation	Intra-articular and intra-bursal	Methylprednisolone acetate / 20, 40, 80 mg/mL	Methylprednisolone acetate, PEG 3350, Polysorbate 80, Monobasic sodium phosphate, Dibasic sodium phosphate, Benzyl alcohol
Dexycu	Postoperative inflammation	Intraocular injection	Dexamethasone / 9%	Acetyl triethyl citrate and WFI
EYSUVIS	Signs and symptoms of dry eye disease	Ophthalmic	Loteprednol etabonate / 0.25%	Benzalkonium chloride 0.01%, glycerin, sodium citrate dihydrate, sodium chloride, Poloxamer 407, edetate disodium dihydrate, citric acid, and WFI
Ryanodex	Malignant hyperthermia	Intravenous injection	Dantrolene sodium / 250 mg / vial	125 mg mannitol, 25 mg polysorbate 80, 4 mg povidone K12 and sufficient sodium hydroxide or hydrochloric acid for pH adjustment
SIMBRINZA	Elevated intraocular pressure (IOP)	Ophthalmic	Brinzolamide/brimonidine tartrate / 1%/0.2%	Benzalkonium chloride 0.03 mg, propylene glycol, carbomer 974P, boric acid, mannitol, sodium chloride, tyloxapol and purified water
Zyprexa Relprevv	Schizophrenia	Intramuscular injection	Olanzapine Pamoate / 210, 300, 405 mg	Carboxymethylcellulose sodium, mannitol, polysorbate 80, sodium hydroxide and/or hydrochloric acid for pH adjustment, and WFI
XIPERE	Macular edema associated with uveitis	Suprachoroidal injection	Triamcinolone acetonide / 40 mg/mL	0.55% (w/v) sodium chloride, 0.5% (w/v) carboxymethylcellulose sodium, 0.02% (w/v) polysorbate 80, potassium chloride, calcium chloride (dihydrate), magnesium chloride (hexahydrate), sodium acetate (trihydrate), sodium citrate (dihydrate), and WFI

Information acquired from FDA Orange Book as of January 2023.

Table 5.
FDA approved long-acting parenteral suspension drug products via 505(b)(2).

aripiprazole lauroxil depots has been demonstrated in a randomized, double-blind, placebo-controlled trial in schizophrenia patients [48].

5. Polymer microspheres

Polymer microspheres consist of polymeric materials that encapsulate APIs in a dispersion manner or as an API core surrounded by the polymer shell, achieving controlled release purpose [49]. Over the past decades, research has been focused on degradable polymer microspheres for drug delivery. Such drug delivery systems are advantageous because microspheres can be injected or ingested, and they can be tailored for desired release profiles and sometimes even provide organ-targeted property.

Biodegradable polymers are synthetic or natural and can be degraded *in vivo*, either enzymatically, non-enzymatically or both, to produce biocompatible and toxicologically safe by-products which are further eliminated by the normal metabolic pathways. The number of such materials that are used in controlled drug delivery systems has increased dramatically over the past twenty years. They can be broadly classified as synthetic biodegradable polymers and naturally occurring polymers. Synthetic polymers include polyanhydrides, relatively hydrophobic materials such as polylactic-co-glycolic acid (PLGA), and others. Natural polymers include complex sugars (*e.g.,* chitosan, hyaluronan) and inorganics (*e.g.,* hydroxyapatite). Among these polymers, PLGA is the most attractive and successful one for formulating microspheres [50].

Microspheres can be manufactured via various microencapsulation processes, including solvent evaporation/extraction, coacervation, spray drying, ionic gelation, and others [51]. Solvent evaporation/extraction method is the most commonly used process to produce the commercial polymer microspheres. Briefly, this method involves emulsification of the organic polymer/API solution in an aqueous continuous phase and subsequent precipitation of the polymer/API. The organic solvent used to dissolve the polymer and API should have enough solubility in aqueous phase to partition and thus enable precipitation of the polymer/API [52]. Methylene chloride and chloroform are commonly used organic solvents for preparing PLGA-based microspheres via solvent evaporation/extraction method [53]. The manufacturing process can have impacts on the structure of polymer microspheres and API release. For instance, when microspheres are produced using a solvent evaporation/extraction method, steps such as emulsification and solvent removal can affect particle size, particle size distribution, surface morphology, porosity, and API release profiles of the microspheres. Typically, when the solvent removal goes fast, PLGA quickly transitions from a rubbery state to a glassy state, and loses polymer chain mobility, resulting in larger particle size and lower density compared to microspheres manufactured through a slow solvent removal process.

The *in vivo* API release profiles of polymer microspheres involve multiple mechanisms over different time scales, including API diffusion from the microspheres, penetration of the release media into the microspheres, and polymer degradation. For hydrophilic API, the release profile is usually continuous with or without an initial burst release phase [54]. Burst release is driven by diffusion of the API absorbed on the surface or near the surface of the microspheres. For hydrophobic API, there is typically an initial burst release, followed by a lag phase where no or minimal API is released, and then there is a secondary continuous release phase. The lag phase is the

Product name	Indication	Route of administration	Active substance / Strength	Formulation
Arestin	Gum infection	Subgingival	Minocycline Hydrochloride / 1 mg	PLGA
Bydureon	Type 2 diabetes mellitus	Subcutaneous injection	Exenatide / 2 mg	PLGA 75:25
Firmagon	Prostate cancer	Subcutaneous injection	Degarelix acetate / 240 mg	Peptide self-assembly
LUTRATE DEPOT	Advanced prostate cancer	Intramuscular injection	Leuprolide acetate / 22.5 mg/vial	Polylactic acid (188.4 mg), triethylcitrate (10.4 mg), polysorbate 80 (3.8 mg), mannitol (88.4 mg) and carmellose sodium (25 mg)
Nutropin Depot	GH deficiency	Subcutaneous injection	Somatotropin / 22.5 mg	PLGA
Plenaxis	Prostate cancer	Intramuscular injection	Abarelix / 100 mg	Abarelix/carboxymethylcellulose complex
Risperdal Consta	Schizophrenia, Psychotic disorders	Intramuscular injection	Risperidone /52 mg	PLGA 75:25
Sandostatin LAR	Acromegaly, Carcinoid tumors	Intramuscular injection	Octreotide acetate / 30 mg	PLGA 55/45, star polymer
Somatuline LA	Acromegaly	Intramuscular injection	Lanreotide acetate / 30 mg	PLGA 75:25
Sustol	Vomiting	Subcutaneous injection	Granisetron / 10 mg	Tri(ethylene glycol) poly(orthoester) (TEG-POE), 392 mg, polyethylene glycol monomethyl ether, 98 mg
Trelstar LA	Prostate cancer	Intramuscular injection	Triptorelin pamoate / 22.5 mg	PLGA
Trivaris	Intraocular inflammation	Intravitreal injection	Triamcinolone acetonide / 8 mg	2.3% (w/w) sodium hyaluronate; 0.63% sodium chloride; 0.3% sodium phosphate, dibasic; 0.04% sodium phosphate, monobasic; and WFIf
Vivitrol	Alcohol dependence in adults 18 years and older	Intramuscular injection	Naltrexone / 380 mg/vial	75:25 polylactide-co-glycolide (PLG) at a concentration of 337 mg of naltrexone per gram of microspheres
Zilretta	Pain killer	Intra-articular	Triamcinolone acetonide / 32 mg	PLGA 75:25

Information acquired from FDA Orange Book as of January 2023.

Table 6.
Example of FDA approved polymer microsphere drug products.

time required for polymer degradation and erosion. Once the polymer degrades to certain extent, the microspheres will go through mass loss and matrix erosion, resulting in continuous release of the API until depletion.

Long-acting injectables are crucial for the patient compliance in chronic diseases. Recently, more and more polymer microsphere formulations have been approved by the U.S. FDA and some of them are approved via 505(b)(2) pathway. A few examples are displayed in **Table 6**. For instance, LUTRATE DEPOT is a sterile PLGA microsphere-based formulation to treat the symptoms of Advanced Prostate Cancer, Endometriosis, and Uterine Leiomyomata. Several variants of Lupron Depot® are clinically available containing different amounts of leuprolide acetate, including 7.5, 22.5, 30 and 45 mg that are administered via intramuscular injection route in a dosing interval of 1, 3, 4 and 6 months, respectively [55]. The API in LUTRATE DEPOT is leuprolide acetate, a GnRH agonist, which acts as an inhibitor of gonadotropin secretion. Administration of leuprolide acetate has resulted in inhibition of the growth of certain hormone dependent tumors as well as atrophy of the reproductive organs [56, 57]. LUTRATE DEPOT is stored in a vial containing white to off white sterile lyophilized microspheres together with the corresponding sterile reconstitution diluent in a pre-filled syringe. When LUTRATE DEPOT and the diluent are mixed together, they become a suspension intended as an intramuscular injection.

6. Challenges

Although most of the challenges during the development of a drug product using the advanced technologies are closely related to the formulation discussed in the previous sections, the relatively high attrition rate of the clinical translation of the advanced drug products is no less attributed to other factors, including analytical characterizations, quality assurance of pharmaceutical manufacturing, the suitable assessment of clinical trial and eventually government regulations and intellectual property (IP), etc. [58]

Taking Doxil as an example, as both free and liposomal DOX existed and have different release mechanisms where free DOX almost release instantly once being injected into the patient's body while liposomal DOX releases slowly. Being able to determine and differentiate the two in the formulation is critical to the study and control of the drug product quality. Traditional ways of analysis rely on separating the two first, such as using ultracentrifugation, ultrafiltration, solid-phase extraction (SPE), and gel filtration, followed by quantification with HPLC or CE afterwards. However, each separation method has its own limitations: ultracentrifugation is limited by liposome size; ultrafiltration due to drug adsorption by the device; for gel chromatography it is the separation time and over dilution whereas SPE being the most used method, still suffers from overestimating the free drug due to liposomal drug release during the separation process [59]. In 2011, researchers have developed a method that allows the simultaneous determination of both free and liposomal DOX using CE and laser-induced fluorescence techniques, therefore eliminating the need of preliminary separation and its induced complication. This method was validated for the determination of free DOX only (not for both free and liposomal DOX, due to the liposomal DOX leakage) with a 0.1 μg/mL lower detection limit, which greatly helped future liposomal formulation developments [60].

Another example is the characterization of the degree of branching of poly(lactide-co-glycolide) (PLGA) for polymer-based long-acting injectables. Two kinds of PLGA have been widely used in long-acting injectable formulations approved by the FDA to control the rate of API release: linear PLGA and branched glucose star PLGA (Glu-PLGA) [61]. Comparing to linear PLGA, branched PLGA has more compacted structure, smaller hydrodynamic volume, smaller radius of gyration, lower viscosity, and greater hydrophilicity, resulting in that it behaves differently in terms of release kinetics from linear PLGA even though they might have comparable molecular weight and lactide:glycolide (L:G) ratio. Being able to reliably characterize the degree of branching of PLGA is therefore critical for establishing a drug's bioequivalence. However, until recently, the characterization of PLGA has been limited to measuring its molecular weight and L:G ratio [61]. To address this analytical limitation, researchers from academia, industry and the FDA worked together and developed a method using gel-permeation chromatography with quadrupole detection (GPC-4D), which greatly facilitated the development process of 505(b)(2) products with PLGA embedded RLDs [62], such as Sandostatin® LAR.

In perspective of quality assurance, the issue is usually centered on reproducibility and proper control of these advanced drug products under cGMP manufacturing. More complex the DDSs, more susceptible they are to slight change in the manufacturing process which causes quality variance such as chemical instability or denaturation of the encapsulated compound in the manufacturing process, compromised long-term stability, etc. [63]. Further complications arise when the advanced formulation technologies involve surface modification of a nanodrug with coating and/or ligands.

Challenges are also associated with the increased number of physicochemical variables of these advanced formulations during the assessment of pharmacokinetics (PK), pharmacodynamics (PD) and toxicokinetics (TK) in animal studies [64, 65]. The in depth understanding of the interaction of these nanodrugs with biological tissues and cells require consultation with academia, industry under the regulatory framework [66]. The human clinical trials often face more complexity than conventional formulations as a number of control groups are required to properly evaluate various aspects of the advanced drug product. Furthermore, many drug products may not demonstrate significantly improved efficacy or reduced side effects when compared to their respective approved counterparts.

Last but not the least, considering the complexity of these advanced formulation technologies incorporated into the drug product, associated often with multiple patents, there are also needs for cross-licensing arrangements. The IP practices and protocols could, therefore, be a perplexing issue which requires a simplified pathway from invention to commercialization to reduce time and save cost [67].

7. Conclusion

Over the past three decades since the first FDA approved nanodrug Doxil, the NDA 505(b)(2) have been actively and increasingly utilized as a preferable application pathway, thanks to the emergence of various novel drug delivery formulation technologies. The 505(b)(2) pathway offers well-balanced advantages to researchers, investors, regulatory agents, and ultimately to the patients. It stimulates new drug investigation as well as promotes the improvement of existing drugs. To take advantage of this application route by (re)formulating with advanced technologies, and to expedite the development and approval course, it is important though, for the sponsors to fully understand not only the scientific scope but also regulatory and intellectual affairs.

Conflict of interest

The authors declare no conflict of interest.

Author details

Jiayi Chen, Zhifeng Zhao, Xinyu Wang and Jingjun Huang*
Ascendia Pharmaceuticals, North Brunswick, New Jersey, USA

*Address all correspondence to: j.huang@ascendiapharma.com

References

[1] Guidance for Industry. Applications Covered by Section 505(b)(2). 1999. Available from: https://www.fda.gov/media/72419/download. [Accessed: January 30, 2023]

[2] Rathee P, Tripathy S, Khatter S, Patra B, Murthy P, Dureja H. 505(b)(2) - a smart pathway to differentiate from competitive, low margin environment of generics. Journal of Generic Medicines. 2021;**17**(4):183-194. DOI: 10.1177/1741134320987866

[3] Kumar M, Jethwani H. The 505(b)(2) drug development pathway: When and how to take advantage of a unique American Regulotory pathway. Regulatory Focus. 2010;**505**:9-13

[4] Klein K, Borchard G, Shah VP, Fluhmann B, McNeil SE, de Vlieger JSB. A pragmatic regulatory approach for complex generics through the U.S. FDA 505(j) or 505(b)(2) approval pathways. Annals of the New York Academy of Sciences. 2021;**1502**(1):5-13. DOI: 10.1111/nyas.14662

[5] Darrow J, He M, Stefanini K. The 505(b)(2) drug approval pathway. Food and Drug Law Journal. 2019;**74**:403-439

[6] Research CfDEa. Determining whether to Submit an ANDA or a 505(b)(2) Application. 2019. Available from: https://www.fda.gov/regulatory-information/search-fda-guidance-documents/determining-whether-submit-anda-or-505b2-application. [Accessed: January 30, 2023]

[7] Freije I, Lamouche S, Tanguay M. Review of drugs approved via the 505(b)(2) pathway: Uncovering drug development trends and regulatory requirements. Therapeutic Innovation & Regulatory Science. 2020;**54**(1):128-138. DOI: 10.1007/s43441-019-00036-y

[8] Barenholz Y. Doxil(R)--the first FDA-approved nano-drug: Lessons learned. Journal of Controlled Release. 2012;**160**(2):117-134. DOI: 10.1016/j.jconrel.2012.03.020

[9] Weiss RB. The anthracyclines: Will we ever find a better doxorubicin? Seminars in Oncology. 1992;**19**(6):670-686

[10] Minotti G, Menna P, Salvatorelli E, Cairo G, Gianni L. Anthracyclines: Molecular advances and pharmacologic developments in antitumor activity and cardiotoxicity. Pharmacological Reviews. 2004;**56**(2):185-229. DOI: 10.1124/pr.56.2.6

[11] Beijnen JH, Rosing H, de Vries PA, Underberg WJ. Stability of anthracycline antitumour agents in infusion fluids. Journal of Parenteral Science and Technology. 1985;**39**(6):220-222

[12] Andrews PA, Brenner DE, Chou FT, Kubo H, Bachur NR. Facile and definitive determination of human adriamycin and daunoribicin metabolites by high-pressure liquid chromatography. Drug Metabolism and Disposition. 1980;**8**(3):152-156

[13] Bandak S, Ramu A, Barenholz Y, Gabizon A. Reduced UV-induced degradation of doxorubicin encapsulated in polyethyleneglycol-coated liposomes. Pharmaceutical Research. 1999;**16**(6):841-846. DOI: 10.1023/a:1018869818282

[14] Goren D, Gabizon A, Barenholz Y. The influence of physical characteristics of liposomes containing

doxorubicin on their pharmacological behavior. Biochimica et Biophysica Acta. 1990;**1029**(2):285-294. DOI: 10.1016/0005-2736(90)90165-k

[15] Gabizon A, Papahadjopoulos D. Liposome formulations with prolonged circulation time in blood and enhanced uptake by tumors. Proceedings of the National Academy of Sciences of the United States of America. 1988;**85**(18):6949-6953. DOI: 10.1073/pnas.85.18.6949

[16] Fielding RM. Liposomal drug delivery. Advantages and limitations from a clinical pharmacokinetic and therapeutic perspective. Clinical Pharmacokinetics. 1991;**21**(3):155-164

[17] Maeda H, Bharate GY, Daruwalla J. Polymeric drugs for efficient tumor-targeted drug delivery based on EPR-effect. European Journal of Pharmaceutics and Biopharmaceutics. 2009;**71**(3):409-419. DOI: 10.1016/j.ejpb.2008.11.010

[18] Matsumura Y, Maeda H. A new concept for macromolecular therapeutics in cancer chemotherapy: Mechanism of tumoritropic accumulation of proteins and the antitumor agent smancs. Cancer Research. 1986;**46**(12 Pt 1):6387-6392

[19] Haran G, Cohen R, Bar LK, Barenholz Y. Transmembrane ammonium sulfate gradients in liposomes produce efficient and stable entrapment of amphipathic weak bases. Biochimica et Biophysica Acta. 1993;**1151**(2):201-215. DOI: 10.1016/0005-2736(93)90105-9

[20] Madden TD, Janoff AS, Cullis PR. Incorporation of amphotericin B into large unilamellar vesicles composed of phosphatidylcholine and phosphatidylglycerol. Chemistry and Physics of Lipids. 1990;**52**(3-4):189-198. DOI: 10.1016/0009-3084(90)90114-7

[21] Barenholz Y, Haran G. Inventors; Yissum research development Co of Hebrew University of Jerusalem, assignee. Efficient loading and controlled release of amphipathic molecules. Patent CA1335565C. 16 May 1995

[22] Allen TM, Chonn A. Large unilamellar liposomes with low uptake into the reticuloendothelial system. FEBS Letters. 1987;**223**(1):42-46. DOI: 10.1016/0014-5793(87)80506-9

[23] Woodle MC, Lasic DD. Sterically stabilized liposomes. Biochimica et Biophysica Acta. 1992;**1113**(2):171-199. DOI: 10.1016/0304-4157(92)90038-c

[24] Woodle MC. Surface-modified liposomes: Assessment and characterization for increased stability and prolonged blood circulation. Chemistry and Physics of Lipids. 1993;**64**(1-3):249-262. DOI: 10.1016/0009-3084(93)90069-f

[25] Hunt C, Papahadjopoulous D. Inventors; University of California, assignee. Method for producing liposomes in selected size range. Patent US4529561A. 16 Jul 1985

[26] Gabizon AA, Barenholz Y, Bialer M. Prolongation of the circulation time of doxorubicin encapsulated in liposomes containing a polyethylene glycol-derivatized phospholipid: Pharmacokinetic studies in rodents and dogs. Pharmaceutical Research. 1993;**10**(5):703-708. DOI: 10.1023/a:1018907715905

[27] Dudrick SJ. History of parenteral nutrition. Journal of the American College of Nutrition. 2009;**28**(3):243-251. DOI: 10.1080/07315724.2009.10719778

[28] Hippalgaonkar K, Majumdar S, Kansara V. Injectable lipid emulsions-advancements, opportunities and

challenges. AAPS PharmSciTech. 2010;**11**(4):1526-1540. DOI: 10.1208/s12249-010-9526-5

[29] Lutz O, Meraihi Z, Mura JL, Frey A, Riess GH, Bach AC. Fat emulsion particle size: Influence on the clearance rate and the tissue lipolytic activity. The American Journal of Clinical Nutrition. 1989;**50**(6):1370-1381. DOI: 10.1093/ajcn/50.6.1370

[30] Kurihara A, Shibayama Y, Mizota A, Yasuno A, Ikeda M, Sasagawa K, et al. Enhanced tumor delivery and antitumor activity of palmitoyl rhizoxin using stable lipid emulsions in mice. Pharmaceutical Research. 1996;**13**(2):305-310. DOI: 10.1023/a:1016063719541

[31] Longmire M, Choyke PL, Kobayashi H. Clearance properties of nano-sized particles and molecules as imaging agents: Considerations and caveats. Nanomedicine (London, England). 2008;**3**(5):703-717. DOI: 10.2217/17435889.3.5.703

[32] Fam SY, Chee CF, Yong CY, Ho KL, Mariatulqabtiah AR, Tan WS. Stealth coating of nanoparticles in drug-delivery systems. Nanomaterials (Basel). 2020;**10**(4):787. DOI: 10.3390/nano10040787

[33] Brissos S, Veguilla MR, Taylor D, Balanza-Martinez V. The role of long-acting injectable antipsychotics in schizophrenia: A critical appraisal. Therapeutic Advances in Psychopharmacology. 2014;**4**(5):198-219. DOI: 10.1177/2045125314540297

[34] Hugo Silva M, Kumar A, Hodnett BK, Tajber L, Holm R, Hudson SP. Impact of excipients and seeding on the solid-state form transformation of indomethacin during liquid Antisolvent precipitation. Crystal Growth & Design. 2022;**22**(10):6056-6069. DOI: 10.1021/acs.cgd.2c00678

[35] Merisko-Liversidge E, Liversidge GG. Nanosizing for oral and parenteral drug delivery: A perspective on formulating poorly-water soluble compounds using wet media milling technology. Advanced Drug Delivery Reviews. 2011;**63**(6):427-440. DOI: 10.1016/j.addr.2010.12.007

[36] Schott H. Controlled flocculation of coarse suspensions by colloidally dispersed solids I: Interaction of bismuth subnitrate with bentonite. Journal of Pharmaceutical Sciences. 1976;**65**(6):855-861. DOI: 10.1002/jps.2600650614

[37] Xu M, Liu H, Zhao H, Li W. How to decrease the viscosity of suspension with the second fluid and nanoparticles? Scientific Reports. 2013;**3**:3137. DOI: 10.1038/srep03137

[38] Moghimipour E, Salimi A, Rezaee S, Balack M, Handali S. Influence of flocculating agents and structural vehicles on the physical stability and rheological behavior of nitrofurantoin suspension. Jundishapur Journal of Natural Pharmaceutical Products. 2014;**9**(2):e12716. DOI: 10.17795/jjnpp-12716

[39] Liechty WB, Kryscio DR, Slaughter BV, Peppas NA. Polymers for drug delivery systems. Annual Review of Chemical and Biomolecular Engineering. 2010;**1**:149-173. DOI: 10.1146/annurev-chembioeng-073009-100847

[40] Koshani R, Tavakolian M, van de Ven TGM. Cellulose-based dispersants and flocculants. Journal of Materials Chemistry B. 2020;**8**(46):10502-10526. DOI: 10.1039/d0tb02021d

[41] Akers MJ. Excipient-drug interactions in parenteral formulations. Journal of Pharmaceutical Sciences. 2002;**91**(11):2283-2300. DOI: 10.1002/jps.10154

[42] Kesisoglou F, Wu Y. Understanding the effect of API properties on bioavailability through absorption modeling. The AAPS Journal. 2008;**10**(4):516-525. DOI: 10.1208/s12248-008-9061-4

[43] Joiner JB, King JL, Shrivastava R, Howard SA, Cottrell ML, Kashuba ADM, et al. Effects of injection volume and route of administration on Dolutegravir In situ forming implant pharmacokinetics. Pharmaceutics. 2022;**14**(3):615. DOI: 10.3390/pharmaceutics14030615

[44] Perez A, Hernandez R, Velasco D, Voicu D, Mijangos C. Poly (lactic-co-glycolic acid) particles prepared by microfluidics and conventional methods. Modulated particle size and rheology. Journal of Colloid and Interface Science. 2015;**441**:90-97. DOI: 10.1016/j.jcis.2014.10.049

[45] Ahmed B, Brown CJ, McGlone T, Bowering DL, Sefcik J, Florence AJ. Engineering of acetaminophen particle attributes using a wet milling crystallisation platform. International Journal of Pharmaceutics. 2019;**554**:201-211. DOI: 10.1016/j.ijpharm.2018.10.073

[46] Farzi M, Yarmand MS, Safari M, Emam-Djomeh Z, Mohammadifar MA. Gum tragacanth dispersions: Particle size and rheological properties affected by high-shear homogenization. International Journal of Biological Macromolecules. 2015;**79**:433-439. DOI: 10.1016/j.ijbiomac.2015.04.037

[47] Hard ML, Mills RJ, Sadler BM, Turncliff RZ, Citrome L. Aripiprazole Lauroxil: Pharmacokinetic profile of this long-acting injectable antipsychotic in persons with schizophrenia. Journal of Clinical Psychopharmacology. 2017;**37**(3):289-295. DOI: 10.1097/JCP.0000000000000691

[48] Meltzer HY, Risinger R, Nasrallah HA, Du Y, Zummo J, Corey L, et al. A randomized, double-blind, placebo-controlled trial of aripiprazole lauroxil in acute exacerbation of schizophrenia. The Journal of Clinical Psychiatry. 2015;**76**(8):1085-1090. DOI: 10.4088/JCP.14m09741

[49] Freiberg S, Zhu XX. Polymer microspheres for controlled drug release. International Journal of Pharmaceutics. 2004;**282**(1-2):1-18. DOI: 10.1016/j.ijpharm.2004.04.013

[50] Makadia HK, Siegel SJ. Poly lactic-co-glycolic acid (PLGA) as biodegradable controlled drug delivery carrier. Polymers (Basel). 2011;**3**(3):1377-1397. DOI: 10.3390/polym3031377

[51] Singh MN, Hemant KS, Ram M, Shivakumar HG. Microencapsulation: A promising technique for controlled drug delivery. Research in Pharmaceutical Sciences. 2010;**5**(2):65-77

[52] Butreddy A, Gaddam RP, Kommineni N, Dudhipala N, Voshavar C. PLGA/PLA-based long-acting injectable depot microspheres in clinical use: Production and characterization overview for protein/peptide delivery. International Journal of Molecular Sciences. 2021;**22**(16):8884. DOI: 10.3390/ijms22168884

[53] Shim H, Sah H. Assessment of residual solvent and drug in PLGA microspheres by derivative thermogravimetry. Pharmaceutics. 2020;**12**(7):626. DOI: 10.3390/pharmaceutics12070626

[54] Yoo J, Won YY. Phenomenology of the initial burst release of Drugs from PLGA microparticles. ACS Biomaterials Science & Engineering.

2020;**6**(11):6053-6062. DOI: 10.1021/acsbiomaterials.0c01228

[55] Nkanga CI, Fisch A, Rad-Malekshahi M, Romic MD, Kittel B, Ullrich T, et al. Clinically established biodegradable long acting injectables: An industry perspective. Advanced Drug Delivery Reviews. 2020;**167**:19-46. DOI: 10.1016/j.addr.2020.11.008

[56] Wilson AC, Meethal SV, Bowen RL, Atwood CS. Leuprolide acetate: A drug of diverse clinical applications. Expert Opinion on Investigational Drugs. 2007;**16**(11):1851-1863. DOI: 10.1517/13543784.16.11.1851

[57] Hoda MR, Kramer MW, Merseburger AS, Cronauer MV. Androgen deprivation therapy with leuprolide acetate for treatment of advanced prostate cancer. Expert Opinion on Pharmacotherapy. 2017;**18**(1):105-113. DOI: 10.1080/14656566.2016.1258058

[58] Sercombe L, Veerati T, Moheimani F, Wu SY, Sood AK, Hua S. Advances and challenges of liposome assisted drug delivery. Frontiers in Pharmacology. 2015;**6**:286. DOI: 10.3389/fphar.2015.00286

[59] Jiang W, Lionberger R, Yu LX. In vitro and in vivo characterizations of PEGylated liposomal doxorubicin. Bioanalysis. 2011;**3**(3):333-344. DOI: 10.4155/bio.10.204

[60] Kim HS, Wainer IW. Simultaneous analysis of liposomal doxorubicin and doxorubicin using capillary electrophoresis and laser induced fluorescence. Journal of Pharmaceutical and Biomedical Analysis. 2010;**52**(3):372-376. DOI: 10.1016/j.jpba.2009.06.028

[61] O'Brien MN, Jiang W, Wang Y, Loffredo DM. Challenges and opportunities in the development of complex generic long-acting injectable drug products. Journal of Controlled Release. 2021;**336**:144-158. DOI: 10.1016/j.jconrel.2021.06.017

[62] Hadar J, Skidmore S, Garner J, Park H, Park K, Wang Y, et al. Characterization of branched poly(lactide-co-glycolide) polymers used in injectable, long-acting formulations. Journal of Controlled Release. 2019;**304**:75-89. DOI: 10.1016/j.jconrel.2019.04.039

[63] Narang AS, Chang RK, Hussain MA. Pharmaceutical development and regulatory considerations for nanoparticles and nanoparticulate drug delivery systems. Journal of Pharmaceutical Sciences. 2013;**102**(11):3867-3882. DOI: 10.1002/jps.23691

[64] Teli MK, Mutalik S, Rajanikant GK. Nanotechnology and nanomedicine: Going small means aiming big. Current Pharmaceutical Design. 2010;**16**(16):1882-1892. DOI: 10.2174/138161210791208992

[65] Tinkle S, McNeil SE, Muhlebach S, Bawa R, Borchard G, Barenholz YC, et al. Nanomedicines: Addressing the scientific and regulatory gap. Annals of the New York Academy of Sciences. 2014;**1313**:35-56. DOI: 10.1111/nyas.12403

[66] Allen TM, Cullis PR. Liposomal drug delivery systems: From concept to clinical applications. Advanced Drug Delivery Reviews. 2013;**65**(1):36-48. DOI: 10.1016/j.addr.2012.09.037

[67] Murday JS, Siegel RW, Stein J, Wright JF. Translational nanomedicine: Status assessment and opportunities. Nanomedicine. 2009;**5**(3):251-273. DOI: 10.1016/j.nano.2009.06.001

Section 2

Repurposing and Drug Discovery

Chapter 6

In Silico Drug Repurposing: An Effective Tool to Accelerate the Drug Discovery Process

Kareti Srinivasa Rao and P. Subash

Abstract

Repurposing "old" drugs to treat both common and rare diseases is increasingly emerging as an attractive proposition due to the use of de-risked compounds, with potential for lower overall development costs and shorter development timelines. This is due to the high attrition rates, significant costs, and slow pace of new drug discovery and development. Drug repurposing is the process of finding new, more efficient uses for already-available medications. Numerous computational drug repurposing techniques exist, there are three main types of computational drug-repositioning methods used on COVID-19 are network-based models, structure-based methods and artificial intelligence (AI) methods used to discover novel drug–target relationships useful for new therapies. In order to assess how a chemical molecule can interact with its biological counterpart and try to find new uses for medicines already on the market, structure-based techniques made it possible to identify small chemical compounds capable of binding macromolecular targets. In this chapter, we explain strategies for drug repurposing, discuss about difficulties encountered by the repurposing community, and suggest reported drugs through the drug repurposing. Moreover, metabolic and drug discovery network resources, tools for network construction, analysis and protein–protein interaction analysis to enable drug repurposing to reach its full potential.

Keywords: drug repurposing, protein–protein interaction, drug discovery, COVID-19, pharmacological repositioning

1. Introduction

Drug repurposing, also known as drug repositioning, is a strategy for speeding up the medicine discovery process by identifying a new therapeutic usage for an already-approved drug for a different indication. One of the outcomes of polypharmacology is the increased success and applicability of drug repurposing, which is a manifestation of the transition from a single to multitarget paradigm in drug discovery [1]. COVID-19 has now been labelled a pandemic, necessitating the development of novel medicines as we move beyond containment. It is unrealistic to meet the current global crisis by developing new pharmaceuticals from the ground up because it is a lengthy procedure. Drug repurposing is a new method in which current drugs that have been proven safe in humans are repurposed to treat diseases that are difficult to cure. While taking these repurposed medications alone may not provide a meaningful clinical advantage, strategically combining them into a cocktail could be quite useful [2].

Repositioning previously approved medications is a promising practice since it lowers the cost and length of the drug development pipeline while also lowering the risk of unexpected side effects. The ability to quickly screen candidates in silico and limit the number of prospective repositioning candidates makes computational repositioning particularly interesting. What is not obvious is how effective such strategies are at generating clinically useful repositioning hypotheses is represented in **Figure 1** [3]. The SARS-CoV-2 virus causes a respiratory infection that can lead to pneumonia. COVID-19 has a mortality rate of 2–3.5%, which rises with age and the presence of comorbidities (e.g., hypertension, cardiac insufficiency, diabetes, and asthma). By April 15, 2020, the new coronavirus has infected 2,033,406 people worldwide and killed over 130,000 people [4]. COVID-19 has depleted health systems around the world, leading countries to take drastic measures such as closing land borders and instituting social distancing regulations to halt the disease's spread [5].

The new coronavirus (SARS-CoV-2), which causes COVID-19, has swiftly become a global danger to public health and the economy [5, 6]. SARS-CoV-2, according to recent clinical reports, produces both mild, self-limiting respiratory tract infection and severe progressive pneumonia, which can lead to multiorgan failure and death. Despite the severity of some cases, no pathogen-specific antivirals are currently available to treat this infection. As a result, several studies have looked at the anti-SARS-CoV-2 activity of currently available medicines [7].

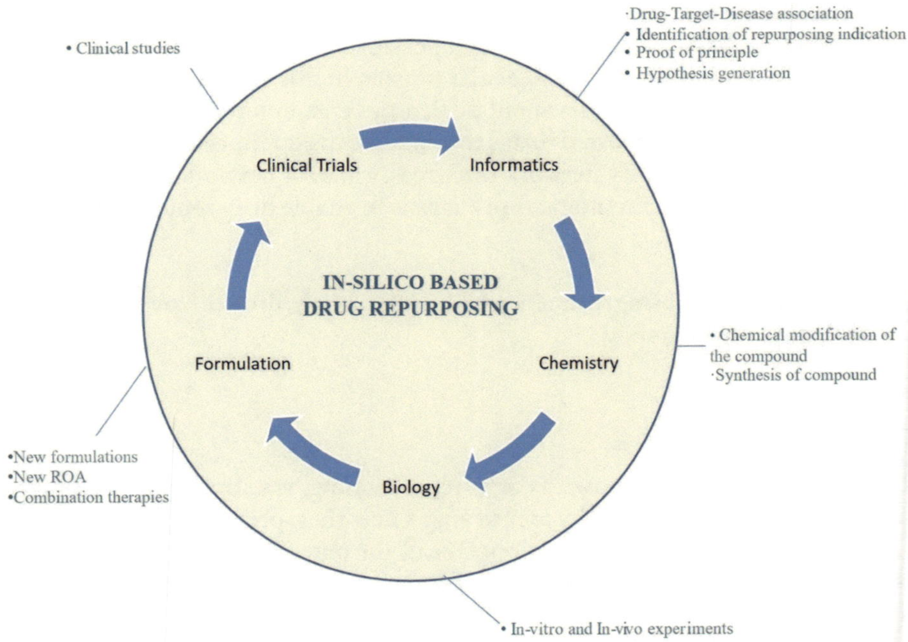

Figure 1.
In silico-based drug repurposing.

2. Faster development times and reduced risks

Attempts to speed up the development of a medication are typically accompanied by an increase in risk. Drug repositioning, on the other hand, offers a solution to the problem. Repositioning candidates have generally gone through numerous phases of clinical development and hence have well-known safety and pharmacokinetic properties, which reduces development risk. Shorter paths to the clinic are also possible because *in vitro* and *in vivo* screening, chemical optimization, toxicity, bulk production, formulation development, and even early clinical development have all been achieved in many situations. In summary, these considerations allow for the reduction of many years from the path to market, as well as major risks and costs (**Figure 2**). As a result, repositioning may provide a superior risk-to-reward ratio than other medication development tactics. These benefits have not gone unnoticed by venture capital firms looking for high value exits for their companies in the near future. Because of the strong response such firms have had from the public equity markets, it is nearly impossible for venture capitalists to invest in a therapeutics company without drug prospects in or approaching clinical trials in 2004. Indeed, repositioning allows for the rapid creation of such a pipeline, and repositioning firms are having little issue with getting venture capital.

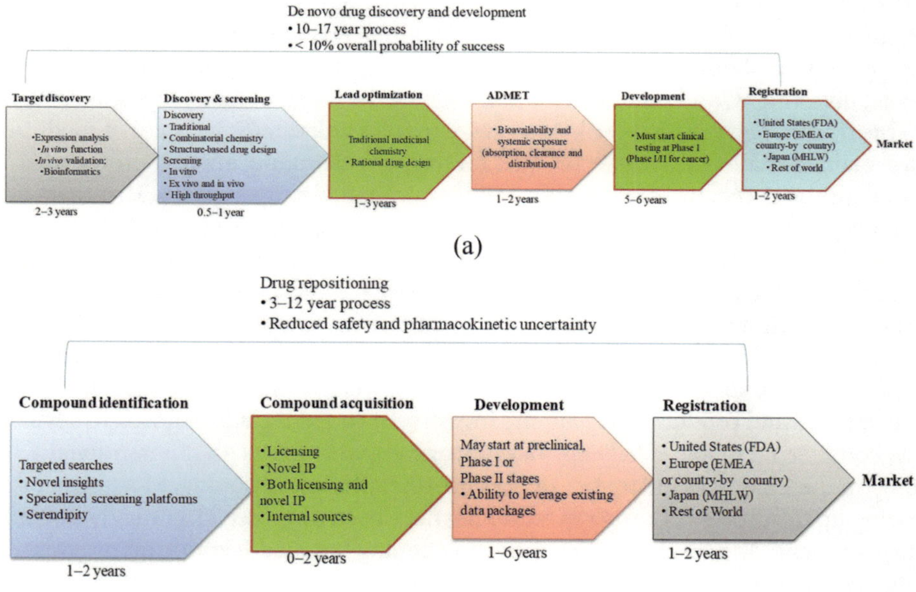

Figure 2.
A comparison of traditional de novo drug discovery and development versus drug repositioning. (a) It is well known that from concept to marketable medicine, de novo drug research and development takes 10–17 years [8]. The probability of success is lower than 10% [9]. (b) because repositioning candidates have frequently gone through numerous phases of development for their initial indication, several phases common to de novo drug discovery and development can be avoided, allowing for a reduction in time and risk. ADMET is an abbreviation for absorption, distribution, metabolism, excretion, and toxicity; EMEA is an abbreviation for European medicines agency; FDA is an abbreviation for Food and Drug Administration; IP is an abbreviation for intellectual property; and MHLW is an abbreviation for Ministry of Health, labour, and welfare.

3. Drug repositioning opportunities

Drug repositioning is a potential approach that is gaining traction among governments and pharmaceutical corporations due to its critical role in decreasing time, cost, and risk in the development of treatments for cancer and other terminal diseases. As this technique became more widely known, multidisciplinary teams of researchers and scientists attempted, with varying degrees of efficiency and success, to computationally study the potential of repositioning drugs to treat other diseases and identify alternative indications, regardless of whether the drug in question was approved, withdrawn, in clinical trials, or failed. Despite the fact that drug repositioning is a relatively new technique, the traditional, costly, and risky de novo drug development process is still necessary for discovering and testing new drugs; however, incorporating some computational drug repositioning models into this process can help to move drugs forward in the development pipeline and ultimately improve drug efficiencies in clinical trials. The potential for drug repositioning to help create the critical medications needed to combat the present coronavirus outbreak cannot be overstated [10].

4. Challenges and opportunities

Traditional drug development strategies are risky, expensive, and prone to failure. As a result, drug repositioning has recently gained attention, and it expedites the release of medications for clinical usage. Drug repositioning, on the other hand, is a complicated process involving a variety of aspects, including technology, business models, patents, investment, and market demands. Despite the fact that many medical databases have been built, determining the best strategy to fully utilise huge volumes of medical data remains a challenge. New techniques for drug repositioning are urgently needed. Another problem that needs to be addressed is intellectual property (IP). IP protection for repositioning medications is minimal [11]. Some novel drug-targeted-disease connections discovered by repositioning researchers, for example, were corroborated by papers or online databases; yet, according to the law, it is difficult to seek IP protection for such associations. Some repositioned medications are unable to enter the market due to intellectual property issues. Furthermore, some repositioning attempts have to be abandoned, wasting both time and money [12]. Because the existing commercial model is serial and produces overlapping investment concerns, it is required to develop a new commercial model. Challenges accompany opportunities. An unintentional finding in the 1920s was the first example of medication repositioning. More ways of speeding up the process of drug repositioning have been proposed after nearly a century of development. As a result, medication repositioning has made significant progress. **Table 1** contains 75 examples of pharmacological repositioning culled from the extensive literature. To increase the performance of drug repositioning in this circumstance, massive machine learning techniques were applied. Experimental procedures, such as target screening approaches, have been developed in addition to computational approaches to provide direct proof of correlations between medications and diseases [11, 12, 24].

5. Drug-based computational approaches

The structure and chemical characteristics of a medicinal compound are clearly linked to its final therapeutic effectiveness. As a result, repositioning options

Drug name	New indication	Origin indication	Mining Approaches	References
Atomoxetine	ADHD	Parkinson's disease	Network Approach	[13, 14]
Allopurinol	Gout	Tumour lysis syndrome	Experiment	[13]
Amphetamine	Hyperkinesis in children (attention deficit hyperactivity disorder, ADHD)	Stimulant	Semantic Approach	[13, 15]
Apomorphine	Erectile dysfunction	Parkinson's disease	Experiment	[16]
Aspirin	Colorectal cancer	Analgesic, antipyretic	Experiment	[16]
Budesonide	Colitis, Ulcerative	Asthma	Computational Approach	[17, 18]
Bupropion	Smoking cessation	Depression	Experiment	[13, 19]
Celecoxib	Colon, colorectal, lung, and breast cancer are all linked to familial adenomatous polyposis.	Osteoarthritis and adult rheumatoid, arthritis	Computational Approach	[17, 20]
Chlorpromazine	Non-sedating tranquillizer	Antiemetic/ antihistamine	Experiment	[17]
Crizotinib	NSCLC	Clinical trials for anaplastic large-cell lymphoma	Experiment	[21]
Cymbalta	Diabetic peripheral neuropathy	Depression	Experiment	[13]
Dapoxetine	Premature ejaculation	Analgesia and depression	Experiment	[13]
Doxepin	Insomnia antipruritic	Antidepressant	Experiment	[19]
Drospirenone	Hypertension	Oral contraceptive	Experiment	[22]
Duloxetine	Stress urinary incontinence, fibromyalgia,	Depression	Computational Approach	[19]
Duloxetine	chronic, musculoskeletal pain, shoulder pain, back pain, osteoa-arthritis knee	Diabetic Neuropathies	Experiment	[17]
Eflornithine	Reduction of unwanted facial hair in women	Anti-infective	Experiment	[17]
Etanercept	Asthma	Rheumatoid arthritis	Network Approach	[22]
Everolimus	Pancreatic neuroendocrine tumours	Immunosuppressant	Text-mining Approach	[21]
Finasteride	Hair loss	Benign prostatic hyperplasia	Experiment	[13, 17]
Fludrocortisone	Hypertension	Cerebral salt wasting syndrome	Experiment	[22]

Drug name	New indication	Origin indication	Mining Approaches	References
Fluoxetine	Premenstrual dysphoric disorder	Depression	Network Propagation	[13]
Furosemide	Bartter syndrome	Edema associated with congestive heart failure	Experiment	[22]
Galantamine	Alzheimer's disease	Polio, paralysis and anaesthesia	Network Approach	[17]
Gemcitabine	Anticancer agent	Antiviral	Experiment	[16]
Hydroxychloroquine	Anti-arthritic systemic lupus erythematosus	Antiparasitic	Experiment	[19]
Imatinib	GIST	BCR-ABL	Experiment	[21]
Imidapril	Cancer cachexia	Hypertension	Experiment	[19]
Infliximab	Different arthritis forms; Alzheimer's disease	Crohn's disease	Experiment	[19]
Leflunomide	Prostate cancer	Rheumatoid arthritis	Network Approach	[16]
Lidocaine	Oral corticosteroid dependent asthma, arrhythmia	Local anaesthesia	Experiment	[13]
Lumigan	Hypotrichosis simplex	Glaucoma	Experiment	[13]
Mecamylamine	ADHD	Moderately severe to severe essential hypertension and uncomplicated cases of malignant hypertension	Experiment	[17]
Metformin	Breast, adenocarcinoma, prostate, colorectal cancer	Diabetes mellitus	Experiment	[16]
Methotrexate	Osteosarcoma, breast cancer, Hodgkin lymphoma	Acute leukaemia	Network Approach	[13]
Methotrexate	Rheumatoid arthritis	Cancer	Experiment	[16]
Mifepristone	Psychotic major depression, Cushing's syndrome	Pregnancy termination	Experiment	[13]
Milnacipran	Fibromyalgia	Depression	Experiment	[13]
Miltefosine	Visceral and cutaneous leishmaniosis	Breast cancer	Experiment	[19]
Minocycline	Ovarian cancer, glioma	Acne	Experiment	[16]
Monoxide	Hair loss	Hypertension	Experiment	[13]
Mycophenolate mofetil	Renal symptoms of systemic lupus erythematosus	Transplanted organ rejection	Experiment	[19]

Drug name	New indication	Origin indication	Mining Approaches	References
Naltrexone	Alcohol withdrawal	Opioid addiction	Experiment	[19]
Nelfinavir	In clinical trials for multiple cancer	AIDS	Network Approach	[21]
Nitroxoline	Bladder, breast cancer	Antibiotic	Experiment	[16]
Noscapine	Multiple cancer types	Antitussive,antimalari al,analgesic	Experiment	[16]
Paclitaxel	Restenosis	Cancer	Network Approach	[13]
Pegvisomant	Hypercholesterolemia	Acromegaly	Experiment	[22]
Perindopril	Alzheimer's disease	Hypertension	Network Approach	[22]
Phentolamine	Impaired night vision, dental anaesthesia reversal agent	Hypertension	Network Approach	[13]
Pioglitazone	Nonalcoholic steatohepatitis	Type 2 diabetes mellitus	Experiment	[23]
Raloxifene	Osteoporosis	Breast and prostate cancer	Experiment	[19]
Rapamycin	Colorectal cancer, lymphoma, leukaemia	Immunosuppressant	Computational Approach	[16]
Requip	Restless legs	Parkinson's disease	Experiment	[13]
Retinoic acid	Acute promyelocytic leukaemia	Acne	Experiment	[19]
Ropinerole	Parkinson's, restless legs syndrome	Hypertension	Experiment	[17]
Sibutramine	Obesity	Depression	Experiment	[13, 16]
Sildenafil citrate	Erectile dysfunction (approved)	Hypertension, angina	Experiment	[13, 19]
Statins	Cancer, leukaemia	Myocardial infarction	Network Approach	[16]
Sunitinib	Pancreatic tumours/ Gastrointestinal Tumour	GIST, renal cell carcinoma	Network Approach	[21]
Tadalafil	Male erectile dysfunction	Inflammation and cardiovascular disease,	Experiment	[17]
Tadalafil	Prostate cancer, hypertension, pulmonary hyperplasia and prostatic hyperplasia	Impotence	Network Approach	[17]
Thalidomide	Moderate to severe erythema nodosum leprosum cutaneous symptoms in leprosy and multiple myeloma	Sedation, nausea and insomnia	Experiment	[17]

Drug name	New indication	Origin indication	Mining Approaches	References
Thalidomide	Leprosy, multiple myeloma	Morning sickness	Network Approach	[13]
Thalidomide	Erythema nodosum leprosum	Anti-emetic	Experiment	[19]
Thiocolchicoside	Leukaemia, multiple myeloma	Muscle relaxant	Network Approach	[16]
Tofisopam	Irritable bowel syndrome	Anxiety-related conditions	Experiment	[17]
Topiramate	Migraine,bulimia	Epilepsy	Experiment	[13]
Trastuzumab	HER2-positive metastatic gastric cancer	HER2-positive breast cancer	Network Approach	[21]
Valproic acid	Solid tumours, Leukaemia	Antiepileptic	Experiment	[16]
Vesnarinone	Oral cancer, leukaemia, lymphoma	Cardioprotective	Experiment	[16]
Wortmannin	Leukaemia	Antifungal	Experiment	[16]
Zidovudine	HIV/AIDS	Cancer	Experiment	[13]
Zoledronic acid	Multiple myeloma, prostate cancer, breast cancer	Anti-bone resorption	Experiment	[16]

Table 1.
Pharmacological repositioning culled from the extensive literature.

for medicinal molecules can be investigated based on chemical similarities. The rationale for this method is based on quantitative connections between chemical structures and biological activity that are well-known (QSAR). Although identical structures in biological systems do not always act the same, computational techniques for drug repositioning can take use of the degrees of resemblance that exist. Chemical similarity techniques work by extracting a set of chemical properties for each drug in a group of medications, then clustering or creating networks based on the recovered features to relate the drugs directly to one another [25]. Simple chemical associations or looking for specific biological traits, such as known drug targets, enriched in the resulting correlations can subsequently be used to infer therapeutic repositioning prospects.

Chemical systems biology is being used to identify new drugs in a network. A unique method of modelling and predicting drug–target interactions is statistical modelling of similarities in chemical structure between medicines and possible ligands [26, 27]. Before and after modelling with chemical drug – ligand interactions, network mapping of a wide range of drugs to protein targets enabled the prediction of new targets, including primary sites of action and off-target proteins as explanations for well-known side effects, with new and unexpected drug binding revealed across major categories of proteins unrelated by sequence or structure. A number of modelling predictions were validated using binding assays, proving the method's efficacy [28]. A generated network of chemogenomic space exhibited a high level of interaction between gene families, giving tractable drug combinations the ability to act on projected targets, by integrating structure – activity data for predicted multiple target binding compounds [29]. This demonstrates how networks can be used as templates for statistical and computational modelling predictions of drug–ligand interactions, and it adds to our understanding of polypharmacology, or the particular binding of a molecule to two or more biological targets [27]. Computational tools for drug discovery are represented in **Table 2**.

Databases	**Functions**	**URL**
BIND	Portal for biomolecular interaction networks	http://bond.unleashedinformatics.com/
BioGRID	A database of physical and genetic interactions of many organisms	http://thebiogrid.org
DIP	A database for experimentally determined protein interactions	http://dip.doe-mbi.ucla.edu/dip/Main.cgi
GWAS	Resource of genome-wide association studies	http://gwas.nih.gov
HPRD	Human proteome database HPID	www.hprd.org/
HPID	A human-protein interaction database	http://wilab.inha.ac.kr/hpid/
IntAct	Open source analysis tools for molecular interaction data	http://www.ebi.ac.uk/intact/
MINT	Database of curated molecular interactions	http://160.80.34.4/mint/
MIPS	Database of mammalian protein–protein interactions that has been manually curated.	http://mips.helmholtz-muenchen.de/proj/ppi/
OMIM	A repository of human genes and genetic diseases.	http://www.ncbi.nlm.nih.gov/omim
STRING	Known and predicted protein–protein interactions database	http://string-db.org/
Metabolic network resources		
BRENDA	A comprehensive enzyme database	www.brenda-enzymes.info/
KEGG	A comprehensive database on metabolic pathways, diseases, drugs, and other topics.	http://www.genome.jp/kegg/
REACTOME	Open access curated pathway database	http://www.reactome.org/ReactomeGWT/entrypoint.html
Drug Discovery Network resources		
CPNM	Context-specific Protein Network Miner	http://www.biotextminer.com/CPNM/index.html
Drug bank	Information on drugs and their targets	http://www.drugbank.ca/
PROMISCUOUS	Resource of drugs, proteins and side effects	http://bioinformatics.charite.de/promiscuous/
STITCH	A database of known and projected drug-protein interactions	http://stitch.embl.de/
ZINC	Chemical compounds that are commercially available are stored in a database	http://zinc.docking.org/

Databases	Functions	URL
Tools for network construction		
Cobweb	A tool for visualising and exploring networks.	http://bioinformatics.charite.de/cobweb/
Cytoscape	Tool for network visualisation and data integration. Many plugins are available for various types of analysis.	http://www.cytoscape.org/
NAViGaTOR	Network visualisation tool	http://ophid.utoronto.ca/navigator/
Tools for network analysis		
Pajek	A large network visualisation and analysis tool	http://vlado.fmf.uni-lj.si/pub/networks/pajek/
Gephi	A dynamic network visualisation tool that also allows for specialising, filtering, navigating, altering, and clustering of network data.	https://gephi.org/
BIANA	Automated network data integration and analysis using other tools such as Cytoscape	http://sbi.imim.es/web/index.php/research/servers/biana?
POINeT	PPI searching, analysis and visualisation tool	http://poinet.bioinformatics.tw/
Network analyser	Plugin for analysing and visualising molecular interaction networks, as well as computing specific network topological metrics.	http://med.bioinf.mpi-inf.mpg.de/netanalyzer/

Table 2.
Tools for protein–protein interaction analysis.

6. Applications of personalised medicine and drug repositioning

The utilisation of personalised medicine methodologies to investigate particular diseases and reposition medications for these diseases has far-reaching diagnostic and therapy implications. Both of these approaches are particularly useful for rare diseases or disease subtypes that are difficult to investigate and conduct clinical trials for due to their rarity [30]. They're also important for patients who are resistant to or have developed resistance to medicines and do not have any other options for treatment. We'll look at how customised medicine and drug repositioning methods can help in these two cases in this section.

7. Orphan or rare diseases

Any disease that affects a small percentage of the population is classified as an orphan or uncommon disease. The majority of known uncommon diseases are genetic in nature, and so they affect people for the rest of their lives. Many manifest early in life, and approximately 30% of children with rare diseases die before reaching the age of five. There is no commonly agreed-upon cut-off figure for determining whether or not a disease is rare. The Rare Disease Act of 2002, for example, defines a rare sickness as any disease or condition that affects fewer than 200,000 people in the United States, whereas in Japan, a rare disease is defined as one that affects fewer than 50,000 people. Rare diseases, on the other hand, are defined by the European Commission on Public Health as those that are life-threatening or chronically debilitating and have such a low prevalence (1 in 2000 individuals) that they require special coordinated efforts to combat. Furthermore, a sickness that is rare in one part of the world or among a specific group of people may be widespread in another. An individual uncommon disease may have a low incidence. However, the 6000 identified rare diseases collectively impact around 25 million Americans, or about 10% of the total [31]. Because rare diseases are defined by therapy availability, resource scarcity, and disease severity, they are now referred to as orphan diseases (ODs), especially since the orphan drug movement began in the United States in 1983. As a result, the United States Orphan Medication Act (1983) covers both rare and non-rare diseases for which there is no reasonable expectation that the cost of developing and commercialising a drug for such a disease in the United States will be recouped via drug sales in the United States. About 6000 rare or OD diseases have been recognised, and the National Institutes of Health's Office of Rare Diseases (ORD) keeps track of them (NIH). While some of the mentioned ODs are well-known (e.g., cystic fibrosis, Huntington's disease), the majority of people are unaware of numerous ODs with patient numbers of less than a hundred. Each year, about 250 new ODs and diseases are characterised [32]. The ODA was created to support the research and marketing of medications (orphan pharmaceuticals) for the treatment of ODs and other disorders. The ODA arose in response to the modest number of orphan medications approved in the United States in the years leading up to the ODA's approval [33]. Unfortunately, the drug research process for ODs is the same as it is for any other disease: it is extremely costly and time-consuming.

8. Discussion and conclusion

After looking at the various ways that computational drug repositioning strategies and models have been used to identify novel therapeutic interactions, we can conclude that each strategy and approach has its own set of benefits and drawbacks, and that combining different strategies and approaches often results in a higher success rate. Despite the fact that we have some excellent computational drug repositioning models, establishing robust models is still a difficult endeavour. Because of the intricacy of mapping such theoretical approaches to imitate actual organisms behaviour, as well as other difficulties such as missing, skewed, and erroneous data, one of the key challenges is bringing theoretical computing ideas into action. For example, reliable gene expression signature profiles may be difficult to define due to a variety of factors, including differences in experimental conditions (e.g., environment variables and patient age) between experiments, which can lead to data discrepancies in gene expression signatures, contributing to biased data. Furthermore, when these genes are employed as medication targets, there may not always be large changes in gene expression, which might lead to erroneous results. Furthermore, when using the chemical structure and molecular information technique, the dearth of high-resolution structural data for drug targets makes it difficult to detect potential drug-target interactions. Another issue that computational drug repositioning models face is the absence of reliable gold-standard datasets with which to evaluate their efficacy.

We offer a brief overview of the subject of computational drug repositioning, with a focus on analytically validating such methods. We cover the three methods of validation that are currently in use, as well as the challenges with consistency and essential assumptions that each of them makes. Finally, we offer an approach for increasing the validity of computational repositioning validation.

Author details

Kareti Srinivasa Rao* and P. Subash
Department of Pharmacy, Indira Gandhi National Tribal University, Amarkantak, MP, India

*Address all correspondence to: ksrao@igntu.ac.in

References

[1] Medina-Franco JL, Giulianotti MA, Welmaker GS, Houghten RA. Shifting from the single to the multitarget paradigm in drug discovery. Drug Discovery Today. 2013;**18**(9-10):495-501

[2] Senanayake SL. Drug repurposing strategies for COVID-19. Future Drug Discovery. 2020;**2**(2):689-706

[3] Brown AS, Patel CJ. A review of validation strategies for computational drug repositioning. Briefings in Bioinformatics. 2018;**19**(1):174-177

[4] Coronavirus E. 13,968 Cases and 223 Deaths: Available from: https://www.worldometers.info/coronavirus/country/ethiopia. Accessed: 2020;27.

[5] Lima WG, Brito JC, Overhage J, Nizer WS. The potential of drug repositioning as a short-term strategy for the control and treatment of COVID-19 (SARS-CoV-2): A systematic review. Archives of Virology. 2020;**165**(8):1729-1737

[6] Rodriguez-Morales AJ, Cardona-Ospina JA, Gutiérrez-Ocampo E, Villamizar-Peña R, Holguin-Rivera Y, Escalera-Antezana JP, et al. Clinical, laboratory and imaging features of COVID-19: A systematic review and meta-analysis. Travel Medicine and Infectious Disease. 2020;**34**:101623

[7] Qu YM, Kang EM, Cong HY. Positive result of Sars-Cov-2 in sputum from a cured patient with COVID-19. Travel Medicine and Infectious Disease. 2020;**34**:101619

[8] Reichert JM. Trends in development and approval times for new therapeutics in the United States. Nature Reviews. Drug Discovery. 2003;**2**(9):695-702

[9] Gilbert J, Henske P, Singh A. Rebuilding big pharma's business model. In vivo-New York then Norwalk. 2003;**21**(10):73-80

[10] Carvalho T, Krammer F, Iwasaki A. The first 12 months of COVID-19: A timeline of immunological insights. Nature Reviews Immunology. 2021;**21**(4):245-256

[11] Oprea TI, Bauman JE, Bologa CG, Buranda T, Chigaev A, Edwards BS, et al. Drug repurposing from an academic perspective. Drug Discovery Today: Therapeutic Strategies. 2011;**8**(3-4):61-69

[12] Roin BN. Unpatentable drugs and the standards of patentability. Texas Law Review. 2008;**87**:503

[13] Novac N. Challenges and opportunities of drug repositioning. Trends in Pharmacological Sciences. 2013;**34**(5):267-272

[14] Yeu Y, Yoon Y, Park S. Protein localization vector propagation: A method for improving the accuracy of drug repositioning. Molecular BioSystems. 2015;**11**(7):2096-2102

[15] Mullen J, Cockell SJ, Tipney H, Woollard PM, Wipat A. Mining integrated semantic networks for drug repositioning opportunities. PeerJ. 2016;**4**:e1558

[16] Gupta SC, Sung B, Prasad S, Webb LJ, Aggarwal BB. Cancer drug discovery by repurposing: Teaching new tricks to old dogs. Trends in Pharmacological Sciences. 2013;**34**(9):508-517

[17] Ashburn TT, Thor KB. Drug repositioning: Identifying and developing new uses for existing drugs.

Nature Reviews. Drug Discovery. 2004;**3**(8):673-683

[18] Ross MK, Yoon J, van der Schaar A, van der Schaar M. Discovering pediatric asthma phenotypes on the basis of response to controller medication using machine learning. Annals of The American Thoracic Society. 2018;**15**(1):49-58

[19] Henriksen K, Christiansen C, Karsdal MA. Serological biochemical markers of surrogate efficacy and safety as a novel approach to drug repositioning. Drug Discovery Today. 2011;**16**(21-22):967-975

[20] Nagaraj AB, Wang QQ, Joseph P, Zheng C, Chen Y, Kovalenko O, et al. Using a novel computational drug-repositioning approach (DrugPredict) to rapidly identify potent drug candidates for cancer treatment. Oncogene. 2018;**37**(3):403-414

[21] Deotarse PP, Jain AS, Baile MB, Kolhe NS, Kulkarni AA. Drug repositioning: A review. International Journal of Pharmacy Research and Review. 2015;**4**:51-58

[22] Wang ZY, Zhang HY. Rational drug repositioning by medical genetics. Nature Biotechnology. 2013;**31**(12):1080-1082

[23] Wang ZY, Quan Y, Zhang HY. Medical genetic inspirations for anticancer drug repurposing. Trends in Pharmacological Sciences. 2014;**35**(1):1-3

[24] Swinney DC, Anthony J. How were new medicines discovered? Nature Reviews. Drug Discovery. 2011;**10**(7):507-519

[25] Eckert H, Bajorath J. Molecular similarity analysis in virtual screening: Foundations, limitations and novel approaches. Drug Discovery Today. 2007;**12**(5-6):225-233

[26] Keiser MJ, Roth BL, Armbruster BN, Ernsberger P, Irwin JJ, Shoichet BK. Relating protein pharmacology by ligand chemistry. Nature Biotechnology. 2007;**25**(2):197-206

[27] Hopkins AL. Network pharmacology: The next paradigm in drug discovery. Nature Chemical Biology. 2008;**4**(11):682-690

[28] Keiser MJ, Setola V, Irwin JJ, Laggner C, Abbas AI, Hufeisen SJ, et al. Predicting new molecular targets for known drugs. Nature. 2009;**462**(7270):175-181

[29] Paolini GV, Shapland RH, van Hoorn WP, Mason JS, Hopkins AL. Global mapping of pharmacological space. Nature Biotechnology. 2006;**24**(7):805-815

[30] Li YY, Jones SJ. Drug repositioning for personalized medicine. Genome Medicine. Mar 2012;**4**(3):1-4

[31] Rados C. Orphan products: Hope for people with rare diseases. FDA Consumer. 2003;**11**:10-15

[32] Wästfelt M, Fadeel B, Henter JI. A journey of hope: Lessons learned from studies on rare diseases and orphan drugs. Journal of Internal Medicine. Jul 2006;**260**(1):1-10

[33] Levitt JA, Kelsey JV. The orphan drug regulations and related issues. Food & Drug LJ. 1993;**48**:525

Chapter 7

Drug Repurposing: Challenges and Successes in the Treatment of SARS-CoV-2

Xolani Henry Makhoba

Abstract

The coronavirus disease 2019 (COVID-19) outbreak resulted in an economic burden, with millions of morbidity and mortality infections, due to the unavailability of treatment and limited resources in many developing countries. Drug repurposing was among the first ways to come up with a solution to combat the COVID-19 outbreak worldwide and save lives. Drug repurposing, well-defined as investigating new hints for approved drugs or progressing formerly considered but unapproved drugs, is the main approach in drug development. It is suggested that at least 30–40% of novel drugs and biologics permitted by the US Food and Drug Administration (FDA) in 2007 and 2009 can be considered repurposed or repositioned products. Here, we discuss some of the proposed and tested drugs as tools to eliminate COVID-19, the challenges and successes of preparing for future pandemics using the drug repurposing approach, and treating other diseases.

Keywords: COVID-19, drug repurposing, challenges, success, preparedness for future

1. Introduction

In 2019, the whole world was hit by the outbreak of severe acute respiratory syndrome coronavirus-2 (SARS-CoV-2) that causes coronavirus diseases 2019 (COVID-19), with a huge economic and social burden to humankind [1]. Many people lost their household income. Many businesses were forced to shut down because of travel restrictions that were imposed to manage this novel disease. Sadly, millions of people lost their lives, and billions of cases were reported worldwide due to this disease. Unfortunately, there was no effective and affordable cure for COVID-19, resulting in the search for urgent treatment of this pandemic. Hence, pharmaceutical and academic institutions came together to develop emergency treatments. Thus, looking at existing drugs for the treatment of closely related diseases to COVID-19 was one of the proposed approaches to combat the scourge of the virus. Vaccines of tested efficacy to stop COVID-19 infection were being investigated vigorously worldwide. Currently, some specific drugs have been authorized for COVID-19, but the improvement of antivirals requires time. Hence, a faster way of treatment is done by drug repurposing [2, 3]. Drug repurposing is a promising approach in disease management because it is fast, easy, and a safe strategy to deal with ever-increasing disease crises because of their previously known applications. Drugs used for managing malaria were proposed for treatment of COVID-19. A study conducted showed that both chloroquine (CQ) and hydroxychloroquine (HCQ), which are known antimalarial medications, were found to have *in vitro* efficacy against SARS-CoV-2 [4]. Various small future studies have shown positive results. However, this outcome has not been declared worldwide, and apprehensions have been elevated due to the indiscriminate use and potential side effects. The clinicians were not in support of the usage of these medications. For example, the correct dose and duration of therapy are unknown. Another conducted study proposed that African countries have since seen low numbers of COVID-19 due to the endemic use of malarial drugs. They investigated the *in vitro* antiviral activity against SARS-CoV-2 of several antimalarial drugs. The outcome of the conducted study showed the following results: chloroquine (EC50 = 2.1 μM and EC90 = 3.8 μM), hydroxychloroquine (EC50 = 1.5 μM and EC90 = 3.0 μM), ferroquine (EC50 = 1.5 μM and EC90 = 2.4 μM), desethylamodiaquine (EC50 = 0.52 μM and EC90 = 1.9 μM), mefloquine (EC50 = 1.8 μM and EC90 = 8.1 μM), pyronaridine (EC50 = 0.72 μM and EC90 = 0.75 μM), and quinine (EC50 = 10.7 μM and EC90 = 38.8 μM) showed *in vitro* antiviral effective activity with IC50 and IC90 compatible with drug oral uptake at doses commonly administered in malaria treatment [5]. The ratio Clung/EC90 ranged from 5 to 59. Lumefantrine, piperaquine, and dihydroartemisinin had IC50 and IC90 too high to be compatible with expected plasma concentrations (ratio Cmax/EC90 < 0.05). With this data, it was then predictable that countries that generally use artesunate-amodiaquine or artesunate-mefloquine account for fewer cases and deaths than those using artemether-lumefantrine or dihydroartemisinin-piperaquine. In recent years, novel coronavirus infections have occurred occasionally in many countries worldwide. Severe acute respiratory syndrome coronavirus (SARS-CoV) arose in 2002, infecting 8,422 people and causing 916 losses during the epidemic. Middle East respiratory syndrome coronavirus (MERS-CoV) was first recognized in 2012. At the end of December 2019, a total of 2499 laboratory-confirmed cases of Middle East respiratory syndrome (MERS), including 861 associated deaths, were reported globally [6]. At the end of 2019, novel coronavirus pneumonia (NCP) appeared in Wuhan and spread speedily. The pathogen was established as a new coronavirus, publicly named COVID-19 by the World Health Organization (WHO). Proteinase is a key enzyme in CoV polyprotein processing. In recent years, research on SARS-CoV and MERS-CoV protease inhibitors has been carried out *in vitro* and *in vivo* Lopinavir (LPV) is a proteinase inhibitor. Both peak (9.6 μg/ml) and trough (5.5 μg/ml) serum concentrations of LPV inhibit SARS-CoV [7]. LPV also blocks a postentry step in the MERS-CoV replication cycle [6]. Ritonavir (RTV) inhibits the CYP3A-mediated metabolism of LPV, thereby increasing the serum concentration of LPV. Lopinavir/Ritonavir (LPV/r) is a combination of lopinavir and ribavirin. The antiviral activity of LPV/r is like that of LPV alone, suggesting that LPV largely drives the effect. Therefore, this review focuses on drug repurposing their success and challenges, and preparedness for future pandemics [8].

2. Different types of human coronaviruses

Coronaviruses (CoVs) are a family of viruses that cause respiratory and intestinal illnesses in humans and animals. They usually cause mild colds in people, but the emergence of the severe acute respiratory syndrome (SARS) epidemic in China in 2002–2003 and the Middle East respiratory syndrome (MERS) on the Arabian Peninsula in 2012 show they can also cause severe disease. In addition to these types of coronaviruses, the whole world has been faced with the highly transmitted type of coronavirus since

December 2019. Severe acute respiratory syndrome coronavirus 2 (SARS-CoV-2), which causes coronavirus disease, was first reported in China in 2019 in Wuhan after some serious pneumonia cases were reported [9]. This disease was first referred to as the 2019 coronavirus but later as COVID-19 by the World Health Organization (WHO). Below, each type of coronavirus is explained briefly and its structure.

2.1 SARS-CoV (the beta coronavirus that causes severe acute respiratory syndrome, or SARS)

Severe acute respiratory syndrome coronavirus was first identified in Southern China around November 2002, and in 2003, it was recognized as global human treatment due to its fast-spreading conditions. For example, this disease was reported in more than 24 countries such as Asia, Europe, Northern America, and Southern America. Despite the reported cases in those areas, in 2004, no cases were reported, and the risk was relatively low [10].

2.2 MERS-CoV (the beta coronavirus that causes Middle East Respiratory Syndrome, or MERS)

Middle East Respiratory Syndrome coronavirus (MERS-CoV) was first reported in Saudi Arabia in 2012 after that reported to some other parts of the countries such as Qatar and Jordan. However, as time passed, in 2018, MERS-CoV infection cases were reported worldwide such as Asia, Europe, America, and African countries. Therefore, more than 2260 confirmed cases and 803 deaths of MERS-CoV-related disease were reported worldwide, with most cases in Saudi Arabia. This disease attracted a lot of attention in pharmaceutical and academic industries due to its high rate of human-to-human transmission and treat to human. Also, to understand its origin and pathophysiology in order to prevent it from spreading father or becoming a human pandemic. Even though health officials were dealing with a relatively new virus with different behavior, they were able to be attended to and controlled quickly, thus reducing its threat to humans [11].

2.3 Human coronavirus (HCoV-NL63)

In Holland in 2004, another novel human coronavirus (HCoV-NL63) was isolated from a seven-month-old infant suffering from respiratory symptoms. This virus has subsequently been identified in various countries, indicating a worldwide distribution. HCoV-NL63 has been shown to infect mainly children and the immune-compromised, who presented with either mild upper respiratory symptoms (cough, fever, and rhinorrhea) or more serious lower respiratory tract involvement such as bronchiolitis and croup, which was observed mainly in younger children. In fact, HCoV-NL63 is the etiological agent for up to 10% of all respiratory diseases.

2.4 SARS-CoV-2 (the novel coronavirus that causes coronavirus disease 2019, or COVID-19)

In 2019 in China Wuhan city, the first reported cases of severe acute respiratory syndrome coronavirus-2 (SARS-CoV-2) were announced as a virus responsible for coronavirus disease 2019 (COVID-19). This disease was then reported in various parts of the world, thereafter, declared as pandemic by World Health Organization (WHO) in 2020 [12, 13]. Millions of infections and millions of fatalities were reported worldwide due to fast spreading of this disease to human-human hosts. Most countries closed their borders to slow the spread of the virus, thus affecting many economies of developed and underdeveloped countries [14]. Current evidence suggests that the virus spreads mainly between people in close contact, for example, at a conversational distance. The virus can spread from an infected person's mouth or nose in small liquid particles when they cough, sneeze, speak, sing, or breathe. Another person can then contract the virus when infectious particles that pass through the air are inhaled at short range (this is often called short-range aerosol or short-range airborne transmission) or if infectious particles come into direct contact with the eyes, nose, or mouth (droplet transmission) (WHO, 2021). Therefore, treatment to combat this disease was needed urgently. Hence, most developed countries invested many in pharmaceutical and academic institutions to foster the research and development of drugs or vaccines to treat millions of infected young and old people from different countries and ethnicities [15]. As a result, the FDA approved the use of various drugs known for treating other diseases, such as malaria. These drugs included famous malaria drugs such as chloroquine, hydroxychloroquine, and others, as shown in **Table 1**. The repurposed drugs target the entry points or strategies used by the virus to enter the human host system. For example, in **Figure 1**, the SARS-CoV-2 viral structure and proteins involved in the virus process are highlighted. Spike glycoprotein is a major role player

Drug name	Structure	Mode of action	References
Chloroquine	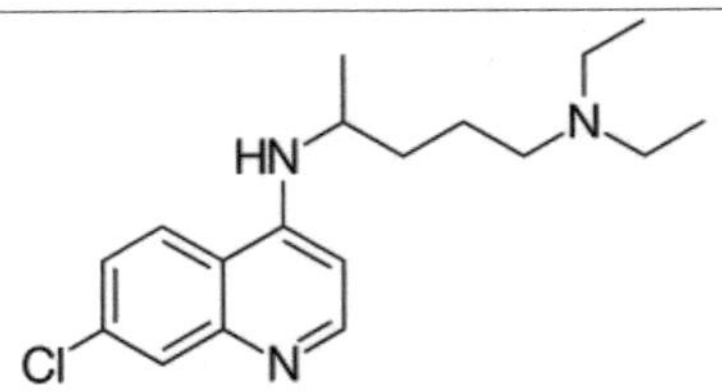	Inhibits the action of heme polymerase in malarial trophozoites, preventing the conversion of heme to hemozoin.	[16]
Hydroxychloroquine	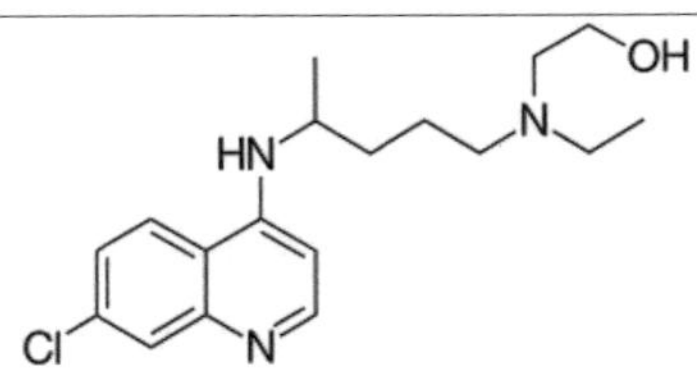	Increase pH within intracellular vacuoles and alter processes such as protein degradation by acidic hydrolases in the lysosome, assembly of macromolecules in the endosomes, and posttranslation modification of proteins in the Golgi apparatus	[17]
Ferroquine	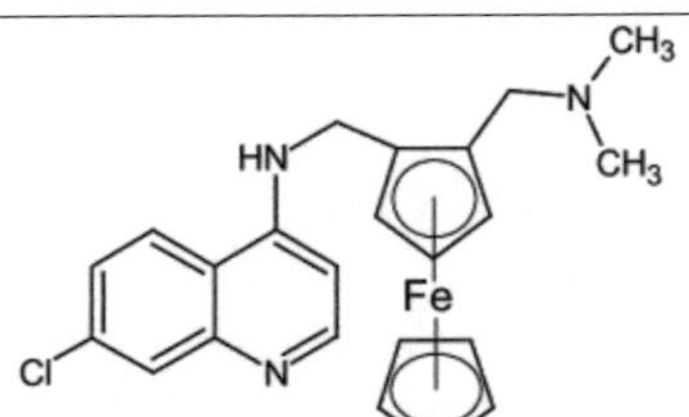	Alters lysosomal pH and induces lysosomal membrane permeabilization	[13]

Drug name	Structure	Mode of action	References
Desethylamodiaquine	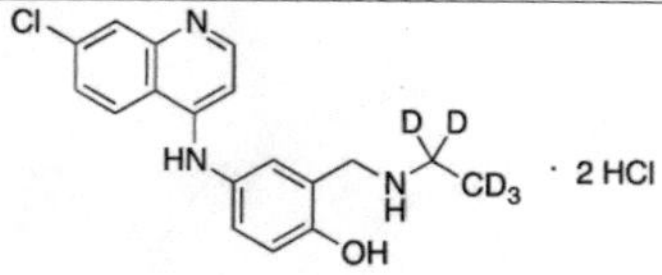	Therapy for the treatment of uncomplicated malaria	[18]
Mefloquine	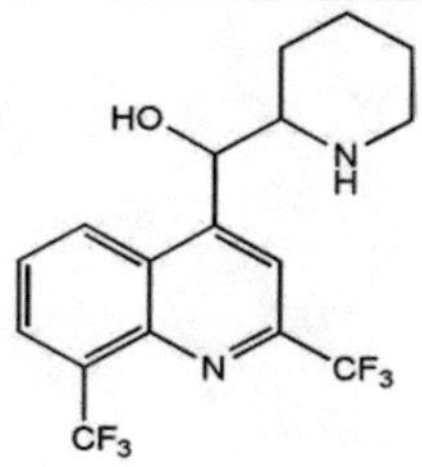	Targets the 80S ribosome of the *Plasmodium falciparum*, inhibiting protein synthesis and causing subsequent schizonticidal effects	[19]
Pyronaridine	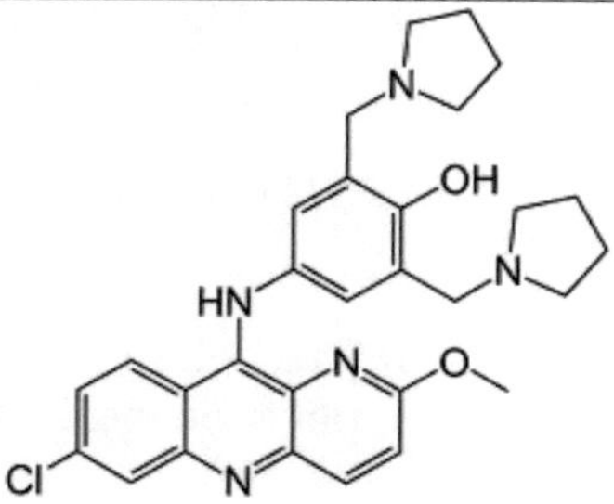	Functions have an inhibitor of hemozoin (biomineral malaria pigment, by-product of hemoglobin digestion) formation, blocking the biopolymerization of β-hematin and thus facilitating the accumulation of toxic hematin into the digestive vacuole of the parasite.	[20]
Quinine	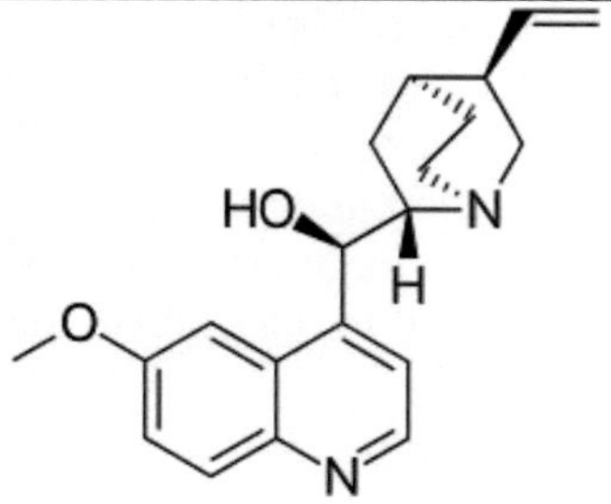	Has rapid schizonticidal action against intra-erythrocytic malaria parasites. It is also gametocytocidal for *Plasmodium vivax* and *Plasmodium malaria*, but not for *Plasmodium falciparum*. Quinine also has analgesic, but not antipyretic properties. The antimalarial mechanism of action of quinine is unknown	[21]

Table 1.
List of some drugs for malarial treatment but considered for COVID-19 treatment.

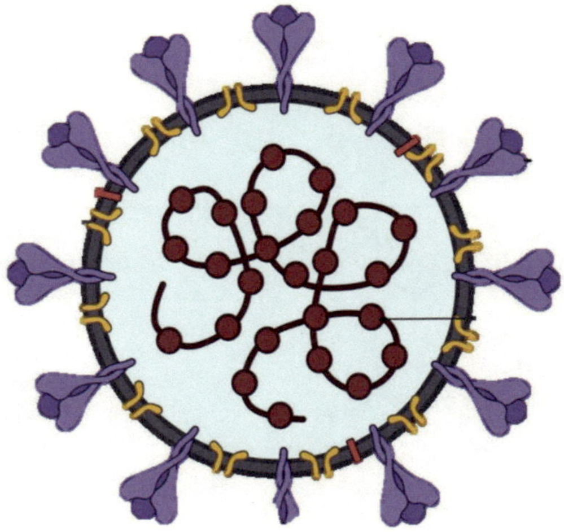

Figure 1.
SARS-CoV-2 virus depicting the location of the nucleocapsid (N), membrane (M), envelope (E), and spike (S) protein. (Adapted from Navhaya et al., 2023 unpublished data).

during viral entry into the human host. Therefore, chloroquine is believed to block the virus's entry into the host and inhibit its replication inside the cellular system [22].

3. Impact of coronaviruses in the past and present

Since the outbreak of the first coronavirus in 2002 (SARS-CoV-1), then the outbreak of influenza A in 2009, which was followed by the MERS-CoV, in 2019, there was an outbreak of SARS-CoV-2 which was declared a global pandemic. SARS-CoV-2 produced the highest number of infections and fatalities compared to the other coronaviruses. It only did not affect the undeveloped countries, but well-developed countries were hit the most. It, therefore, caused a lot of panic in the health system worldwide. These viruses are somehow observed to produce the same symptoms individuals infected by them, from fever, cough, and shortness of breath to sore throats (**Figure 2**). Though there has been a huge drive to develop effective treatment or management of SARS-CoV, it is important to highlight some of the drugs proposed as tools to fight this pandemic [23].

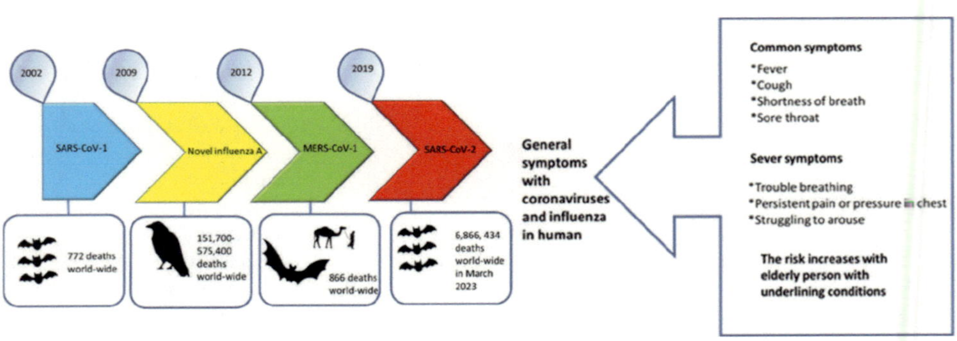

Figure 2.
Summary of the impact of coronaviruses and influenza in the past and present.

4. Summary of malaria and its treatment

Malaria is one of the major causes of death, especially in underdeveloped countries. In Africa, many drugs have been approved to treat or manage malaria, such as chloroquine, hydroxychloroquine, ferroquine, and others, as listed in **Table 1** were developed. However, the outbreak of COVID-19 in 2019 became a major concern as many countries worldwide were affected. The urgent treatment of the virus was needed; therefore, drugs that were meant for the treatment or management of the disease caused by *Plasmodium* parasites were proposed for the treatment of COVID-19. Below are some of the drugs that were tested or meant for the treatment of various types of *Plasmodium* species but repurposed or proposed for the treatment of SARS-CoV-2. Drug repurposing represents an enthusiastic mechanism to use approved drugs outside the scope of their original indication and accelerate the discovery of new therapeutic options [24].

5. Success, challenges, and preparedness for future treatment of COVID-19

Major success stories in the management of the COVID-19 were seen, and evidence is the scraping of travel regulations due to the decrease in the transmissions of the disease. The emergency approval of various vaccines, such as Pfizer, messenger RNA vaccine, protein subunit vaccine, MORDENA, and Johnson and Johnson vaccine, give hope to many people. However, challenges were reported regarding the intake of the vaccine in various parts of the world due to hesitations. This resulted in the slow intake of the vaccines and the boosters. As a result, various types of SARS-CoV-2 variants were developed in various countries, such as the United Kingdom, South Africa, and the United States just to mention but a few. One of the most important things to prepare for a future pandemic is the availability of accurate information. Proper education at all levels of age, in order to prepare better for what may come [25].

6. Cancer and HIV drugs repurposing for COVID-19 treatment

Both cancer and HIV are the pauses a huge threat to human life worldwide. With cancer, it is difficult to avoid because it can be inherently detected, but with HIV, it is documented that it can be transferred from human-to-human through

Drug name	Cancer/HIV	Action	Ref
Ruxolitinib	Cancer	Reduction of hyperinflammation during cytokine storm	[26]
Bevacizumab	Cancer	Vascular permeability inhibition	[27]
Carmofur	Cancer	Blockade of viral replication	[28]
Lopinavir	HIV	inhibits the activity of an enzyme critical for the HIV viral lifecycle	[28]
Ritonavir	HIV	binds to the protease active site and inhibits the activity of the enzyme	[29]
Indinavir	HIV	binds to the protease active site and inhibits the activity of the enzyme	[30]
Saquinavir	HIV	binds to the protease active site and inhibits the activity of the enzyme	[31]

Table 2.
A list of some drugs for cancer and HIV treatment but repurposed for COVID-19 treatment.

unprotected sex and through sharing needles with someone who has the virus in their system. There is no effective cure for both diseases; however, there are management approaches. The outbreak of COVID-19 presented the opportunity for drug repurposing from both cancer and HIV drugs to treat the pandemic. **Table 2** summarizes some drugs that are known for either cancer or HIV management but were tested for COVID-19 and were reported to be promising tools for this disease.

7. Conclusions and future perspectives

Drug repurposing is a promising tool in addressing various diseases, especially those that are still under study. The recent COVID-19 has taught us many lessons, from understanding its biology to drug development. Different types of drugs are being repurposed from the known disease to use against the treatment of coronavirus 2019. This approach has given many researchers and pharmaceutical industries to prepare for future pandemics using the same method to treat future pandemics.

Acknowledgements

This work was supported by South African Medical Research Council Self-Initiated Research (SIR) grants.

Author details

Xolani Henry Makhoba
Department of Biochemistry, Microbiology and Biotechnology, University of Limpopo, Sovenga, South Africa

*Address all correspondence to: xolani.makhoba@ul.ac.za

References

[1] Rubin R. COVID-19 vaccines vs variants - determining how much immunity is enough. Journal of the American Medical Association. 2021;**325**:1241-1243. DOI: 10.1001/jama.2021.3370

[2] Richman DD. Antiviral drug discovery to address the COVID-19 pandemic. mBio. 2020;**2020**:11. DOI: 10.1128/mBio.02134-20 e02134-20

[3] Chavda VP, Vora L, Vihol D. COVAX-19® Vaccine: Completely blocks virus transmission to non-immune individuals. Clinical Complementary Medicine Pharmacology. 2021;**1**(1):100001-100004. DOI: 10.1016/j.ccmp.2021.100004 In this issue

[4] Villamagna AH, Gore SJ, Lewis JS, Doggett JS. The need for antiviral drugs for pandemic coronaviruses from a global Health perspective. 2020. DOI: 10.3389/fmed.2020.596587

[5] Achan J, Talisuna AO, Erhart A, Yeka A, Tibenderana JK, Baliraine FN, et al. Quinine, an old anti-malarial drug in a modern world: Role in the treatment of malaria. Malaria Journal. 2011;**10**:144

[6] Kondratskyi A, Kondratska K, Abeelen FV, Gordienko D, Dubois C, Toillon RA, et al. Ferroquine, the next generation antimalarial drug, has antitumor activity. Nature Scientific Reports. 2017;7:15986. DOI: 10.1038/s41598-017-16154-2

[7] Anyorigiya TA, Castel S, Mauf K, Atuguba F, Ogutu B, Oduro A, et al. Pharmacokinetic profle of amodiaquine and its active metabolite desethylamodiaquine in Ghanaian patients with uncomplicated falciparum malaria. Malaria Journal. 2021;**20**:18. DOI: 10.1186/s12936-020-03553-6

[8] Wong W, Bai XC, Sleebs BE, Triglia T, Brown A, Thompson JK, et al. The antimalarial Mefloquine targets the Plasmodium falciparum 80S ribosome to inhibit protein synthesis. Nature Microbiology. 2017;**2**:17031. DOI: 10.1038/nmicrobiol

[9] Rijken MJ, McGready R, Jullien V, Tarning J, Lindegardh N, Phyo AP, et al. Pharmacokinetics of amodiaquine and desethylamodiaquine in pregnant and postpartum women with Plasmodium vivax Malaria. Antimicrobial Agents and Chemotherapy. 2011;**2011**:4338-4342. DOI: 10.1128/AAC.00154-11

[10] Wani WA, Jameel E, Baig U, Mumtazuddin S, Hun LT. Ferroquine and its derivatives: New generation of antimalarial agents. European Journal of Medicinal Chemistry. 2015;**101**:534e551. DOI: 10.1016/j.ejmech.2015.07.009

[11] Fox RI. Mechanism of action of hydroxychloroquine as an antirheumatic drug. Seminars in Arthritis and Rheumatism. 1993;**1993**:82-91. DOI: 10.1016/s0049-0172(10)80012-5

[12] Coban C. The host targeting effect of chloroquine in malaria. Current Opinion in Immunology. 2020;**66**:98-107

[13] Dyall J, Coleman CM, Hart BJ, et al. Repurposing of clinically developed drugs for treatment of Middle East respiratory syndrome coronavirus infection. Antimicrobial Agents and Chemotherapy. 2014;**58**(8):4885-4893. DOI: 10.1128/AAC.03036-14

[14] Dyall J, Gross R, Kindrachuk J, et al. Middle East respiratory syndrome and severe acute respiratory syndrome: Current therapeutic options and potential targets for novel therapies.

Drugs. 2017;**77**(18):1935e66. DOI: 10.1007/s40265-017-0830-1

[15] El Bairi K, Amrani M, Afqir S. Starvation tactics using natural compounds for advanced cancers: Pharmacodynamics, clinical efficacy, and predictive biomarkers. Cancer Medicine. 2018;7(6):2221-2246. DOI: 10.1002/cam4.1467

[16] Huang F, Zhang C, Liu Q, Zhao Y, Zhang Y, Qin Y, et al. Identification of amitriptyline HCl, flavin adenine dinucleotide, azacitidine and calcitriol as repurposing drugs for influenza A H5N1 virus-induced lung injury. PLoS Pathogens. 2020;**16**(3):e1008341. DOI: 10.1371/journ al.ppat.1008341

[17] Scherman D, Fetro C. Drug repositioning for rare diseases: Knowledge-based success stories. Thérapie. 2020;**75**:161-167. DOI: 10.1016/j.therap.2020.02.007

[18] Sertkaya A, Birkenbach A, Berlind A, Eyraud J. Examination of clinical trial costs and barriers for drug development. US Department of Health and Human Services, office of the assistant secretary for planning and evaluation report. 2014;**1**:1-92

[19] Yeu Y, Yoon Y, Park S. Protein localization vector propagation: A method for improving the accuracy of drug repositioning. Molecular BioSystems. 2015;**11**:2096-2102. DOI: 10.1039/c5mb0 0306g

[20] Hodos RA, Kidd BA, Shameer K, Readhead BP, Dudley JT. In silico methods for drug repurposing and pharmacology. Wiley Interdisciplinary Review in Systematic Biology. 2016;**8**(3):186-210. DOI: 10.1002/wsbm.1337

[21] Harrison C. Coronavirus puts drug repurposing on the fast track. Nature Biotechnology. 2020;**38**(4):379-381. DOI: 10.1038/d41587-020-00003-1

[22] El Bairi K, Amrani M, Kandhro AH, Afqir S. Prediction of therapy response in ovarian cancer: Where are we now? Critical Review in Clinical Laboratory Science. 2017;**54**(4):233e66. DOI: 10.1080/10408363.2017.1313190

[23] El Bairi K, Atanasov AG, Amrani M, Afqir S. The arrival of predictive biomarkers for monitoring therapy response to natural compounds in cancer drug discovery. Biomedical Pharmacotherapy. 2019;**109**:2492-2498. DOI: 10.1016/j.biopha.2018.11.097

[24] El Bairi K, Jabi R, Trapani D, et al. Can the microbiota predict response to systemic cancer therapy, surgical outcomes, and survival? The answer is in the gut. Expert Review in Clinical Pharmacology. 2020;**13**(4):403-421 [Published online ahead of print]

[25] Woodhead M, Ewig S, Torres A. Severe acute respiratory syndrome (SARS). European Respiratory Journal. 2003;**21**:739-740. DOI: 10.1183/09031936.03.00035403

[26] Woo PC, Huang Y, Lau SK, Yuen KY. Coronavirus genomics and bioinformatics analysis. Viruses. 2010;**2**:1804-1820. DOI: 10.3390/v2081803

[27] Drexler JF, Gloza-Rausch F, Glende J, Corman VM, Muth D, Goettsche M, et al. Genomic characterization of severe acute respiratory syndrome-related coronavirus in European bats and classifcation of coronaviruses based on partial RNA-dependent RNA polymerase gene sequences. Journal of Virology. 2010;**2010**(84):11336-11349. DOI: 10.1128/JVI.00650-10

[28] LeDuc JW, Barry MA. SARS, the frst pandemic of the 21st century. Emerging Infectious Diseases. 2004;**10**:e26. DOI: 10.3201/eid1011.040797_02

[29] Zhou P, Yang XL, Wang XG, Hu B, Zhang L, Zhang W, et al. A pneumonia outbreak associated with a new coronavirus of probable bat origin. Nature. 2020;**579**:270-273. DOI: 10.1038/s41586-020-2012-7

[30] Benvenuto D, Giovanetti M, Ciccozzi A, Spoto S, Angeletti S, Ciccozzi M. The 2019-new coronavirus epidemic: Evidence for virus evolution. Journal of Medical Virology. 2020;**92**:455-459. DOI: 10.1002/jmv.25688

[31] Shield C. Coronavirus: From bats to pangolins, how do viruses reach us? Deutsche Welle. 2020;**84**:104493

Chapter 8

Perspective Chapter: Appraisal of Paclitaxel (Taxol) Pros and Cons in the Management of Cancer – Prospects in Drug Repurposing

John Oluwafemi Teibo, Chioma Ejiro Irozuru, Titilade Kehinde Ayandeyi Teibo, Olabode Ebenezer Omotoso, Ahmad O. Babalghith and Gaber El-Saber Batiha

Abstract

Paclitaxel (Taxol) is potent natural anticancer drug that has evolved over the years. It has been useful in the management of many cancers. Hence, this review aims to appraise the pros and cons of paclitaxel in the management of cancers using literature. Paclitaxel acts by obstructing mitotic spindle formation attributed to clamp-down of mitotic clampdown hence arresting the cell cycle at the G_2/M phase. Some of the notable side effects of paclitaxel usage include: hair loss, numbness, bone marrow suppression, muscle pain, allergic reactions, diarrhea, etc. Among the mechanism of paclitaxel resistance are P-glycoprotein efflux pumps, mutation in tubulin and alterations in binding regions of β-tubulin, altered function of cytokine expression as well as apoptotic Bcl-2 and p53. Combination of paclitaxel with cisplatin clearly improves the duration of progression-free survival and of overall survival of breast cancer. Paclitaxel which is a valuable natural anticancer drug seems promising in the management of non-cancer diseases such as COVID-19, renal and hepatic fibrosis, inflammation, skin disorders, axon regeneration, limb salvage, and coronary artery restenosis. With the advancement of technology, it is expected that the biosynthesis, chemo-resistance as well as its targeted delivery would unfold and perhaps open new uses and vista to the old drug of about five decades ago.

Keywords: paclitaxel, cancer management, mechanism of action, resistance, repurposing

1. Introduction

One of the World Health Organization (WHO) list of essential medicine is paclitaxel which is also known as Taxol and belongs to the taxane family (**Figure 1**). It's an approved drug used to treat some cancers which include: breast, ovarian, lung, esophageal, cervical among other, it has a total market value of over $1 billion per year [1, 2]. Some of the notable side effects of paclitaxel usage include: hair loss, numbness, bone marrow suppression, muscle pain, allergic reactions, diarrhea, etc. [3].

One of the remarkable natural anticancer drugs—paclitaxel was first extracted from the Pacific yew tree, *Taxus brevifolia* in 1971. The yield from the bark of the yew tree was 0.01–0.05% which was low and this prompted the search for alternative means of synthesis which range from microbial fermentation, chemical synthesis, tissue, and cell culture [4]. It acts by obstructing mitotic spindle formation attributed to clampdown of mitotic clampdown hence arresting the cell cycle at the G_2/M phase [5].

Among the mechanism of paclitaxel resistance are P-glycoprotein efflux pumps, mutation in tubulin and alterations in binding regions of β-tubulin, altered function of cytokine expression as well as well as apoptotic Bcl-2 and p53 [6]. Combination of paclitaxel with cisplatin clearly improves the duration of progression-free survival and of overall survival of breast cancer [7].

Earlier development shows that the combination of nab-paclitaxel and gemcitabine significantly improved the survival of patients with metastatic pancreatic cancer [8]. Recently, low-dose paclitaxel seems promising in treating non-cancer diseases, such as skin disorders, renal and hepatic fibrosis, inflammation, axon regeneration, limb salvage, and coronary artery restenosis. Future studies would help to understand the mechanisms underlying these effects in order to design therapies with specificity [9].

Nanocarrier systems including nanoparticles, liposomes, micelles, bioconjugates, and dendrimers have been employed in order to improve paclitaxel solubility and eliminate undesired side effects [10].

In the review, we examined the history, synthesis and biosynthesis of paclitaxel and also highlight the usage in the treatment of various cancers. We also presented the mechanism of action, combination with other drugs and well as the side effects and

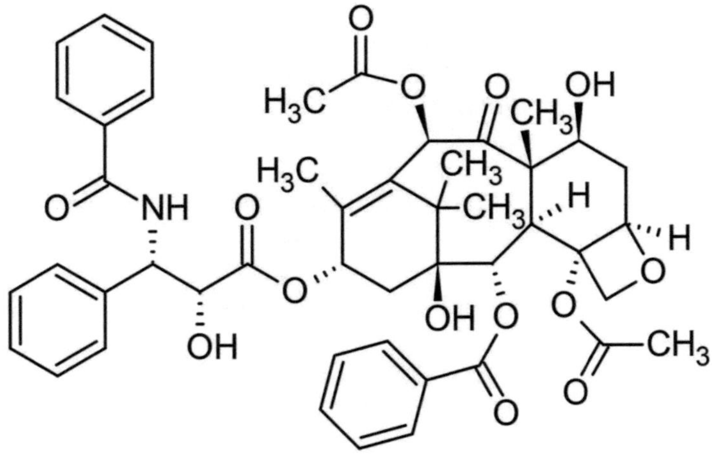

Figure 1.
Structure of paclitaxel.

mechanisms of resistance. Hence, we concluded and provided future directions on paclitaxel with increasing evidence in the management of other disease other than cancer.

2. Materials and methods

2.1 Literature search

Literature search was done across many databases such as Google Scholar, PubMed, Embase, and Scopus using the keywords "Paclitaxel" and "Cancer." A lot of research article was obtained as this area has been explored for the past 50 years. Preprints that have not been peer-reviewed; non-cancer studies were excluded as well as gray literature. This was filtered with abstract, title and full text to identify relevant articles that can be integrated to assess the appraisal of paclitaxel (Taxol) in the management of cancers. The other articles were excluded by abstract, title or full text after the authors have read the abstract or articles and discovered the articles do not adhere to the objectives of our review.

3. History and synthesis

Paclitaxel has been previously extracted from the bark of the Pacific Northwest yew tree which is one of eight varieties of Taxus species specifically the *Taxus brevifolia* [1, 11]. The yew tree has been historically used in the production spear points and other weapons, household implements and diverse tools [12, 13]. The active compound in paclitaxel was identified by Mansukh Wani and Monroe Wall in 1971 [14–16]. The drug was also selected that same year by the NCI as a candidate for preclinical development and took the crucial step of entering into an agreement with the National Forest Service to ensure a harvest of the yew [17, 18]. A breakthrough in the development of paclitaxel occurred in 1979 when Dr. Susan Horwitz at Albert Einstein Medical College in New York identified the drug's unique mechanism of action as a promoter of microtubule assembly and its cytostatic activity on many types of tumors, thus increasing scientific interest in studying the drug [19, 20]. According to the National Cancer Institute (NCI), the *Taxus brevifolia* has a very poor Taxol content of only about 0.06% in the bark making it incapable of meeting the market and research's needs [21, 22]. It was then concluded that the slow growth rate and high cost of production of paclitaxel made production impractical, non-environmentally conscious and financially burdening resulting in its insufficiency as a natural source of paclitaxel [23, 24]. The isolation of Taxol from endophytic fungus was also used to produce Taxol [11, 25]. This is done by the chemical conversion of 10-deacetylbaccatin-III to Taxol using synthetic and semi-synthetic methods [25]. Fermentation is also used to produce paclitaxel from microorganisms but it produces a small yield of between 24 ng and 70 μg per liter and it is very unstable [26].

3.1 Biosynthesis

Paclitaxel can be synthesized from the isoprenoid precursors, including IPP (isopentenyl pyrophosphate) and its isomer DMAPP (dimethylallyl pyrophosphate) utilized by organisms in the biosynthesis of terpenes and terpenoids, which can be produced through the MVA (mevalonate) pathway and the MEP (methylerythritol phosphate) pathway [4] as shown in **Figure 2**.

3.2 Mechanism of action

Paclitaxel is a chemotherapeutic drug functioning as a mitotic inhibitor that is used to treat common cancers [21, 25]. Paclitaxel is known to be the earliest microtubule-stabilizing agent that is able to arrest the cell cycle in the G_2/M phase and also promote apoptotic cell death [27, 28]. In preclinical *in vitro* studies, Taxol with concentrations as low as 0.05 μmol/L have been shown to promote microtubule assembly by decreasing the lag time for the microtubule assembly, and also to shift its equilibrium in favor of microtubule formation [29, 30]. It performs this role by interrupting the normal function of microtubule growth by hyper-stabilizing the structure, preventing the dissociation of microtubules, blocking cell cycle progression, preventing mitosis, and inhibiting the growth of cancer cells [31, 32]. In essence, Taxol reduces the concentration of tubulin that is needed for the assembly of microtubule in the presence or absence of factors that are usually essential for this function, such as exogenous GTP or microtubule-associated proteins [33]. Microtubules treated with Taxol are known to be stable even after a short period of treatment with calcium or low temperatures, conditions that easily promote disassembly [27]. This unusual stability results in the inhibition of the normal dynamic reorganization of the microtubule network [34]. Specifically, paclitaxel binds to the Taxol-binding domain of the β subunit of tubulin which is the "building block" of microtubules, and the binding of paclitaxel locks these building blocks in place preventing their depolymerization [35]. The complex compound formed (microtubule/paclitaxel) is unable to disassemble, thus reducing the critical concentration of the assembled tubulin subunits and increases the percentage of assembled tubulin subunits (shortening and lengthening) blocking the progression to mitosis [2]. As an anticancer drug, the microtubules in the prophase stage forms a spindle that pulls the chromosomes away from the equator to the poles [36]. During later stages, they depolymerize and the spindle structure dissolves [29] and the exposure to cold temperatures and calcium ions can also trigger depolymerization of microtubules [37]. The binding site of paclitaxel has been shown to be different from that for guanosine triphosphate, vinca alkaloids, colchicine, or

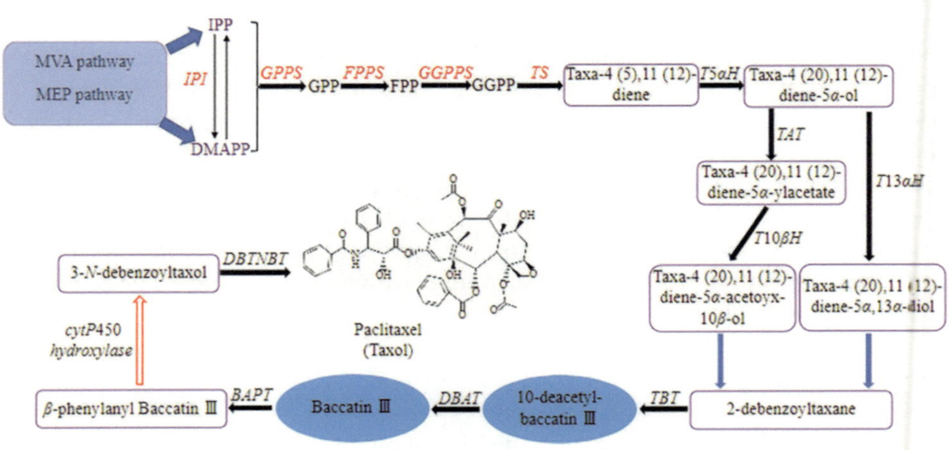

Figure 2.
Biosynthetic pathway of paclitaxel [4].

podophyllotoxin and is present on the microtubule rather than tubulin dimers [38]. The mechanism of action of paclitaxel has been proposed on the basis of its effective action as a chemotherapeutic drug for different types of cancers.

3.3 Repurposing of paclitaxel for possible therapeutic outcomes

Drug repurposing has become an economical as it saves money and time, it also overcomes development risk associated with new drugs. Great benefits that exist with drug repurposing has already been outlined especially the knowledge of the mechanism of actions of the drugs that has been studied using new methods such as genomic expression and *in vitro* drug screening and target verification. Paclitaxel has been studied to show its effects in different types of cancers. Currently, new studies have also shown its involvement in non-cancer diseases also such as fibrosis. Zhang et al. [9] indicated that signal transducer and activator of transcription 3 (STAT3) were reduced in mice and *in vitro* in a dose dependent manner. They hypothesized that the administration of low doses of paclitaxel administration, may block the STAT3 (signal transducer and activator of transcription 3). This singular activity is responsible the attenuation of fibrous that has unilateral ureteral obstruction.

3.4 Appraisal of treatment effects/success

Rowinsky and collaborators [25] reported an excellent review on the preclinical and early clinical trials with paclitaxel and observed that 30% of the patients with ovarian achieved a complete remission [39]. Shortly after the original report of activity in ovarian cancer, three additional clinical trials provided confirmation that responses are observed (mostly partial remissions) in 20–50% of the patients with this disease.

Sparano et al. [40] experimentally depicted that paclitaxel significantly improves overall survival. There was also a 32% reduction in the hazard ratio for death afforded by weekly paclitaxel which was observed in a similar administration of anthracycline-containing chemotherapy. Sparano et al. [40] results are in consonant with studies of metastatic breast cancer that demonstrated a beneficial administration of paclitaxel weekly. Zhu et al. [41] explained in his journal that paclitaxel in combination with immunotherapy can increase the efficacy of treatment against breast cancer by inhibiting the normal function of Tregs and thus reversing the immune escape of tumors.

O'Shaughnessy et al. [42] performed a randomized clinical trial including 139 patients and suggested that paclitaxel in combination with alisertib improves progression-free survival observed in patients with ER-positive, ERBB2-negative or triple-negative metastatic breast cancer which had been pretreated with endocrine therapy. Markman et al. [43] evaluated the activity of single agent weekly paclitaxel in patients with both platinum and paclitaxel (delivered every 3 weeks)—resistant ovarian cancer. Forty-eight patients with platinum and paclitaxel-resistant ovarian cancer received single agent weekly paclitaxel (80 mg/m^2/week). It was observed that the weekly administration of paclitaxel can be a useful management approach in women with both platinum and paclitaxel (given every 3 weeks)-resistant ovarian cancer.

4. Combinations with other drugs

Studies have shown that combination chemotherapy produces faster response rates and longer progression-free survival than single agents [39, 44, 45]. They remain the mainstay of therapy for patients with advanced breast cancer, and these regimens often include the anthracycline doxorubicin. When paclitaxel and MG1 were combined experimentally, their combination improved the efficacy of all of the breast cancer models tested, demonstrates greater efficiency in murine tumor models, greater tumor killing in vivo and thus is a promising alternative approach for the treatment of patients with refractory breast cancer [39]. Kawiak et al. [46] experimental study indicated that plumbagin increases the sensitivity of breast cancer cells to paclitaxel. The role of ERK (a component of mitogen-activated protein kinases that controls cell proliferation and survival) in plumbagin-mediated sensitization of breast cancer cells to paclitaxel was shown through the enhancement of the synergistic effect between compounds in cells with decreased ERK expression. These results imply that plumbagin can inhibit the activation of ERK in breast cancer cells and this plays a vital role in the sensitization of cells to paclitaxel-induced cell death [46].

Elserafi et al. demonstrated experimentally that the combination chemotherapy of paclitaxel and cisplatin provided similar response rate, lower toxic effect and overall survival when compared sequentially and in combination [44]. Also, Steuer et al. [45] showed that the combination of carboplatin-paclitaxel had a more favorable toxic-effect profile when compared to the combination of cisplatin-etoposide [45]. An experiment was carried out by Shroff et al. to evaluate the association between progression-free survival and the addition of nanoparticle albumin-bound (nab)-paclitaxel to gemcitabine-cisplatin for the treatment of patients with advanced biliary tract cancer. The result indicated that the treatment with nab-paclitaxel in addition to gemcitabine-cisplatin prolonged median progression-free survival, response rate and overall survival when compared to controls treated with gemcitabine-cisplatin alone [47, 48].

A combination of chemotherapeutic drugs doxorubicin and paclitaxel are known to be active in the treatment of advanced breast cancer. However, earlier studies indicated that this combination had a high incidence of congestive heart failure which was caused by increased exposure to doxorubicin and its metabolite doxorubicinol [49, 50]. Limitations of the paclitaxel-doxorubicin-cisplatin (TAP) regimen in the treatment of endometrial cancer include tolerability and cumbersome scheduling [51, 52]. In a phase 3 study of the efficacy and safety of the albumin-bound paclitaxel (nab-paclitaxel) plus gemcitabine versus gemcitabine monotherapy in patients with metastatic pancreatic cancer, the combination drug significantly improved overall survival, progression-free survival, and response rate [53, 54]. Combination therapy resulted both in a superior overall response rate and a superior time to treatment failure, two frequent measures of efficacy in metastatic chemotherapy trials [55].

5. Side effects/toxicity in organs

Traditional paclitaxel has a very poor solubility in water, and their solvents are likely to cause serious adverse effects [56]. There is evidence in the literature to suggest that paclitaxel effects are concentration-dependent. Adverse effects associated with paclitaxel administration include the peripheral neuropathy, hypersensitive reactions, myelosuppression, hepatotoxicity, bradycardia, cardiotoxicity, myalgias, hypotension, diarrhea, arthralgias, nausea, mucositis, gastrointestinal toxicity, and alopecia [57].

5.1 Myelosuppression

A major dose-limiting side effect of the administration of paclitaxel is myelosuppression which is known as bone marrow suppression that results in the decrease in the production of blood cells [57]. Specifically, paclitaxel administration results in grade IV leukopenia and neutropenia in about 26 and 68% of patients, respectively [58].

5.2 Hypersensitivity reactions

Hypersensitive reactions are mostly encountered either during or shortly after infusion with paclitaxel and the onset is usually very rapid, and seen within a few minutes of starting the infusion [59, 60]. Studies have shown that the solvent for paclitaxel (Cremophor EL®, castor oil vehicle) plays a very crucial role in hypersensitivity reactions such as anaphylactoid hypersensitivity reactions, abnormal lipoprotein patterns, hyperlipidemia, aggregation of erythrocytes and peripheral neuropathy which has been mediated by kinetic interference [61–63].

5.3 Neuropathy

Paclitaxel is known to cause weakness, cold sensitivity, numbness, pain from muscle and nerve damage to the hands and feet. Higher doses of paclitaxel are associated with an increased incidence of neuropathy, in fact, grade 3 or 4 neutropenia was observed in 68% [64, 65]. The effect of paclitaxel on microtubule assembly and disassembly reduces the normal axonal transport system leading to a length-dependent sensorimotor axonal neuropathy [66].

5.4 Renal and hepatic toxicities

Renal as well as hepatic toxicities are also a clinical concern in the administration of paclitaxel because they may compromise essential organ functions, impair renal excretion and reduce metabolism which lead to increased risk of other severe adverse effects [67]. This toxicity may be related to germline variations, such as single-nucleotide polymorphisms (SNPs) in genes that affect the pharmacokinetics and/or pharmacodynamics of paclitaxel [68].

5.5 Myalgias and arthralgias

Paclitaxel causes a syndrome characterized by diffuse myalgias and arthralgias, which can be resistant to opioids and other pain medications. Patients have reported pain that typically starts between day 2 and day 7 of administration and peaks on days 3–4 but remains consistent in intensity and duration with continuation of drug administration [58].

5.6 Dermatological adverse effects

Photosensitivity, pustular eruptions, folliculitis, extravasation, dorsal hand-foot syndrome, hair and nail changes, fixed erythrodysesthesia and also pigmentary changes are all caused by prolonged administration of paclitaxel [61].

6. Resistance

Drug resistance still remains the fundamental limiting factor to achieving cures to patients with cancer. Paclitaxel has been established as the first-line chemotherapeutic treatment drug for breast cancer [69, 70]. Mechanisms of drug resistance include over-expression of P-glycoprotein efflux pump, alterations in binding regions of β-tubulin and tubulin mutations, reduced function of significant apoptosis proteins (such as Bcl-2 and p53), alterations in cytokine expression (such as Interleukin-6), paclitaxel detoxification mediated by CYP [6], altered expression of regulatory proteins. These proteins include keratin 17 (KRT17) in cervical cancer cells, which may increase cell migration and PTX survival, or fibronectin type III domain-containing protein 5 (FNDC5), which could promote paclitaxel sensitivity by inhibiting NF-κB/MDR1 signaling in NSCLC [71], as well as microtubule specific effects with mutated β-tubulin, varied levels of β-tubulin isotypes, and chemical modification of tubulin [72]. Experimentally using indirect immunofluorescence and electron microscopy, acquired Taxol resistance in Chinese hamster ovary cell lines possessed altered α-tubulin or β-tubulin and required Taxol in the medium for normal growth have demonstrated that these resistant cells have mutations in tubulin, resulting in impaired microtubule assembly. In essence, continuous exposure to Taxol is required for polymerization to proceed normally, thereby promoting the formation of functional microtubules.

The ABC transporters are well known to be energy dependent transporters that exist across the cell membrane and transfer substrate across the cells using hydrolysis of ATP [32, 72]. Increased expression of ABC transporters such as ABCB1, ABCB4, and ABCG2 mRNA resulted in efflux of anticancer drug paclitaxel (pumping drug out the cell), leading to reduction in their efficacy and development of multidrug resistance (MDR) cells [73]. ABCB1 belongs to ABC transporter family and encodes a membrane protein P-glycoprotein, which is a well-known efflux pump responsible for Multi drug resistance [74]. Cells resistant to paclitaxel showed cross-resistance to other hydrophobic drugs and exhibited increased level of P-glycoprotein [64].

7. Conclusion and future direction

Plant-based medicines has shown potent anti-cancer, anti-diabetic, anti-viral and neuroprotective effect [75–77]. Notable pros of paclitaxel's have been its usage in many cancers, high success rate from preclinical and clinical trial data, its combinatorial properties with other drugs. Also, it has also been shown to be promising in treating non-cancer diseases such as renal and hepatic fibrosis, inflammation, skin disorders, axon regeneration, limb salvage, and coronary artery restenosis [9] Further research would be needful to show insight to the mechanistic mode of action in various diseases processes. It was recently reported by [78] that through protein-protein network analysis (bioinformatic and proteomics data analysis). Paclitaxel was the most potent candidate showcasing anti-cancer as well as anti-viral property. More wet lab research is needed to validate and enhance its repurposing strategy.

Also, notable cons about paclitaxel that would be improved in the incoming years include: utilization of biotechnology to improve biosynthesis of paclitaxel will unfold with improved technologies and technological application. Overcoming the chemo-resistance associated with paclitaxel would enhance its usage in many other diseases as well as novel combination with other drugs/therapies will uncover faster response and survival in patients. Modification with targeted deliveries like novel liposomes and magnetic particle preparations would ensure prompt pharmacological action. Alternating the formulation approach to minimize its toxicity as a result of Cremophor. This assessment of the pros and cons of paclitaxel is discussed in this chapter (**Figure 3** below).

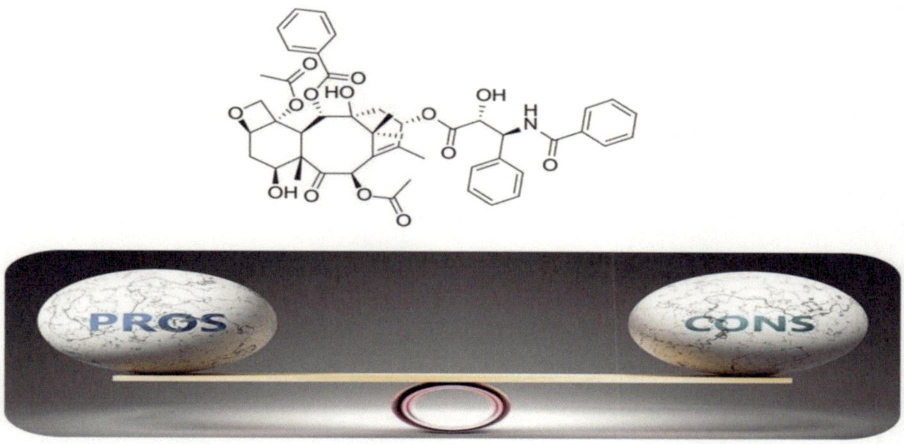

Figure 3.
Overview of the pros and cons of paclitaxel in cancer management.

Researchers envisages more development and improvement in the near future for synthesis, overcoming chemo-resistance, combination with other drugs and repurposing and application in non-cancer diseases of the compound extracted from the bark of pacific yew tree some five decades ago.

Conflict of interest

The authors declare no conflict of interest.

Author details

John Oluwafemi Teibo[1*], Chioma Ejiro Irozuru[2], Titilade Kehinde Ayandeyi Teibo[3], Olabode Ebenezer Omotoso[2], Ahmad O. Babalghith[4] and Gaber El-Saber Batiha[5]

1 Department of Biochemistry and Immunology, Ribeirão Preto Medical School, University of São Paulo, São Paulo, Brazil

2 Department of Biochemistry, Faculty of Basic Medical Sciences, University of Ibadan, Ibadan, Nigeria

3 Department of Maternal-Infant and Public Health Nursing, College of Nursing, University of São Paulo Ribeirão Preto, São Paulo, Brazil

4 Medical Genetics Department, College of Medicine, Umm al-qura University, Makkah Saudi Arabia

5 Department of Pharmacology and Therapeutics, Faculty of Veterinary Medicine, Damanhour University, Damanhour, AlBeheira, Egypt

*Address all correspondence to: johnteibo@usp.br

References

[1] Cragg GM. Paclitaxel (Taxol®): A success story with valuable lessons for natural product drug discovery and development. Medicinal Research Reviews. 1998;**18**:315-331

[2] Howat S, Park B, Oh IS, Jin YW, Lee EK, Loake GJ. Paclitaxel: Biosynthesis, production and future prospects. New Biotechnology. 2014;**31**(3):242-245

[3] Khanna C, Rosenberg M, Vail DM. A review of paclitaxel and novel formulations including those suitable for use in dogs. Journal of Veterinary Internal Medicine. 2015;**29**(4):1006-1012

[4] Yang Y, Mao J, Tan X. Research progress on the source, production, and anti-cancer mechanisms of paclitaxel. Chinese Journal of Natural Medicines. 2020;**18**(12):890-898

[5] Brito DA, Yang Z, Rieder CL. Microtubules do not promote mitotic slippage when the spindle assembly checkpoint cannot be satisfied. The Journal of Cell Biology. 2008;**182**(4):623-629

[6] Ding J, Li M, Deng L, Li T. Study on biological characteristics and mechanism of paclitaxel induced drug resistance in endometrial carcinoma cells. BioMed Research International. 2018;**2018**:8372085

[7] Hájek R. Paclitaxel (Taxol) [paclitaxel (Taxol)]. Casopís Lékařů Ceských. 1996;**135**(12):393-396

[8] Ma WW, Hidalgo M. The winning formulation: The development of paclitaxel in pancreatic cancer. Clinical Cancer Research. 2013;**19**(20):5572-5579

[9] Zhang D, Yang R, Wang S, Dong Z. Paclitaxel: New uses for an old drug. Drug Design, Development and Therapy. 2014;**208**:279-284

[10] Nehate C, Jain S, Saneja A, Khare V, Alam N, Dubey RD, et al. Paclitaxel formulations: Challenges and novel delivery options. Current Drug Delivery. 2014;**11**(6):666-686

[11] Rowinsky EK, Donehower RC. Paclitaxel (Taxol). The New England Journal of Medicine. 1995;**332**(15):1004-1014

[12] Walker FE. Paclitaxel (TAXOL®): Side effects and patient education issues. Seminars in Oncology Nursing. 1993;**9**(4):6-10

[13] Qiao W, Ling F, Yu L, Huang Y, Wang T. Enhancing Taxol production in a novel endophytic fungus, *Aspergillus aculeatinus* Tax-6, isolated from *Taxus chinensis* var. *mairei*. Fungal Biology. 2017;**121**(12):1037-1044

[14] Wani MC, Taylor HL, Wall ME, Coggon P, McPhail AT. Plant antitumor agents. VI. The isolation and structure of Taxol, a novel antileukemic and antitumor agent from *Taxus brevifolia*. Journal of the American Chemical Society. 1971;**93**(9):2325-2327

[15] Li D, Fu D, Zhang Y, Ma X, Gao L, Wang X, et al. Isolation, purification, and identification of Taxol and related taxanes from Taxol-producing fungus *Aspergillus niger* subsp. taxi. Journal of Microbiology and Biotechnology. 2017;**27**(8):1379-1385

[16] Żwawiak J, Zaprutko L. A brief history of Taxol. Journal of Medical Sciences. 2014;**83**(1):47-52

[17] Wang T, Li L, Zhuang W, Zhang F, Shu X, Wang N, et al. Recent research progress in Taxol biosynthetic pathway and acylation reactions mediated by Taxus acyltransferases. Molecules. 2021;**26**(10)

[18] Gennari C, Carcano M, Donghi M, Mongelli N, Vanotti E, Vulpetti A. Taxol semisynthesis: A highly enantio- and diastereoselective synthesis of the side chain and a new method for ester formation at C-13 using thioesters. The Journal of Organic Chemistry. 1997;**62**(14):4746-4755

[19] Schiff PB, Fant J, Horwitz SB. Promotion of microtubule assembly in vitro by Taxol. Nature. 1979;**277**(5698):665-667

[20] Kumar S, Mahdi H, Bryant C, Shah JP, Garg G, Munkarah A. Clinical trials and progress with paclitaxel in ovarian cancer. International Journal of Women's Health. 2010;**2**:411-427

[21] Abu Samaan TM, Samec M, Liskova A, Kubatka P, Busselberg D. Paclitaxel's mechanistic and clinical effects on breast cancer. Biomolecules. 2019;**9**(12):789

[22] Walsh V, Goodman J. Cancer chemotherapy, biodiversity, public and private property: The case of the anti-cancer drug. Social Science & Medicine. 1999;**49**(9):1215-1225

[23] Holton RA, Kim HB, Somoza C, Liang F, Biediger RJ, Boatman PD, et al. First total synthesis of Taxol. 2. Completion of the C and D rings. Journal of the American Chemical Society. 2002;**116**(4):1599-1600

[24] Much JK. Ethical issues and paclitaxel (TAXOL®) administration. Seminars in Oncology Nursing. 1993;**9**(4):16-20

[25] Rowinsky EK, Cazenave LA, Donehower RC. Taxol: A novel investigational antimicrotubule agent. Journal of the National Cancer Institute. 1990;**82**(15):1247-1259

[26] Stierle A, Strobel G, Stierle D. Taxol and taxane production by *Taxomyces andreanae*, an endophytic fungus of Pacific yew. Science. 1993;**260**(5105):214-216

[27] Band HS. Mechanism of action of Taxol. Trends in Pharmacological Sciences. 1992;**13**:134-136

[28] Kundranda MN, Niu J. Albumin-bound paclitaxel in solid tumors: Clinical development and future directions. Drug Design, Development and Therapy. 2015;**9**:3767-3777

[29] Branine M, Bazzicalupo A, Branco S. Biology and applications of endophytic insect-pathogenic fungi. PLoS Pathogens. 2019;**15**(7):e1007831

[30] Bernabeu E, Cagel M, Lagomarsino E, Moretton M, Chiappetta DA. Paclitaxel: What has been done and the challenges remain ahead. International Journal of Pharmaceutics. 2017;**526**(1-2):474-495

[31] Fukaya K, Kodama K, Tanaka Y, Yamazaki H, Sugai T, Yamaguchi Y, et al. Synthesis of paclitaxel. 2. Construction of the ABCD ring and formal synthesis. Organic Letters. 2015;**17**(11):2574-2577

[32] Stavraka C, Blagden S. The La-related proteins, a family with connections to cancer. Biomolecules. 2015;**5**(4):2701-2722

[33] Arnst J. When Taxol met tubulin. The Journal of Biological Chemistry. 2020;**295**(41):13994-13995

[34] Weaver BA. How Taxol/paclitaxel kills cancer cells. Molecular Biology of the Cell. 2014;**25**(18):2677-2681

[35] Suresh G, Kokila D, Suresh TC, Kumaran S, Velmurugan P, Vedhanayakisri KA, et al. Mycosynthesis of anticancer drug Taxol by *Aspergillus oryzae*, an endophyte of *Tarenna asiatica*, characterization, and its activity against a human lung cancer cell line. Biocatalysis Agricultural Biotechnology. 2020;**2020**:24

[36] Fu Y, Li S, Zu Y, Yang G, Yang Z, Luo M, et al. Medicinal chemistry of paclitaxel and its analogues. Current Medicinal Chemistry. 2009;**16**(30):3966-3985

[37] Falah M, Rayan M, Rayan A. A novel paclitaxel conjugate with higher efficiency and lower toxicity: A new drug candidate for cancer treatment. International Journal of Molecular Sciences. 2019;**20**(19):4965

[38] Wen G, Qu XX, Wang D, Chen XX, Tian XC, Gao F, et al. Recent advances in design, synthesis and bioactivity of paclitaxel-mimics. Fitoterapia. 2016;**110**:26-37

[39] Bourgeois-Daigneault MC, St-Germain LE, Roy DG, Pelin A, Aitken AS, Arulanandam R, et al. Combination of paclitaxel and MG1 oncolytic virus as a successful strategy for breast cancer treatment. Breast Cancer Research. 2016;**18**(1):83

[40] Sparano JA, Wang M, Martino S, Jones V, Perez EA, Saphner T, et al. Weekly paclitaxel in the adjuvant treatment of breast cancer. The New England Journal of Medicine. 2008;**358**(16):1663-1671

[41] Zhu L, Chen L. Progress in research on paclitaxel and tumor immunotherapy. Cellular & Molecular Biology Letters. 2019;**24**:40

[42] O'Shaughnessy J, McIntyre K, Wilks S, Ma L, Block M, Andorsky D, et al. Efficacy and safety of weekly paclitaxel with or without oral Alisertib in patients with metastatic breast cancer: A randomized clinical trial. JAMA Network Open. 2021;**4**(4):e214103

[43] Markman M, Blessing J, Rubin SC, Connor J, Hanjani P, et al. Phase II trial of weekly paclitaxel (80 mg/m^2) in platinum and paclitaxel-resistant ovarian and primary peritoneal cancers: A Gynecologic Oncology Group study. Gynecologic Oncology. 2006;**101**(3):436-440

[44] Elserafi MM, Zeeneldin AA, Abdelsalam IM, Nassar HR, Moneer MM, Buhoush WH. First-line paclitaxel and cisplatin used sequentially or in combination in metastatic breast cancer: A phase II randomized study. Journal of the Egyptian National Cancer Institute. 2018;**30**(1):13-20

[45] Steuer CE, Behera M, Ernani V, Higgins KA, Saba NF, Shin DM, et al. Comparison of concurrent use of thoracic radiation with either carboplatin-paclitaxel or cisplatin-etoposide for patients with stage III non-small-cell lung cancer: A systematic review. JAMA Oncology. 2017;**3**(8):1120-1129

[46] Kawiak A, Domachowska A, Lojkowska E. Plumbagin increases paclitaxel-induced cell death and overcomes paclitaxel resistance in breast cancer cells through ERK-mediated apoptosis induction. Journal of Natural Products. 2019;**82**(4):878-885

[47] Shroff RT, Javle MM, Xiao L, Kaseb AO, Varadhachary GR, Wolff RA, et al. Gemcitabine, cisplatin, and

nab-paclitaxel for the treatment of advanced biliary tract cancers: A phase 2 clinical trial. JAMA Oncology. 2019;**5**(6):824-830

[48] Perri G, Prakash L, Qiao W, Varadhachary GR, Wolff R, Fogelman D, et al. Response and survival associated with first-line FOLFIRINOX vs gemcitabine and nab-paclitaxel chemotherapy for localized pancreatic ductal adenocarcinoma. JAMA Surgery. 2020;**155**(9):832-839

[49] Perez EA. Doxorubicin and paclitaxel in the treatment of advanced breast cancer: Efficacy and cardiac considerations. Cancer Investigation. 2001;**19**(2):155-164

[50] Gaitanis A, Staal S. Liposomal doxorubicin and nab-paclitaxel: Nanoparticle cancer chemotherapy in current clinical use. Methods in Molecular Biology. 2010;**624**:385-392

[51] Jiang Y, Zhou Y, Zhang CY, Fang T. Co-delivery of paclitaxel and doxorubicin by pH-responsive prodrug micelles for cancer therapy. International Journal of Nanomedicine. 2020;**15**:3319-3331

[52] Li Y, Hou H, Zhang P, Zhang Z. Co-delivery of doxorubicin and paclitaxel by reduction/pH dual responsive nanocarriers for osteosarcoma therapy. Drug Delivery. 2020;**27**(1):1044-1053

[53] Von Hoff DD, Ervin T, Arena FP, Chiorean EG, Infante J, Moore M, et al. Increased survival in pancreatic cancer with nab-paclitaxel plus gemcitabine. The New England Journal of Medicine. 2013;**369**(18):1691-1703

[54] Sahai V, Catalano PJ, Zalupski MM, Lubner SJ, Menge MR, Nimeiri HS, et al. Nab-paclitaxel and gemcitabine as first-line treatment of advanced or metastatic cholangiocarcinoma: A phase 2 clinical trial. JAMA Oncology. 2018;**4**(12):1707-1712

[55] Sledge GW, Neuberg D, Bernardo P, Ingle JN, Martino S, Rowinsky EK, et al. Phase III trial of doxorubicin, paclitaxel, and the combination of doxorubicin and paclitaxel as front-line chemotherapy for metastatic breast cancer: An intergroup trial (E1193). Journal of Clinical Oncology. 2003;**21**(4):588-592

[56] Bi Z, Chen P, Liu YB, Zhao T, Sun X, Song XR, et al. Efficacy and safety analysis of paclitaxel, docetaxel and liposomal paclitaxel after neoadjuvant therapy in breast cancer. Breast Cancer Research and Treatment. 2020;**184**(2):397-405

[57] Bisch SP, Sugimoto A, Prefontaine M, Bertrand M, Gawlik C, Welch S, et al. Treatment tolerance and side effects of intraperitoneal carboplatin and dose-dense intravenous paclitaxel in ovarian cancer. Journal of Obstetrics and Gynaecology Canada. 2018;**40**(10):1283-7 e1

[58] Bjorn N, Jakobsen Falk I, Vergote I, Green H. ABCB1 variation affects myelosuppression, progression-free survival and overall survival in paclitaxel/carboplatin-treated ovarian cancer patients. Basic & Clinical Pharmacology & Toxicology. 2018;**123**(3):277-287

[59] Feldweg AM, Lee CW, Matulonis UA, Castells M. Rapid desensitization for hypersensitivity reactions to paclitaxel and docetaxel: A new standard protocol used in 77 successful treatments. Gynecologic Oncology. 2005;**96**(3):824-829

[60] Castells MC, Tennant NM, Sloane DE, Hsu FI, Barrett NA, Hong DI, et al. Hypersensitivity reactions to chemotherapy: Outcomes and safety

of rapid desensitization in 413 cases. The Journal of Allergy and Clinical Immunology. 2008;**122**(3):574-580

[61] Sibaud V, Leboeuf NR, Roche H, Belum VR, Gladieff L, Deslandres M, et al. Dermatological adverse events with taxane chemotherapy. European Journal of Dermatology. 2016;**26**(5):427-443

[62] Lenz HJ. Management and preparedness for infusion and hypersensitivity reactions. The Oncologist. 2007;**12**(5):601-609

[63] Picard M. Management of hypersensitivity reactions to taxanes. Immunology and Allergy Clinics of North America. 2017;**37**(4):679-693

[64] Tahara M, Kiyota N, Yokota T, Hasegawa Y, Muro K, Takahashi S, et al. Phase II trial of combination treatment with paclitaxel, carboplatin and cetuximab (PCE) as first-line treatment in patients with recurrent and/or metastatic squamous cell carcinoma of the head and neck (CSPOR-HNO2). Annals of Oncology. 2018;**29**(4):1004-1009

[65] Kim JY, Lee S, Kim Y, Jeong EJ, Lee IH, Son MH, et al. Subacute toxicity and toxicokinetics study of DHP107, an oral paclitaxel formulation with once-weekly dosing in mice. Regulatory Toxicology and Pharmacology. 2019;**103**:196-204

[66] Marupudi NI, Han JE, Li KW, Renard VM, Tyler BM, Brem H. Paclitaxel: A review of adverse toxicities and novel delivery strategies. Expert Opinion on Drug Safety. 2007;**6**(5):609-621

[67] Sahni V, Choudhury D, Ahmed Z. Chemotherapy-associated renal dysfunction. Nature Reviews. Nephrology. 2009;**5**(8):450-462

[68] Boso V, Herrero MJ, Santaballa A, Palomar L, Megias JE, de la Cueva H, et al. SNPs and taxane toxicity in breast cancer patients. Pharmacogenomics. 2014;**15**(15):1845-1858

[69] Liu S, Zhang K, Zhu Q, Shen Q, Zhang Q, Yu J, et al. Synthesis and biological evaluation of paclitaxel and vorinostat co-prodrugs for overcoming drug resistance in cancer therapy in vitro. Bioorganic & Medicinal Chemistry. 2019;**27**(7):1405-1413

[70] Ashrafizadeh M, Zarrabi A, Hashemi F, Moghadam ER, Hashemi F, Entezari M, et al. Curcumin in cancer therapy: A novel adjunct for combination chemotherapy with paclitaxel and alleviation of its adverse effects. Life Sciences. 2020;**256**:117984

[71] Galletti E, Magnani M, Renzulli ML, Botta M. Paclitaxel and docetaxel resistance: Molecular mechanisms and development of new generation taxanes. ChemMedChem. 2007;**2**(7):920-942

[72] Liu Y, Cai Q, Bao PP, Su Y, Cai H, Wu J, et al. Tumor tissue microRNA expression in association with triple-negative breast cancer outcomes. Breast Cancer Research and Treatment. 2015;**152**(1):183-191

[73] Nemcova-Furstova V, Kopperova D, Balusikova K, Ehrlichova M, Brynychova V, Vaclavikova R, et al. Characterization of acquired paclitaxel resistance of breast cancer cells and involvement of ABC transporters. Toxicology and Applied Pharmacology. 2016;**310**:215-228

[74] Samli H, Samli M, Vatansever B, Ardicli S, Aztopal N, Dincel D, et al. Paclitaxel resistance and the role of miRNAs in prostate cancer cell lines. World Journal of Urology. 2019;**37**(6):1117-1126

[75] Teibo J, Bello S, Olagunju A, Olorunfemi F, Ajao O, Fabunmi O. Functional foods and bioactive compounds: Roles in the prevention, treatment and management of neurodegenerative diseases. GSC Biological Pharma Science. 2020;**11**(2):297-313

[76] Teibo JO, Akinfe OA, Olagunju AS, Olorunfemi FG, Teibo TKA, Olaoba OT, et al. Chemo-preventive roles of medicinal foods against environmental carcinogens-induced cancers. Cancer Research Journal. 2021;**2021**:e2101

[77] Teibo JO, Ayinde KS, Olaoba OT, Adelusi TI, Teibo TKA, Bamikunle MV, et al. Functional foods' bioactive components and their chemoprevention mechanism in cervical, breast, and liver cancers: A systematic review. Functional Foods in Health and Disease. 2021;**11**(11):559-585

[78] Al-Motawa MS, Abbas H, Wijten P, de la Fuente A, Xue M, Rabbani N, et al. Vulnerabilities of the SARS-CoV-2 virus to proteotoxicity-opportunity for repurposed chemotherapy of COVID-19 infection. Frontiers in Pharmacology. 2020;**9**(11):585408

Chapter 9

Drug Repurposing: Scopes in Herbal/Natural Products-based Drug Discovery and Role of in silico Techniques

Manisha Kotadiya

Abstract

Natural products and their derivatives are the most promising and prolific resources in identifying the therapeutic small compounds with potential therapeutic activity. Nowadays, working with herbal or natural products can be boosted by collecting the data available for their chemical, pharmacological, and biological characteristics properties. Using in silico tools and methods, we can enhance the chances of getting a better result in a precise way. It can support experiments to emphasis their sources in fruitful directions. Though due to their limitations with respect to current knowledge, quality, quantity, relevance of the present data as well as the scope and limitations of cheminformatics methods, herbal product-based drug discovery is limited. The pharmaceutical re-profiling is done with the main objective to establish strategies by using approved drugs and rejected drug candidates in the diagnosis of new diseases. Drug repurposing offers safety lower average processing cost for already approved, withdrawn drug candidates. In silico methods could be oppressed for discovering the actions of un-investigated phytochemicals by identification of their molecular targets using an incorporation of chemical informatics and bioinformatics along with systems biological approaches, hence advantageous for small-molecule drug identification. The methods like rule-based, similarity-based, shape-based, pharmacophore-based, and network-based approaches and docking and machine learning methods are discussed.

Keywords: docking, molecular simulation, bioinformatic tools, machine learning, target identification, databases

1. Introduction

Herbal or natural products and their derivatives have an ancient status in using them as traditional medicines to treat ailments and various diseases. However, in today's era, they become a prolific resource for identifying small therapeutic molecules as an inspiration. With regard to it, around two-thirds of small-molecule medicines or drugs approved in between 1981 and 2019. William C. Campbell, Satoshi Omura, and

Youyou Tu got noble prize for the discovery of two natural products such as **avermectin and artemisinin**, and they are used in the treatment of parasitic diseases caused by parasites [1].

Due to these evolutionary processes, natural compounds consist of various biological activities in different races. Because of these characteristics, the wide range of products from natural resources are identified as privileged structural molecules [2, 3]. They are highly diverse with respect to structure, pharmacological, and physiological properties. Some are having good ADME and physicochemical properties, and some are clearly beyond and generally recognized as small drug-like chemical space [4–6]. Almost all phytochemicals and other compounds from natural origin have complex molecular structure with respect to their 3D molecular shape, geometry, stereochemistry, ring complexity, and conformations like more number of rotatable bonds and absence of aromaticity [7–9]. This includes numerous basic obstacles to 3D cheminformatics methodologies, which is why the creation of force fields and algorithms for the prediction and identification of protein-bound conformations of such complex compounds remains the most actively pursued research period in cheminformatics and bioinformatics [10–15].

In silico methods can contribute to natural product small-molecule discovery and can also became a backbone to experimentalists throughout the lead identification [16–19]. They are not only used for identifying bioactive molecule but also used to prioritize material for testing [20, 21]. In silico methods are also adopted as follows:

i. data curation and dereplication,

ii. chemical space analysis, visualization, and comparison,

iii. accentuation of product-likeness,

iv. prediction of ADME properties and safety profiling.

A high-performance computer facility on-site is no longer required. Calculations may now be conducted at extremely large sizes in the cloud at a cheap cost and complexity. Simply paying software license fees is a significant cost component that has steadily climbed in recent years. Simultaneously, we are seeing an increase in the number of sophisticated open-source tools, similar to what has been widely used in the area of bioinformatics. Some of the best softwares in this category are as follows:

i. RDKit and CDK [22, 23]

ii. KNIME [24, 25] (an open-source analytics platform), and

iii. Scikit-learn (an open-source Python module for machine learning) [26]

This summarizes the methods and in silico tools for repurposing to provide a concise but comprehensive overview of the scope and limitations for herbal or other natural origin-based drug discovery in a format that is accessible to researchers from different areas with an interest in drug discovery. The conversation covers a huge number of methods in cheminformatics, bioinformatics as well as data resources relevant to natural product-based drug discovery.

2. Herbal/natural product databases and computational methods/tools

Most databases also provide free bulk download, allowing for virtual screening and other uses. According to these studies, the total number of natural compounds whose structures can be obtained via bulk download from free databases exceeds 250 k, approaching 300 k. Unfortunately, many databases have a brief half-life; just a handful are sustainably managed and under continuous improvement. Data quality is always an issue, but when it comes to phytoconstituents, extra care should be taken, especially when integrating the data with computational methods that rely on correct depiction of 3D molecular structures. This is because of that stereochemical information on phytocompounds is frequently erroneous. Virtual databases can be distinguished into following:

i. encyclopedic and natural product/herbal data sources,

ii. databases augmented with phytoconstituents used in traditional medicines,

iii. specialized databases dedicated to certain ecosystems, geographical locations, animals, pharmacological activities, or even their classes.

Super Natural II [27] is the most comprehensive free database, with over 325 k substances. The database may be queried using a chemistry-aware online interface; however, mass download is not supported. A handful of the best free, downloadable materials are described below:

i. **Universal Natural Products Database** (UNPD) [5], which lists more than 200 k compounds;.

ii. In addition, major databases such as the TCM database-Taiwan [28], which has information on over 60 k compounds discovered in Chinese medicinal plants, natural product Atlas [29], which contains information on over 25 k chemicals found in bacteria and fungus; and

iii. The Collective Molecular Activities of Useful Species (CMAUP) database [30, 31], which has information on over 47 k chemicals from over 5600 plants;

iv. We discovered that only around 16% of our collection of roughly 250 k compounds were available in the ChEMBL database and by overlapping our set with the whole ChEMBL database (a database offering bioactivity data on approximately 2 million compounds) [32, 33];

v. Similarly, when we compared the dataset to all small-molecule ligands documented in the Protein Data Bank (PDB), we discovered that only roughly 2000 molecules have at least one co-crystallized X-ray structure of excellent quality [6].

3. In silico analysis, physicochemical studies, and structural properties of natural products

Computational chemistry has been playing a key role in the characterization of compounds by their physicochemical and structural properties. Phytocompounds cover a much lots of chemical space than synthetic [34]. The structural uniqueness (and complexity) of some phytocompounds and other natural compounds from other sources could allow them to target macromolecules. They are on average heavier and more hydrophobic than synthetic drugs and synthetic, drug-like compounds. Their structural complexity is also often higher, in particular with regard to stereochemistry (commonly quantified by the number of chiral centers [35], the number of fractions of Csp3 atoms, and or the number of bridge head atoms in ring systems and 3D molecular shape) [36]. All natural compounds show an enormous diversity of ring systems, in particular of aliphatic systems. One study showed that 83% of core ring scaffolds of natural products are absent in commercially available screening databases [37]. Compounds from natural sources from different kingdoms have distinct physicochemical and structural properties. For example, natural compounds with macrocycles or long aliphatic chains are more commonly to marine species than terrestrial species. Bacteria also manufacture a large number of macrocyclic natural chemicals. Natural compounds have a large number of heteroatoms and, as a result, a wide range of functional groups [38]. Computational Methods for Assessing the Institutional Variety of Herbal Compounds are unparalleled in terms of the structural diversity, which is expressed on a fragment level [39]. The majority of studies comparing the diversity of compounds with that of chemical drugs use the idea of biochemical structures (scaffolds) presented by Bemis and Murcko [40]. A powerful tool for the intuitive visual analysis of the structural diversity of sets of compounds is Scaffold Hunter [41]. Some of the methods are enlist as below:

The open-source, Java-based program has a graphical interface and different clustering techniques.

Scaffold Hunter is based on the concept of molecular scaffold hierarchical representation and categorization ("scaffold tree").

An early prototype of this instrument served as the foundation for the structural categorization of bioactive substances (SCONP), a technique for mapping compounds' chemical space [42].

Principal component analysis (PCA) is one of the most widely used approaches for modeling the chemical space [43], which projects high-dimensional data into a low-dimensional space for improved interpretability, while keeping information loss to a minimum. Natural compounds have been used in several studies for mapping the chemical space of small molecules [44], for mode of action prediction and for the analysis of structure-activity relationships. Despite significant variations in chemical structure, these studies reveal a high degree of similarities between natural substances and synthesized pharmaceuticals in terms of pharmacophore characteristics [45]. T-distributed algorithms are another effective way for reducing dimensionality.

Stochastic Neighbor Embedding (t-SNE) [46], as well as the recently announced Uniform Manifold Approximation and Projection for Dimension Reduction (UMAP) [47], generates plots in which comparable things are clustered together and dissimilar ones are represented by distant points. Although t-SNE can provide graphics that seem to be superior to those produced by PCA, the approach does not really scale well with dataset size.

UMAP is theoretically similar to t-SNE and yields comparable results, but it is quicker. Medina-research Franco's group has been working on many techniques for such intuitive characterization, visualization, and comparison of chemical collections, with an emphasis on their databases producing similar result faster (**Figure 1**).

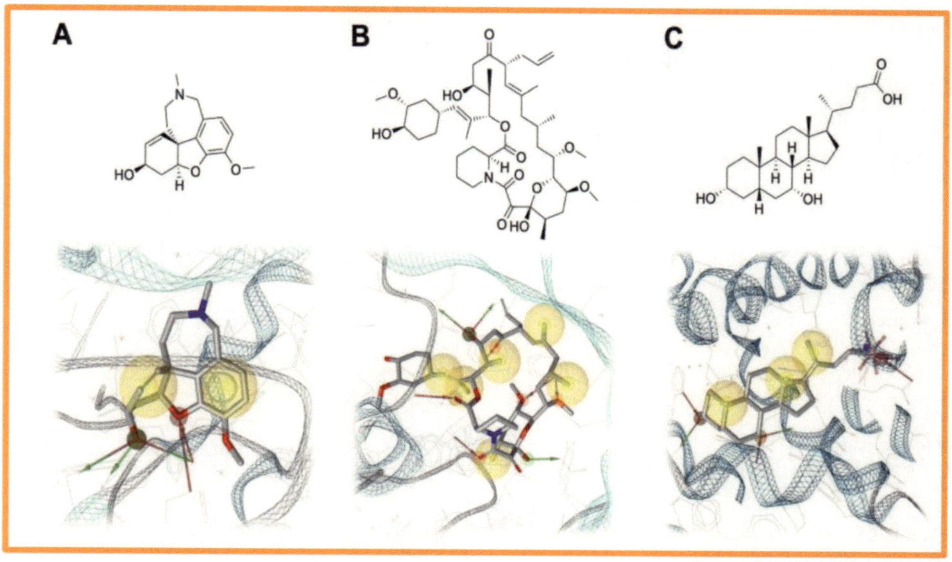

Figure 1.
Examples of approved drugs and interaction of drugs to their target proteins: (A) (−)-galantamine, an ACEs inhibitor used for the treatment of Alzheimer's disease (PDB: 1DX6), (B) tacrolimus, a macrocyclic immunosuppressant (PDB: 1FKF) and (C) chenodeoxycholic acid for the treatment of hypocholesterolaemia (PDB: 6HL1) [39].

4. Computational methods for the analysis of natural compounds and their drug-likeness prediction

Computational tools are able to discriminate natural compounds and natural-like compounds from synthetic compounds with high. Accuracy, and they are also able to quantify the natural compound-likeness of compounds. As such, they are frequently used in compound design, library design, natural compound selection (and their derivatives and analogs) among heterogeneous compound collections, and compound prioritizing [48]. The Natural Products-Likeness Score created by Ertl is one of the most well-established techniques [49]. This score measures the chemicals based on the resemblance of their fragment from those of existing natural compounds using Bayesian statistics. The Natural Product-Likeness Score has been re-implemented with certain changes in various tools and platforms [50]. Additional techniques include a theoretically comparable method based on extended connectivity fingerprinting (ECFPs) and a **rule-based approach** [50].

More recently, we developed Natural Product-Scout, a tool for identifying NPs and NP-like compounds in large sets of molecules. Arbitrary forest classification techniques are trained and tested database of known biologically active compounds.

On a sample test set, a classifier based on Molecular ACCess System keys achieved an area under the characteristics curve (AUC) of 0.997 as well as the Matthews correlation coefficient (MCC) of 0.960. Similarity maps are used by NP-Scout to identify locations in a compound that help to the identification of a compound as NP and synthetic chemical (**Figure 2**). NP-Scout may be accessed via a free online service [52].

Recently, the Natural Compounds Molecular Fingerprint (**NC-MFP**) was presented as a novel method of defining the structural properties of natural compounds in term of the scaffold and fragments they are made up of [53]. It has been

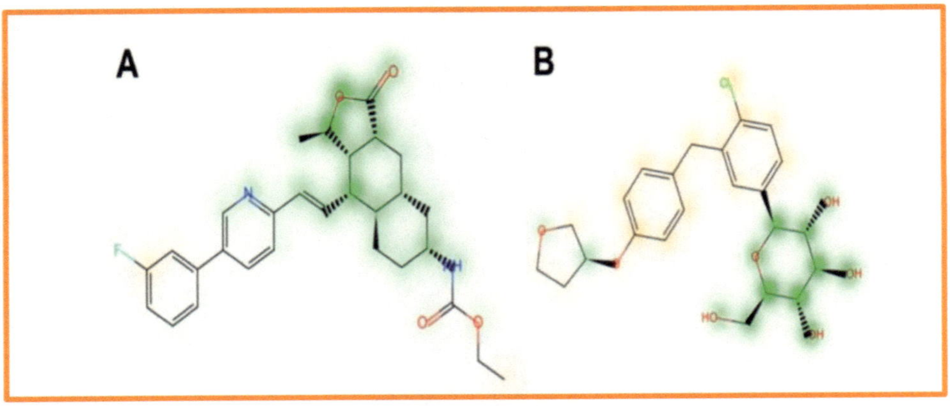

Figure 2.
Similarity maps of (A) vorapaxar and (B) empagliflozin [51].

demonstrated that the NC-MFP outperforms existing fingerprints in distinguishing natural substances from manufactured ones.

5. Computational identification of natural products likely to interfere with biological activities

Computational techniques have a robust track record in the identification of bioactive natural origin compounds.

For their research, they used a wide range of virtual screening methods, from simple, fast methods based on 2D molecular fingerprint similarity to more complex.

Machine learning algorithms have lately become a standard in screening for pharmacological active natural compounds [54].

The structural properties of many NPs, including such greater levels of conformational flexibility, the complexity of about their shapes and ring system (particularly macrocycles), inadequacies of molecular force fields primarily model defined for synthetic substances, and uncertainly related to protonation states, tautomerism, and oxidation states pose particular challenges to 3D virtual screening techniques. One method for reducing the spatial structure of natural substances is to eliminate sugars and sugar-like substances that are not required for bioactive components on a target of interest [55]. This can be done, for example, by use of defined (**SMARTS**) patterns. Given the sparsity of available structural data, docking of natural compounds to the structures of macromolecules can pose a profound challenge. This is because of **docking algorithms** and scoring functions are highly sensitive even to very small changes in 3D structure such as commonly induced by ligand binding method (including solvent effects). However, also this hurdle may be overcome by the prudent use of homology modeling techniques, induced fit docking approaches, and molecular dynamics simulations. In case of extremely flexible proteins, docking against multiple, protein structures (“**ensemble docking**”) may be a good way onward (not only for screening but also for binding area prediction) [56, 57]. Diligence and patience will certainly be required and, above all, checks of the plausibility of a hypothesis using all available information can help to piece the puzzle together. More often than in virtual screening, docking algorithms produce good results in binding mode prediction [58]. Provided that the natural compounds of interest is not excessively large or flexible (as a rough guide, not exceeding 35 heavy atoms or eight rotatable bonds), that the ligand binding site is well defined (i.e., not overly shallow, not solvent-exposed), and that the interaction between the binding partners involves two or more directed interactions, and there is a good chance that a satisfactorily accurate binding pose can be obtained that offers crucial insights for the development of optimization strategies. Binding posture prediction is more practicable than virtual screening, since that allows researchers to ignore the most difficult component of docking, which is grading compounds based on their ligand binding, and it allows them to focus their efforts on a single ligand-target combination. Docking, particularly in the context of NP research, allows for the rationalization of stereoselectivity in ligand binding (and other processes, such as metabolism). The significance of incorporating accurate conformational information with 3D techniques, particularly docking, cannot be emphasized. In the following paragraphs, we will examine several exemplary investigations in which virtual screening has been effectively used to identify bioactive chemicals. Using katsumadain A, a diarylheptanoid inhibiting influenza neuraminidase, as a template for 3D molecular shape-based screening, a number of structurally distinct NPs were identified that inhibit the viral enzyme with IC50 values in the sub-micromolar to low-micromolar range (for example, artocarpin (1), which is depicted in **Figure 3**) [59]. In another study, pharmacophore-based virtual screening was combined with a shape-based approach in order to identify activators of the G protein-coupled bile acid receptor 1 **(GPBAR1)** [51]. In addition to several NP databases, a collection of synthetic compounds was screened. Among the 14 selected NPs, eight (57%) obtained a measured receptor activation of at least 15% at 20 μM concentration.

Two of these compounds, (1) farnesiferol B (2) and microlobidene (3), are based on molecular scaffolds that had not yet been associated with GPBAR1 modulation. Both compounds were reported to have EC50 values of approximately 14 μM. Among all 19 selected compounds, only two were active (applying the identical activity threshold).

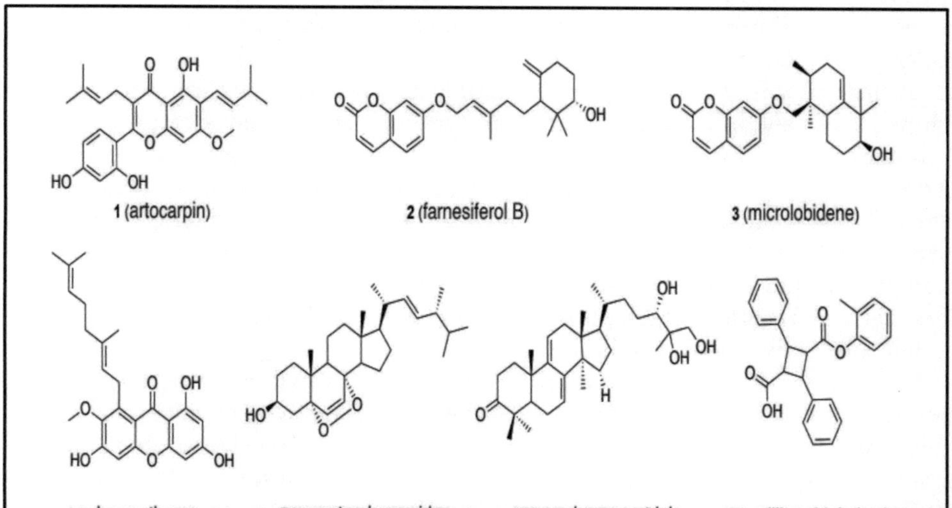

Figure 3.
Natural compound and their derivatives identified by virtual screening method.

6. In silico prediction of the therapeutic targets of natural products

Identifying the receptors of small compounds is critical for assessing the pharmacological activity and safety of drugs, as well as their future development. However, the method of action of a significant percentage of marketed medications is uncertain or very loosely understood.

Target prediction in silico is a large-scale use of virtual screening [60], in which one, many, or even several molecules are assessed against the broadest collection of macromolecules conceivable. A number of techniques including models have been released in recent years [61], and they have emerged as valuable tools in earlier drug discovery. The majority of target prediction strategies are ligand-based, which is connected to the issues with docking and structure-based methods.

Ligand-based methodologies range from simple similarity-based approaches to advanced machine learning as well as network-based approaches. Surprisingly, despite the variety of computer tools for target prediction available today, our understanding of their utility under real-world situations remains restricted [62]. This is largely due to the (in practice) exorbitant expenses associated with the practical, scientific, proactive evaluation of such models, but it is also due to the often used inadequate, superficial retrospective validation techniques [63]. To the best of our knowledge, the only computational technique that has received rigorous experimental validation is the well-established Similarity Ensemble Approach (SEA) [64]. One may argue that testing models using current data tends to an exaggeration of how effectively a model would perform in real-world scenarios.

It is more likely that **phenotypic test** readouts with different types of cells or information for structurally similar drugs would be obtained. By merging all available information, some false-positive predictions are likely to be eliminated, leaving many fewer prospective targets to be studied experimentally. In a recent in-depth study of the behavior and scope of a similarity-based approach and a machine learning approach for estimating the targets of small molecules, we display that the reliability of either approach's predictions is strongly influenced by the structural relationship between the compounds of interest and compounds represented in the training set. This issue must be carefully examined while working with natural substances, considering that target prediction algorithms are largely intended for, and with natural chemicals, given that target prediction algorithms are largely built for and trained on synthetic compound measurement data. In the same investigation, we discovered that, surprisingly, the similarity-based strategy outscored the machine learning technique using the already available data. While a meaningful correlation of these two methods should be approached with caution for several reasons, the results indicate that the basic similarity-based strategy is a solid choice, particularly when model interpretability is considered. This is also shown in the high performance of other well-known, similarity-based models, like Swiss Target Prediction [65].

The majority of the compounds differ structurally from more common, synthetic chemicals that account for the majority of the observed activity data. More complicated similarity-based approaches that examine molecules based on their 3D molecular structure are supposed to identify such distant structural similarities, but how effectively these methods would function in practice was unknown until recently. We investigated the capability of ROCS [66].

ROCS, a premier shape-based screening engine which also takes chemical feature distributions into consideration, was used to discover the biomolecules targets of "complex" molecules using a knowledge and understanding of "non-complex" molecules with measured bioactivity data [67].

We designated molecules as "complex" for this work if they are either (extremely) large in size (45 to 55 heavier atoms) or macrocyclic. We classified compounds as "non-complex" when they were tiny in size (15 to 30 heavy atoms). A collection of 28 pharmacologically important targets were investigated. A diversified set of 10 complicated small molecules was created automatically for each one of the targets. Each of these molecules had a single low-energy conformation that was used as a query for ROCS screening against a multi-conformational knowledge base. The knowledge base has 3642 targets and 272,640 non-complex molecules. This study discovered that ROCS accurately rated at least one known target in the top 10 spots (out of 3642) for up to 37% of the 280 complicated small compounds used as queries. This result is amazing given the dissimilarity of the queries and compounds in the knowledge base. It suggests that target prediction is achievable for a large number of difficult complicated compounds. It should be noted that, in many circumstances, researchers will be able to significantly limit the number of target candidates based on specialist knowledge and accessible information. There were at least 31 identified complex molecules and natural product-like molecules among the 280 complicated small molecules. The top-10 rate of success for these compounds was lower (23% vs. 37%). This is due to the fact that the median Tanimoto coefficient between the complex NP (or NP-like substance) and the nearest simple molecules in the knowledge base is only 0.13. For pairings of compounds with such a minimal degree of similarity, it is reasonable to predict that the respective binding interaction possess will be unique, which is normally outside the reach of ligand-based approaches.

In addition to 3D similarity-based techniques, 3D pharmacophore-based methodologies are commonly utilized for prediction of target protein in the context of natural substances research. A profiling investigation, for example, evaluated secondary metabolites extracted from the medicinal plant Ruta graveolens against a battery of over 2000 pharmacophore models spanning over 280 targets.

Arborinine was found as an antagonist of Angiotensin-converting enzymes (ACEs) (measured IC50 = 35 M) results from in silico screening, among many other bioactive chemicals and interactions. Machine learning-based methods for natural chemical target prediction have sparked the greatest attention in recent years. Some of examples for online tools are given below:

i. SPIDER,

ii. TIGER, and

iii. Starfish

Spider employs self-organizing maps in conjunction with "fuzzy" chemical descriptors, allowing it to be extended to NPs. The model proved useful in identifying 5-lipoxygenase, peroxisome proliferator-activated receptors, steroid receptors, prostaglandin E2 synthase 1, and Farnesoid X receptor as therapeutic targets of the archazolid A, and it accurately predicted prostanoid receptor 3 as a molecular target for doliculide, which is a 16-membered depsipeptide [68]. SPIDER has effectively discovered the targets of other fragment-like natural compounds, such as Sparteine, for which the kappa opioid receptor, p38 mitogen-activated protein kinase, and muscarinic and nicotinic receptors were clinically verified as targets [3]. DL-goitrin, whose targets have been experimentally proven to be receptor pregnane X and the cholinergic receptor,

Graveolinine acts on cyclooxygenase-2, serotonin 5HT2B receptors were clinically verified as targets, isomacroin acts on adenosine A3, and platelet growth factor receptors were clinically identified as targets.

DEcRyPT uses random forest regression to build a revised list of possible macromolecule targets based on predictions obtained from spider, the Target-Drug Relationship Predictor. DEcRyPT was used to successfully identify 5-lipoxygenase for which ortho-naphthoquinone-lapachone is well-known substrate. Lapachone hydroquinone was shown as inhibitor of 5-lipoxygenase.

TIGER is thematically connected to SPIDER. However, it utilizes updated Cats descriptors and employs a different technique for assessing expected targets. The, glucocorticoid, Orexin as well as cholecystokinin receptor were effectively discovered as therapeutic hit for marine NP (±) marinopyrrole A by TIGER. Among other proteins, the model correctly predicted estrogen receptors and as binding biomolecule of the stilbenoid resveratrol [69]. Starfish is a stacked ensemble approach for target prediction trained on synthetic compounds.

As a component of the development process, various machine learning methods were investigated. The authors determined the optimum stacking strategy by feeding molecular fingerprints into k-nearest neighbor's model and a random forest model. The probability predicted by such models in which each of the therapeutic targets are employed as input for a logistic regression-based meta-classifier (level 1). On a test set of NPs, the stacking technique performed much better than the separate models (ROC AUC 0.94; BEDROC score 0.73). Network techniques for predicting biological targets of natural chemicals have also been published. Cheng and colleagues, for example, created statistical models in order to bind natural compounds to cancer targets and their protein involved in disorders like aging. Neural networks system was recently trained on clinical indication data and applied to discover favored molecular scaffold in natural products. Based on these models' predictions, a unique template database for 100 indications were created, which may be used as a preliminary step for NP-based drug development. The reader is directed to reference for further information on this subject. Natural compounds that are likely to disrupt with biological experiments can be identified computationally. The proclivity of compounds to interfere with biological assays remains a significant challenge in compound screening experiments. The flavonoid quercetin, a well-known pan assay interference compound, exemplifies the scope of the issue: since about 28 July 2020, and the PubChem Bioassay repository identified quercetin as conclusively bioactive in over 800 separate bioassays, representing a hit rate of more than 50%. The most typically seen method of test interference is aggregation formation, which happens under certain assay circumstances. Covalent binding, redox cycling, interference with spectroscopy assay, metal chelation, membrane rupture, and breakdown in buffers are further significant processes [70].

7. Computational identification of natural products likely to interfere with biological assays

The development of computer techniques to address this challenge has been gradual. Until recently, the tools available to users comprised numerous rule sets, a few similarity-based techniques, and a statistical method. The most well-known method and widely used rule set is pan assay interference components (pains) rule set. Despite the unambiguous declarations of its creators, operators of the PAINS rules set all too frequently overlook the significant drawbacks of its scope, applicability, and trustworthiness. Other relevant rule sets here include rapid elimination of swill rules as well as a set of rules generated from an Nuclear magnetic resonance-based approach in detecting tiny compounds that give false-positive test results owing to interaction (ALARM NMR) [71]. Aggregator Advisor is a useful similarity-based technique that identifies compounds with similar structural structures. Aggregator Advisor is a handy similarity-based technique that indicates compounds that have a close structural affinity to identified aggregators based on molecular scaffolds.

Hit Dexter 2.0 is the second generation of a series of machine learning models meant to identify compounds that are likely to exhibit prolific hitter behavior in primary screening and/or confirmatory dose-response tests, independent of the underlying (interference) mechanism. All of these methods are generated from databases dominated by synthetic chemicals. As we demonstrate in our work on Hit Dexter 2.0, the training set, although comprising of around 250 k compounds, covers just a tiny proportion (approximately 15%) of the active compounds with molecules that are structurally related to the model to make credible predictions. This means that, once again, discretion is required when employing any of these techniques, specifically in the area of NPs.

8. In silico prediction of ADME and safety profiles of natural products

The biodistribution and safety characteristics of NPs are frequently a source of difficulty in NP-based drug development. The hERG channel (whose blockage has been associated with potentially deadly cardiac arrhythmia), cytochrome P450 enzymes (which can induce drug-drug interactions and toxicity), and P-glycoprotein are some of the most well-known anti-targets tackled by NPs (an efflux pump with broad substrate specificity that can effectively cause drug resistance). A wide range of computational models (e.g., pharmacophore models, statistical models, docking machine learning models, etc.) are also used to handle these and many additional anti-targets and end points. However, because of the data available, these and many other in silico methods are tested/tested using substances that are mainly of synthetic origin. For example [72, 73],

i. Hit Dexter 2.0's application to natural compounds is restricted. The fidelity of Hit Dexter's estimations has been proven to decline significantly beyond a given distance from the training data, since the training data is mostly constituted of synthetic substances.

ii. In contrast, FAME3, a theoretically comparable machine learning model for predicting metabolic sites of small compounds, has been demonstrated to function well on natural compounds, despite the fact that the bulk of chemicals in the training set are synthetic. The reason for the FAME3 models' high robustness and good result on molecules is that the liability of atom locations in compounds is described based on their determinative atom surroundings, and these proximate neighborhoods are much more excessive among compounds and synthetic substances than their worldwide molecular similarity (**Table 1**).

Sr. No.	Purpose	
1	Docking	Glide, Auto dock, Tar Fish Dock, Flare
2	Binding site prediction	Sitemap, Computed Atlas of Surface Topography of proteins (Castp), Findsite, LigASite
3	Pathway analysis	Therapeutic Performance Mapping System
4	Drug design	Forge, Spark
5.	Pharmacokinetic parameters	Swiss ADME
6	Genomics	Connectivity map (CMap), Directionality map (DMAP)
7	Molecular simulation	Imods, Gromacs

Table 1.
Available software for in silico drug repurposing.

9. Conclusions

NPs provide remarkable hurdles to both experimentalists and theorists, yet data on recently approved small-molecule medications demonstrate that NP research is worthwhile and can deliver useful, new therapeutics. Modern in silico approaches can contribute significantly to the speeding and non-risking of natural drug development. However, model applicability must be carefully monitored, especially when dealing with NPs, because computational approaches are often created for and trained on data for synthesized chemicals. Unfortunately, even recently established models sometimes lack rigorous definitions of the application area and do not appropriately notify users about compounds with unreliable predictions. Researchers, in fact, may be attracted to use one of the numerous free, user-friendly web applications. Obviously, the idea holds true for these web applications as well: in the absence of solid indications of the trustworthiness of individual forecasts, these estimates are not to be believed. Given the renewed interest in NP research, the increasing availability of biological, chemical, advances in algorithms, and structural data, and improvements in algorithms, modeling techniques, as well as computing capability, the future will see the sustained connectivity of computational techniques in natural compound-based drug development pipelines.

Conflict of interest

Authors declare that there is no conflict of interest.

Author details

Manisha Kotadiya
Department of Pharmaceutical Chemistry, S.M. Shah Pharmacy College, Mehemdabad, Gujarat, India

*Address all correspondence to: manishakotadiya3@gmail.com

References

[1] Newman D, Cragg G. Natural products as sources of new drugs over the nearly four decades from 01/1981 to 09/2019. Journal of Natural Products. 2020;**83**:770-803

[2] Cragg G, Newman J. Biodiversity: A continuing source of novel drug lead. Pure and Applied Chemistry. 2005;**77**:7-24

[3] Rodrigues T, Reker D, Schneider P, Schneider G. Counting on natural products for drug design. Nature Chemistry. 2016;**8**:531-541

[4] Atanasov G, Waltenberger B, Pferschy-Wenzig E, Linder T, Wawrosch C, Uhrin P, et al. Discovery and resupply of pharmacologically active plant-derived natural products: A review. Biotechnology Advances. 2015;**33**:1582-1614

[5] Gu J, Gui J, Chen L, Yuan G, Lu H, Xu X. Use of natural products as chemical library for drug discovery and network pharmacology. PLoS One. 2013;**8**:e62839

[6] Chen Y, de Lomana M, Friedrich N, Kirchmair J. Characterization of the chemical space of known and readily obtainable natural products. Journal of Chemical Information and Modeling. 2018;**58**:1518-1532

[7] Clemons P, Bodycombe N, Carrinski H, Wilson J, Shamji WB, Koehler A, et al. Small molecules of different origins have distinct distributions of structural complexity that correlate with protein-binding profiles. Proceedings of the National Academy Science USA. 2010;**107**:8787-18792

[8] Chen H, Engkvist O, Blomberg N, Li J. A comparative analysis of the molecular topologies for drugs, clinical candidates, natural products, human metabolites and general bioactive compounds. Medical Chemistry. 2012;**3**:312-321

[9] David B, Grondin A, Schambel P, Vitorino M, Zeyer D. Plant natural fragments, an innovative approach for drug discovery. Phytochemical Review. 2019;**2019**. DOI: 10.1007/s11101-019-09612-4

[10] Friedrich N, Flachsenberg F, Meyder A, Sommer K, Kirchmair J, Rarey M. Conformator: A novel method for the generation of conformer ensembles. Journal of Chemical Information and Modeling. 2019;**59**:731-742

[11] Friedrich N, de Bruyn KC, Flachsenberg F, Sommer K, Rarey M, Kirchmair J. Benchmarking commercial conformer ensemble generators. Journal of Chemical Information and Modeling. 2017;**57**:2719-2728

[12] Olgac A, Orhan I, Banoglu B. Benchmarking commercial conformer ensemble generators. Future Medicinal Chemistry. 2017;**9**:1665-1686

[13] Ikram N, Durrant J, Muchtaridi M, Zalaludin A, Purwitasari N, Mohamed N, et al. Molecular docking and 3D-pharmacophore modelling to study the interactions of Chalcone derivatives with estrogen receptor alpha. Journal of Chemical Information and Modeling. 2015;**55**:308-316

[14] Grienke U, Mihaly-Bison J, Schuster D, Afonyushkin T, Binder M, Guan S, et al. Pharmacophore-based discovery of FXR-agonists. Part II: Identification of bioactive triterpenes from *Ganoderma lucidum*. Bioorganic & Medicinal Chemistry. 2011;**19**:6779-6791

[15] Landrum G. "RDKit," can be found under www.rdkit.org

[16] Steinbeck C, Han Y, Kuhn S, Horlacher O, Luttmann E, Willighagen E. The chemistry development kit (CDK): An open-source Java library for chemo- and bioinformatics. Journal of Chemical Information and Computer Sciences. 2003;**43**:493-500

[17] "KNIME j Open for Innovation," can be found under https://www.knime.com/

[18] Pedregosa F, Varoquaux G, Gramfort A, Michel V, Thirion B, Grisel O, et al. Scikit-learn: Machine learning in Python. Journal of Machine Learning Research. 2011;**12**:2825-2830

[19] Banerjee P, Erehman J, Gohlke B, Wilhelm T, Preissner R, Dunkel M. Super natural II-a database of natural products. Nucleic Acids Research. 2014;**43**:935

[20] Chen C. TCM database@Taiwan: The World's largest traditional Chinese medicine database for drug screening in silico. PLoS One. 2011;**6**:e15939

[21] "Natural Products Atlas (2019)," can be found under https://www.npatlas.org

[22] Wolber G, Langer T. Ligand Scout: 3-D pharmacophores derived from protein-bound ligands and their use as virtual screening filters. Journal of Chemical Information and Modeling. 2005;**45**:160-169

[23] Ertl P, Schuffenhauer A. Cheminformatics analysis of natural products: Lessons from nature inspiring the design of new drugs. Progress in Drug Research. 2008;**66**:219-235

[24] Chen Y, Stork C, Hirte S, Kirchmair J. NP-scout: Machine learning approach for the quantification and visualization of the natural product-likeness of small molecules. Biomolecules. 2019;**9**:43

[25] Lucas X, Gruning B, Bleher S, Gunther S. Journal of Chemical Information and Modeling. 2015;**55**:915-924

[26] Hert J, Irwin J, Laggner C, Keiser M, Shoichet B. Quantifying biogenic Bias in screening libraries. Nature Chemical Biology. 2009;**5**:479-483

[27] El-Elimat T, Zhang X, Jarjoura D, Moy F, Orjala J, Kinghorn A, et al. Chemical diversity of metabolites from Fungi, Cyanobacteria, and plants relative to FDA-approved anticancer agents. ACS Medicinal Chemistry Letters. 2012;**3**:645-649

[28] Muigg P, Rosen J, Bohlin L, Backlund A. Marine natural products: A source of novel anticancer drug. Phytochemistry Reviews. 2013;**12**:449-457

[29] Chavez-Hernandez A, Sanchez-Cruz N, Medina-Franco J. A fragment library of natural products and its comparative Chemoinformatic characterization. Molecular Informatics. 2020;**39**:2000050

[30] Zeng X, Zhang P, Wang Y, Qin C, Chen S, He W, et al. CMAUP: A database of collective molecular activities of useful plants. Nucleic Acids Research. 2019;**47**:1118

[31] Bemis G, Murcko M. The properties of known drugs. 1. Molecular frameworks. Journal of Medicinal Chemistry. 1996;**39**:2887-2893

[32] Bento A, Gaulton A, Hersey A, Bellis L, Chambers J, Davies M, et al. The ChEMBL bioactivity database: An update. Nucleic Acids Research. 2014;**42**:1083-1090

[33] Schafer T, Kriege N, Humbeck L, Klein K, Koch O, Mutzel P. Scaffold hunter: A comprehensive visual analytics framework for drug discovery. Journal of Cheminformatics. 2017;**9**:28

[34] Koch M, Schuffenhauer A, Scheck M, Wetzel S, Casaulta M, Odermatt A, et al. Charting biologically relevant chemical space: A structural classification of natural products (SCONP). Proceedings of the National Academic Science USA. 2005;**102**:17272-17277

[35] Saldivar-Gonzalez F, Pilon-Jimenez A, Medina-Franco J. BIOFACQUIM: A Mexican compound database of natural products. Physical Science Review. 2019;**4**:2018-0103

[36] Frederick R, Bruyere C, Vancraeynest V, Reniers J, Meinguet C, Pochet L, et al. Novel trisubstituted harmine derivatives with original in vitro anticancer activity. Journal of Medicinal Chemistry. 2012;**55**:6489-6501

[37] Rosen J, Rickardson L, Backlund A, Gullbo J, Bohlin L, Larsson R, et al. QSAR and Combinatorial Science. 2009;**28**:436-446

[38] Van der Maaten L, Hinton G. Visualizing Data using t-SNE. Journal of Machine Learning Research. 2008;**9**:2579-2605

[39] McInnes L, Healy J, Melville J. UMAP: Uniform Manifold Approximation and Projection for Dimension Reduction, arXiv e-prints 2018, 1802.03426v2

[40] Yu M. Knowledge-based approach to de novo design using reaction vectors. Journal of Chemical Information and Modeling. 2011;**51**:541-557

[41] Ertl P, Rogg S, Schuffenhauer A. Knowledge-based approach to de novo design using reaction vectors. Journal of Chemical Information and Modeling. 2008;**48**:68-74

[42] Jayaseelan K, Moreno P, Truszkowski A, Ertl P, Steinbeck C. Natural product-likeness score revisited: An open-source, open-data implementation. BMC Bioinformatics. 2012;**13**:106

[43] Zaid H, Raiyn J, Nasser A, Saad B, Rayan A. Physicochemical properties of natural based products versus synthetic chemical. Open Nutraceuticals Journal. 2010;**3**:194-202

[44] "NP-Scout," can be found under https://nerdd.zbh.uni-hamburg.de/npscout/

[45] Seo M, Shin H, Myung Y, Hwang S, T. No K. Development of natural compound molecular fingerprint (NC-MFP) with the dictionary of natural products (DNP) for natural product-based drug development. Journal of Cheminformatics. 2020;**12**:6

[46] Kirchweger B, Rollinger J. In: Filho VC, editor. Natural Products as Source of Molecules with Therapeutic Potential. 2018. pp. 333-364

[47] Kirchweger B, Rollinger M. A strength-weaknesses opportunities-threats (SWOT) analysis of cheminformatics in natural product research. Progress in the Chemistry of Organic Natural Products. 2019;**110**:239-271

[48] Grienke U, Schmidtke M, Kirchmair J, Pfarr K, Wutzler P, Durrwald R, et al. Antiviral potential and molecular insight into neuraminidase inhibiting diarylheptanoids from *Alpinia katsumadai*. Journal of Medicinal Chemistry. 2010;**53**:778-786

[49] Amaro R, Baudry J, Chodera J, Demir O, McCammon J, Miao Y, et al. Ensemble docking in drug discovery. Biophysical Journal. 2018;**114**:2271-2278

[50] Warren G, Andrews C, Capelli A, Clarke B, LaLonde J, Lambert M, et al. A critical assessment of docking programs

and scoring functions. Journal of Medicinal Chemistry. 2006;**49**:5912-5931

[51] "ROCS. Open Eye Scientific Software," can be found under https://www.eyesopen.com

[52] Kirchweger B, Kratz J, Ladurner A, Grienke U, Langer T, Dirsch V, et al. In Silico workflow for the discovery of natural products activating the G protein-coupled bile acid receptor 1. Frontiers in Chemistry. 2018;**6**:242

[53] Grisoni F, Merk D, Friedrich L, Schneider G. Design of Natural-Product-Inspired Multitarget Ligands by machine learning. ChemMedChem. 2019;**14**:1129-1134

[54] Cereto-Massague A, Ojeda M, Valls C, Mulero M, Pujadas G, Garcia-Vallve S. Tools for in silico target fishing. Methods. 2015;**71**:98-103

[55] Mathai N, Chen Y, Kirchmair J. Validation strategies for target prediction methods. Briefings Bioinference. 2019;**21**:791-802

[56] Mathai N, Kirchmair J. Similarity-based methods and machine learning approaches for target prediction in early drug discovery: Performance and scope. International Journal of Molecular Sciences. 2020;**21**:3585

[57] Keiser M, Setola V, Irwin J, Laggner C, Abbas A, Hufeisen S, et al. Predicting new molecular targets for known drugs. Nature. 2009;**462**:175-181

[58] Lounkine E, Keiser M, Whitebread S, Mikhailov D, Hamon J, Jenkins J, et al. Large-scale prediction and testing of drug activity on side-effect targets. Nature. 2012;**486**:361-367

[59] Gfeller D, Grosdidier A, Wirth M, Daina A, Michielin O, Zoete V. Swiss target prediction: A web server for target prediction of bioactive small molecules. Nucleic Acids Research. 2014;**42**:32-38

[60] Chen Y, Mathai N, Kirchmair J. Scope of 3D shape-based approaches in predicting the macromolecular targets of structurally complex small molecules including natural products and macrocyclic ligands. Journal of Chemical Information and Modeling. 2020;**60**:2858-2875

[61] Rollinger J, Schuster D, Danzl B, Schwaiger S, Markt P, Schmidtke M, et al. In silico target fishing for rationalized ligand discovery exemplified on constituents of *Ruta graveolens*. Planta Medica. 2009;**75**:195-204

[62] Reker D, Rodrigues T, Schneider P, Schneider G. Identifying the macromolecular targets of de novo-designed chemical entities through self-organizing map consensus. Proceedings of the National Academy of Sciences. 2014;**111**:4067-4072

[63] Schneider P, Schneider G. De-orphaning the marine natural product (±)-marinopyrrole A by computational target prediction and biochemical validation. Chemical Communications. 2017;**53**:2272-2274

[64] Cockroft N, Cheng X, Fuchs J. Starfish: A Stacked Ensemble Target Fishing Approach and its Application to Natural Products. Chemical Communications. 2019;**9**:4906-4920

[65] Reker D, Perna A, Rodrigues T, Schneider P, Reutlinger M, Monch B, et al. Revealing the macromolecular targets of complex natural products. Nature Chemistry. 2014;**6**:1072-1078

[66] Schneider G, Reker D, Chen T, Hauenstein K, Schneider P, Altmann K, et al. DE orphaning the macromolecular

targets of the natural anticancer compound Doliculide. Chemical International Edition England. 2016;**55**:12408-12411

[67] Walters W, Stahl M, Murcko M. Virtual screening—An overview. Drug Discovery Today. 1998;**3**:160-178

[68] Huth J, Mendoza R, Olejniczak E, Johnson R, Cothron D, Liu Y, et al. ALARM NMR: A rapid and robust experimental method to detect reactive false positives in biochemical screens. Journal of the American Chemical Society. 2005;**127**:217-224

[69] Irwin J, Duan D, Torosyan H, Doak A, Ziebart K, Sterling T, et al. An aggregation advisor for ligand discovery. Journal of Medicinal Chemistry. 2015;**58**:7076-7087

[70] Yang J, Ursu O, Lipinski C, Sklar L, Oprea T, Bologa C. Badapple: Promiscuity patterns from noisy evidence. Journal of Cheminformatics. 2016;**8**:29

[71] Stork C, Chen Y, Sicho M, Kirchmair J. Hit Dexter 2.0: Machine-learning models for the prediction of frequent hitters. Journal of Chemical Information and Modeling. 2019;**59**:1030-1043

[72] Kirchmair J, Goller A, Lang D, Kunze J, Testa B, Wilson D, et al. Predicting drug metabolism: Experiment and/or computation? Nature Reviews Drug Discovery. 2015;**14**:387-404

[73] Sicho M, Stork C, Mazzolari A, de Bruyn KC, Pedretti A, Testa B, et al. FAME 3: Predicting the sites of metabolism in synthetic compounds and natural products for phase 1 and phase 2 metabolic enzymes. Journal of Chemical Information and Modeling. 2019;**59**:3400-3412

Chapter 10

Computational Approaches in Drug Repurposing

Christabel Chikodi Ekeomodi, Kingsley Ifeanyi Obetta, Mmesoma Linus Okolocha, SomtoChukwu Nnacho, Martins Oluwaseun Isijola and InnocentMary IfedibaluChukwu Ejiofor

Abstract

Drug repurposing is a term applied to finding a new therapeutic and pharmacological indication for an existing drug molecule with a known indication. Repurposing existing drugs to treat both rare and widespread ailments is more and more compelling due to the use of less risky compounds, which may result in lower entire development costs and quicker development timelines. This is due to the high attrition rates, high cost, and slow new drug discovery and development pace. The introduction of computational techniques and their advancements in drug design, discovery, and development has provided a platform for scientists to kick-start drug repurposing with ease. Computational approaches have provided rationality in drug repurposing, reducing the chances of failure in drug repurposing attempts. In this chapter, we present techniques for drug repurposing that are both conventional and computational, talk about the difficulties faced by scientists who attempt drug repurposing, and suggest creative solutions to these difficulties to help drug repurposing reach its full potential.

Keywords: drug, repurposing, computational, diseases, in-silico

1. Introduction

Drug repurposing simply means the science and technology of assigning new indications to exist molecules or medications with known therapeutic usage and safety profiles, most stemming from serendipitous discoveries [1]. According to the drug bank library of drug molecules, there are 4302 approved drugs [2–5]. Though these drugs have been classified based on the target enzymes and pharmacological/therapeutic effects, they might still have the potential to activate or inhibit other enzymatic pathways, leading to different impacts on the body. Drug repurposing is all about utilizing and studying other possible enzymatic pathways or effects an already known drug can activate or inhibit, leading to pharmaceutical or pharmacological importance.

The traditional method of developing drugs is time-consuming and expensive; repurposing known drugs is a viable and promising alternative [6]. Developing a new drug involves studying its effectiveness, toxicity, pharmacokinetic, and pharmacodynamic profiles in cell- and animal-based investigations and its effectiveness and safety in humans in clinical trials. It typically takes 13 years and 2–3 billion dollars to develop a new drug from bench to bedside [7]. Drug discovery and development is a less attractive business for funding because of the rising costs and length of time. On the other hand, drug repurposing aims to identify new medical uses for an approved or experimental drug. Clinical trials can be hastened because the drug's dosing and safety have been thoroughly investigated, considerably cutting the time and money needed for development [8].

Due to the high rates of illness and death associated with certain emerging diseases, repurposing drugs may be the most effective approach for addressing these

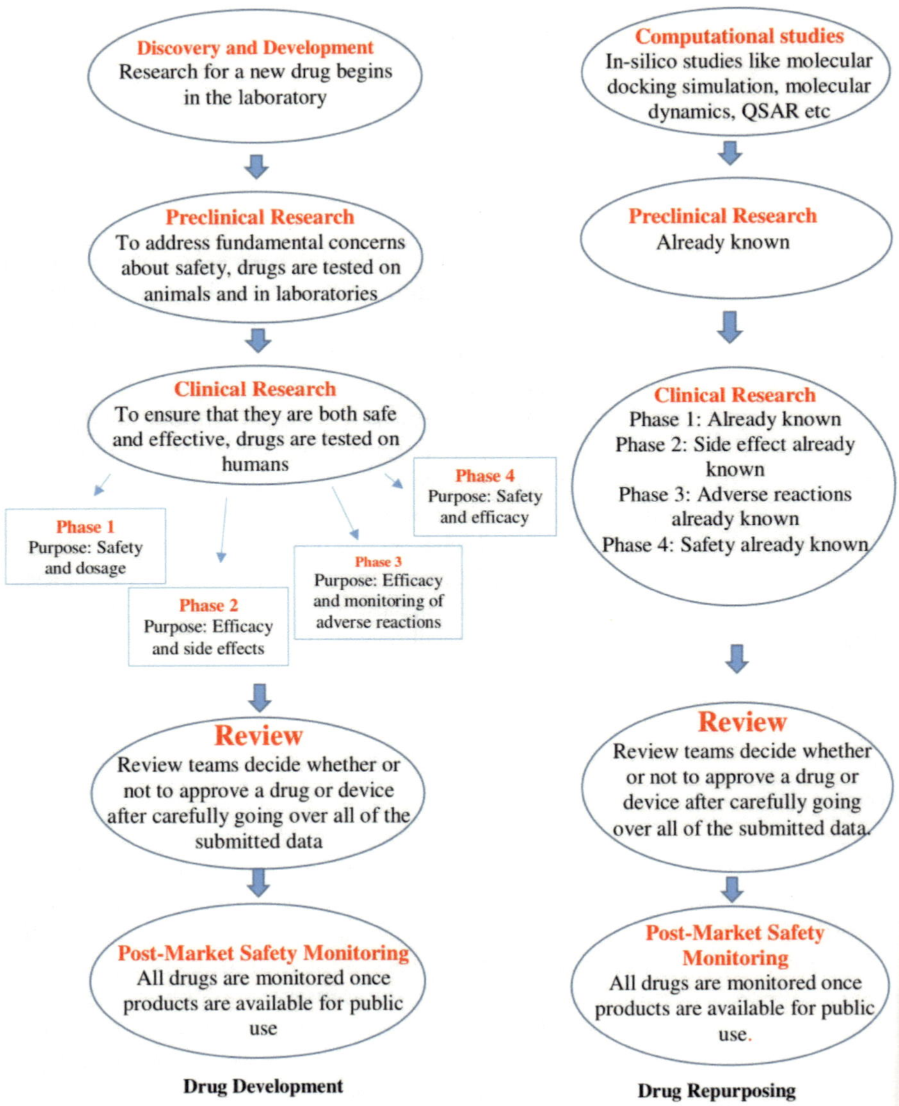

Figure 1.
Drug development vs. drug.

conditions. When there is an urgent need to develop new medications and treatments during an outbreak, such as was the case with the COVID-19 pandemic, the strategy of quickly repurposing existing drugs has a significant advantage as it has the potential to identify medications that could be used to address the situation [9].

With current R&D costs, developing de novo drug therapies for more than 8000 rare diseases is inconceivable; nevertheless, drug repositioning, based on finding hidden associations or building connections between a drug and disease, holds promise for orphan drug disease therapy [10]. Furthermore, evaluating approved medications to determine new indications assists pharmaceutical companies in extending the patent life of drugs through application to adjacent diseases and in protecting IP against competitors [1].

Compared to the conventional drug development procedure, as shown in **Figure 1**, the advent of computation methods in medicinal research has provided a lesser expensive and less time-consuming approach to finding other disease conditions that can be treated using already approved or experimental drugs.

2. Repurposing principles

There are typically two main repositioning principles for drugs. First, because many diseases are interdependent, medications for one condition may also be effective for treating other disorders. Second, because medicines are naturally confusing, they can be linked to various targets and pathways. According to the source of the findings, drug repositioning research can be divided into two groups:

a. Drug-based tactics, in which discoveries are based on drug-related knowledge.

b. Disease-based strategies, in which discoveries are based on disease-related knowledge [9].

3. Repurposing techniques

In-silico approaches using existing data to find new drug-disease linkages and experimental screening approaches are the two main categories of systematic repurposing techniques.

3.1 Experimental screening approaches

Experimental screening approaches are used as a source of hits for drug discovery and drug repurposing, with notable differences in their application and outcomes. Searches in drug discovery programs are typically done for de novo candidate hits, fuelled by an HTS campaign, which requires highly specialized screening facilities and compound libraries containing several million compounds. Repurposing programs focus on advanced known molecules that either approved or failed with some knowledge of their safety or MoA available, led by in-depth screening and with smaller compound libraries. Typically approved compound libraries containing 500–2000 compounds and a similar number of existing but unapproved compounds are thought to be available.

3.2 *In-silico* approaches

In-silico repurposing techniques analyze data already in existence using sophisticated analytical methods to discover new possible connections between a drug and a disease [1]. The capacity to predict the conformation of small-molecule ligands inside the proper target binding site with a high degree of accuracy makes molecular docking one of the most commonly used in silico processes; after the creation of the first algorithms in the 1980s, molecular docking became a crucial tool in drug discovery. For example, investigations can be conveniently performed involving important molecular events, including ligand binding modes and the corresponding intermolecular interactions that stabilize the ligand-receptor complex. Furthermore, molecular docking algorithms execute quantitative predictions of binding energetics, providing rankings of docked compounds based on the binding affinity of ligand-receptor complexes [11]. Identifying the most likely binding conformations requires two steps: (i) exploration of an ample conformational space representing various potential binding modes; (ii) accurate prediction of the interaction energy associated with each of the predicted binding conformations. Molecular docking programs perform these tasks through a cyclical process in which the ligand conformation is evaluated by specific scoring functions [11].

In-silico approaches can broadly be divided into molecular techniques and real-world data approaches.

3.2.1 Molecular approaches

The molecular approaches are based on understanding drug activity and disease pathophysiology. They are often powered by large-scale molecular data known as omic data, including genomic, transcriptomic, or proteomic data and data based on drug targets and chemical structure. Due to the availability of datasets on drugs and diseases, as well as the robustness and reproducibility of the data, transcriptomics, and genomics are the two data types most widely used to support drug repurposing [12]. Transcriptomics studies the expression levels of thousands of genes, often accomplished by quantifying RNA using RNASeq or gene expression microarrays. One approach to using transcriptomics for drug repurposing is based on the idea that reversing gene expression signatures may result in a clinical benefit [1].

3.2.2 Real-world data approaches

The Real-world data approach focuses on identifying unknown and sometimes unexpected relationships between drugs and diseases or their symptoms. They are data based on individuals' health, habits, and behavior captured without environmental intervention or bias introduced by data collection methodologies [1]. The real-world data approaches include network-based drug repurposing, ligand-based drug repurposing, structure-based drug repurposing, and machine-learning techniques [13].

3.2.2.1 Network-based drug repurposing

Network-based computational biology has become more prevalent in recent times. It integrates the relationship between biological molecules into networks to discover newly discovered properties at the network level and investigate how cellular systems induce different biological phenotypes under other conditions. A network can be represented as a connected graph in the network pharmacology framework, with each node representing either an individual molecular entity, its biological target, a modifier molecule within a biological process, or a target pathway, and each edge representing either a direct or indirect interaction between two connected nodes. An instance of this approach was demonstrated in 2009 by Hu and Agarwal, who utilized publicly available gene expression profiles from NCBI Gene Expression Omnibus (GEO) to construct a network that showed the similarity between different diseases. They then integrated this network with molecular profiles and knowledge of drugs and drug targets, which enabled them to identify opportunities for drug repositioning, as well as to propose molecular targets and mechanisms underlying drug effects [14]. In 2012, Jin et al. also devised a new method for repurposing drugs for cancer therapeutics that takes advantage of off-target effects that may affect critical cancer cell signaling pathways [15]. A hybrid model composed of a network component called cancer-signaling bridges and a Bayesian factor regression model was used to identify off-target effects of drugs on signaling proteins [13]. The main limitation of network-based approaches is that many biological aspects of the disease still need to be discovered, and network-based approaches may fail to produce promising drug candidates; also, biological elements interact with one another to form a complex system. As a result, this class of methods may have more practical effects [16].

3.2.2.2 Ligand-based drug repurposing

Ligand-based approaches are evaluated because similar compounds have similar biological properties. These methods have been widely used in drug repurposing to analyze and predict the activity of ligands for new targets. The number of publicly accessible compound records (more than a hundred million provided only by PubChem) is far greater than the number of deposited protein crystal structures (as of today, less than 150,000 in the Protein Data Bank) [17, 18]. Ligand-based methods rely on the chemical space coverage of already-known molecules. Deep learning and multi-task learning have been successfully used in ligand chemogenomic benchmark studies. When target and drug similarities were considered, the algorithm better predicted new drug-target associations. Machine-learning approaches play an essential role in silico Chemogenomics [13].

3.2.2.3 Structure-based drug repurposing

Structure-based similar protein structures increase the likelihood of performing similarly and identifying related ligands. Protein comparison is a technique used in medication repurposing to find secondary targets for a medicine that has already been licensed [19]. Proteins can be compared on a broad scale based on how similar their sequences are. The kinome is the most often-used example of a phylogenetic tree constructed using protein sequences [20]. In this tree, proteins from the same family are more likely to detect substrates or ligands that share similar functions, as in the case of dual inhibitors of the EGFR and ErbB2 receptors for an epidermal growth factor [21]. Sequence alignments work best when proteins have a high level of sequence identity. In contrast, local protein comparison works better when proteins share a low level of sequence identity to uncover unknown targets of known ligands [22]. It has become more crucial to compare protein binding sites to find local similarities [19]. This process is frequently followed by computing several descriptors that help determine a similarity score to locate cavities on the protein surface and compare binding sites. It is important to note that, when available, ligand binding modes are a valuable tool for finding new targets. Putting a focus on target-ligand interactions is one method of modeling molecular recognition. Several techniques, like structure-based pharmacophores or interaction fingerprints, can accomplish this. When the protein-ligand complex's structure is unknown, one can predict hot spots in the binding site using computational approaches [23]. The viability of crystallographic structures of protein-ligand complexes is a prerequisite for structure-based techniques. The level of specificity that can be used to represent a binding site depends on resolution and sensitivity to atomic coordinates. While a protein's static model can be seen in its crystallographic structure, conformational variations can cause the appearance of additional pockets [13].

3.2.2.4 Machine learning approaches

Although machine learning methods produce better prediction models, they are more data-dependent. Combining machine learning methods and other techniques can make an effective treatment plan for COVID-19 [16]. The general approach has been to fuse the structure-based and ligand-based screening methods with AI algorithms to build prediction models. AI and ML algorithms like deep learning, support vector machine (SVM), random forest (RF), Naive Bayesian, and neural networks have been extensively used for high throughput screening with lots of dataset molecules. In recent years, the development of next-generation computational methods using Artificial Intelligence (AI), Machine Learning (ML), and network medicine approaches has positively impacted the different stages of drug development [24].

4. Success stories in computational drug repurposing

The field of data science is blooming, and its role in detecting potential candidates for drug repurposing has yet to be explored. There are various approaches to drug repurposing, but the computational approach is unique in the way it utilizes neither in-vivo nor in-vitro techniques. It is known as in-silico drug repurposing—an expediting, cost-friendly, and reliable process [25]. This method relies heavily on data from diverse sources like electronic health records (EHRs) comprising disease diagnoses, lab test results, medical prescriptions, genetic data from biobanks, chemogenomic data, and proteomic data [26]. These data sources, when collated and analyzed, are then capable of producing valuable insights. A few instances:

Given widespread tuberculosis and its extensive resistance mechanisms to current anti-infective treatment, Kleandrova et al. performed a study on computational drug repurposing for antituberculosis therapy by creating a multi-condition model based on quantitative structure–activity-relationship (QSAR) [27]. This sought to find potential antituberculosis agents capable of acting as inhibitors of multiple strains of the bacteria. The model utilized a combination of perturbation theory concepts and machine learning techniques to screen large data repositories for chemical structures with the potential to inhibit Mycobacterium tuberculosis, the causative organism. The dataset comprised 8898 agency-regulated chemicals, including investigational and FDA-approved drugs. After that, stipulated metrics were used to rank these agents, with priority given to those exhibiting the highest values. Top of the list was macozinone, BTZ-043, and niclosamide, but niclosamide is a popularly known antihelminthic. This drug is believed to have anti-parkinsonian, anti-diabetic, and antiviral properties [28]. It is also important to mention that through computationally identifying drugs that can increase the mRNA expression of downregulated genes in hepatocellular carcinoma (HCC) and decrease the mRNA expression of upregulated genes, the antitumor activity of niclosamide and its ethanolamine salt (NEN) was discovered. The antiproliferative activity of niclosamide and NEN in different HCC cell lines and primary human hepatocytes was then evaluated in vitro. This was further confirmed by in vivo testing against two mouse models (genetically induced liver tumors and patient-derived xenografts [PDXs]) for HCC to show a substantial reduction in the cancer progression after oral administration of NEN compared to niclosamide [29].

Similarly, Zhang et al. performed thorough data mining to identify drugs with anti-Alzheimer properties [30]. Their study revealed seven drugs inhibiting acetylcholinesterase, a known drug target of most anti-Alzheimer conventional medicines. These drugs, which have never been used in the management of Alzheimer's, can be used in the future for cognitive deficiency therapy in patients with the disease. Zhang et al. previously conducted an identical study for drugs that can be used for anti-diabetic treatment [31]. Using data mining and pathogenesis information, their study repurposed 58 drugs, out of which nine were prioritized for having higher potential in treating diabetes. Among these nine drugs were four (diflunisal, nabumetone, niflumic acid, and valdecoxib) used in rheumatoid arthritis, osteoarthritis, and pain management. Connectivity map analysis showed that cells treated with these four drugs had similar gene expression as cells treated with conventional anti-diabetic medications like metformin and glimepiride. Evidence from Koren et al., 2019 also suggests that a different class of drugs, the alpha-1 adrenergic antagonists, might have a potential impact on diabetes control [32]. These success stories, though sparse in their numbers, hold a promise for the future. Diseases like diabetes often last for a lifetime, and an estimated 400 million people [33] worldwide suffer from it; therefore, integrating the results of this expediting approach to drug discovery into clinical practice will revolutionize modern medicine.

5. Limitations

Drug repurposing by pharmaceutical companies faces many challenges. There is a need to create a business model to support the use of existing molecules as therapeutics for new indications and repurposing drug pathways. There is also a need to demonstrate the effectiveness and recover the investment required to bring recycled products to market [1]. Furthermore, this methodology is based on structural files and cannot be used immediately when identifying a new or orphan target [24]. This is because a more extensive collection of records may not be achieved since there is no defining identifier to connect data [16]. This can be seen in the Artificial Intelligence, Machine Learning, and network medicine approaches of computational drug repurposing, which require large amounts of data to train models. Lack of access to structured, standardized data related to analytics and clinical trials can impair the tool's predictive ability. Furthermore, the majority of developed models are local models; that is, they are specific to one problem, and there is no global model or suite that helps in solving or querying the wide range of problems drug discovery teams may encounter [24].

All computational-based drug repurposing methods heavily depend on data. Existing databases pose lots of challenges for researchers. The volume of data in some databases needs to be increased to generate a suitable model, and there is no determinant identifier to connect data to collect more comprehensive datasets. Data descriptions could be clearer, making it easier to understand them. The databases also contain data for a specific purpose rather than complete data. Lastly, introducing new Active Pharmaceutical Compounds (API) commands has made them difficult to learn and use. Existing databases have some limitations that can be overcome using software engineering techniques [16]. In terms of improving efficacy and reducing the time and cost of a drug discovery project, computational-based approaches may produce more acceptable results than others. Every computational drug repurposing method has advantages and disadvantages and heavily depends on data [16].

The computational approach is auspicious and effective in other domains. Natural language processing, for example, has proven helpful in translation, spell-checking, and other applications. However, AI/ML-based techniques necessitate a large amount of data to train the models. The inaccessibility of structured and standardized data associated with assays and clinical trials may jeopardize the tools' predictive ability. Furthermore, most developed models are local, which means they are specific to one problem. No global model or suite can help resolve or query a wide range of issues that a drug discovery team may frequently encounter [24].

6. Opportunities in the computational repurposing of drugs

Although sciences and technology have progressed rapidly, de novo drug development has been costly and time-consuming over the past decades. Given these circumstances, "drug repurposing" (or "drug repositioning") has appeared as an alternative tool to accelerate the drug development process by seeking new indications for already approved drugs rather than discovering de novo drug compounds, nowadays accounting for 30% of newly marked medications in the U.S [34]. Even though the application of computational methodologies to drug repurposing has yielded some positive results and has been propounded to repurpose drugs on a large scale by utilizing available high-throughput data, due to the failure of the current drug regimen, many more diseases need urgent attention in terms of new drug therapies. There are increasing number of deaths from Neglected tropical diseases. The World Health Organization (WHO) describes neglected tropical diseases (NTDs) as a diverse group of communicable diseases that prevail in tropical and subtropical conditions [35]. Neglected Tropical Diseases include Buruli ulcer, Chagas disease, dengue and chikungunya, dracunculiasis (Guinea-worm disease), echinococcosis, foodborne trematodiases, African human trypanosomiasis (sleeping sickness), leishmaniasis, leprosy (Hansen's disease), lymphatic filariasis, mycetoma, chromoblastomycosis, and other deep mycoses, onchocerciasis (river blindness), rabies, scabies, and other ectoparasitoses, schistosomiasis, soil-transmitted helminthiases, snakebite envenoming, taeniasis/cysticercosis, trachoma, and yaws and other endemic treponematoses [35]. According to WHO, NTDs cause about 200,000 deaths yearly [35]. A person may become severely disabled, disfigured, blind, or malnourished after contracting an NTD and frequently acquire multiple NTDs at once. If new drugs have to be developed for these conditions through conventional means, many deaths must have been recorded before the drugs get to market.

According to Nigeria Centre for Disease Control (NCDC), in 2021 and 2022, Cholera killed more people in Nigeria than COVID-19 [36]. Even though there are standard treatment guidelines for this condition, the death rate keeps rising. Globally, lives are being lost from different types of cancers, even with all the treatments currently available. Lives are also being lost from various other diseases affecting mankind. Computational drug repurposing will go a long way in providing within a short time a possible better treatment and management options for these diseases and all other diseases challenging mankind.

7. Conclusion

The utilization of existing drugs to identify other potential therapeutic indications can be done more quickly and with less expense through computational drug repurposing. This approach is facilitated by the use of protein and chemical databases, which have been developed to support computational techniques. These databases enable existing drugs to be acquired in the necessary formats for computational studies. There is now a broad selection of available computational tools, with more currently under development, which can help to advance the application of computational approaches in drug repurposing. With access to these tools and databases, any researcher with an interest in this area can begin to explore drug repurposing. The effective use of computational drug repurposing has the potential to improve treatment and management options for a wide range of diseases affecting humanity.

Acknowledgements

The authors express their gratitude to the CURIES research group, whose support and encouragement have been invaluable.

Conflict of interest

The authors declare no conflict of interest.

Author details

Christabel Chikodi Ekeomodi*, Kingsley Ifeanyi Obetta, Mmesoma Linus Okolocha, SomtoChukwu Nnacho, Martins Oluwaseun Isijola and InnocentMary IfedibaluChukwu Ejiofor
Faculty of Pharmaceutical Sciences, Nnamdi Azikiwe University, Awka, Nigeria

*Address all correspondence to: cc.ekeomodi@stu.unizik.edu.ng

References

[1] Cha Y, Erez T, Reynolds IJ, Kumar D, Ross J, Koytiger G, et al. Drug repurposing from the perspective of pharmaceutical companies. British Journal of Pharmacology. 2018;**175**(2):168-180. DOI: 10.1111/bph.13798

[2] Wishart DS, Feunang YD, Guo AC, Lo EJ, Marcu A, Grant JR, et al. DrugBank 5.0: A major update to the DrugBank database for 2018. Nucleic Acids Research. 2017;**2017**. DOI: 10.1093/nar/gkx1037

[3] Wishart DS, Knox C, Guo AC, Cheng D, Shrivastava S, Tzur D, et al. DrugBank: A knowledgebase for drugs, drug actions and drug targets. Nucleic Acids Research. 2008;**36**:D901-D906

[4] Knox C, Law V, Jewison T, Liu P, Ly S, Frolkis A, et al. DrugBank 3.0: A comprehensive resource for 'omics' research on drugs. Nucleic Acids Research. 2011;**39**:D1035-D1041

[5] Wishart DS, Knox C, Guo AC, Cheng D, Shrivastava S, Tzur D, et al. DrugBank: A knowledgebase for drugs, drug actions and drug targets. Nucleic Acids Research. 2008;**36**:D901-D906

[6] Kumar S, Kovalenko S, Bhardwaj S, Sethi A, Gorobets NY, Desenko SM. Poonam, Rathi B. drug repurposing against SARS-CoV-2 using computational approaches. In Drug Discovery Today. 2022;**27**(7):2015-2027. DOI: 10.1016/j.drudis.2022.02.004

[7] Yella JK, Yaddanapudi S, Wang Y, Jegga AG. Changing trends in computational drug repositioning. Pharmaceuticals (Basel, Switzerland). 2018;**11**(2):57. DOI: 10.3390/ph11020057

[8] Pushpakom S, Iorio F, Eyers PA, Escott KJ, Hopper S, Wells A, et al. Drug repurposing: Progress, challenges and recommendations. Nature Reviews. Drug Discovery. 2019;**18**(1):41-58. DOI: 10.1038/nrd.2018.168

[9] Jarada TN, Rokne JG, Alhajj R. A review of computational drug repositioning: Strategies, approaches, opportunities, challenges, and directions. Journal of Chemistry. 2020;**12**(1). DOI: 10.1186/s13321-020-00450-7

[10] Sardana D, Zhu C, Zhang M, Gudivada RC, Yang L, Jegga AG. Drug repositioning for orphan diseases. Briefings in Bioinformatics. 2011;**12**(4):346-356. DOI: 10.1093/bib/bbr021

[11] Ferreira LG, Dos Santos RN, Oliva G, Andricopulo AD. Molecular docking and structure-based drug design strategies. Molecules. 2015;**20**(7):13384-11342. DOI: 10.3390/molecules200713384

[12] Menden MP, Iorio F, Garnett M, McDermott U, Benes CH, Ballester PJ, et al. Machine learning prediction of Cancer cell sensitivity to drugs based on genomic and chemical properties. PLoS One. 2013;**8**:4. DOI: 10.1371/journal.pone.0061318

[13] March-Vila E, Pinzi L, Sturm N, Tinivella A, Engkvist O, Chen H, et al. On the integration of In Silico drug design methods for drug repurposing. Frontiers in Pharmacology. 2017;**8**:298. DOI: 10.3389/fphar.2017.00298

[14] Hu G, Agarwal P. Human disease-drug network based on genomic expression profiles. PLoS One. 2009;**4**(8):e6536. DOI: 10.1371/journal.pone.0006536

[15] Jin G, Fu C, Zhao H, Cui K, Chang J, Wong STC. A novel method of transcriptional response analysis to facilitate drug repositioning for cancer therapy. Cancer Research. 2012;**2012**(72):33-44. DOI: 10.1158/0008-5472.CAN-11-2333

[16] Masoudi-Sobhanzadeh Y. Computational-based drug repurposing methods in COVID-19. BioImpacts: BI. 2020;**10**(3):205-206. DOI: 10.34172/bi.2020.25

[17] Berman HM, Westbrook J, Feng Z, Gilliland G, Bhat TN, Weissig H, et al. The protein data bank. Nucleic Acids Research. 2000;**28**(1):235-242. DOI: 10.1093/nar/28.1.235

[18] Wang X, Liu C, Wang J, Fan Y, Wang Z, Wang Y. Proton pump inhibitors increase the chemosensitivity of patients with advanced colorectal cancer. Oncotarget. 2017;**8**:58801-58808. DOI: 10.18632/oncotarget.18522

[19] Ehrt C, Brinkjost T, Koch O. Impact of binding site comparisons on medicinal chemistry and rational molecular design. Journal of Medicinal Chemistry. 2016;**59**:4121-4151. DOI: 10.1021/acs.jmedchem.6b00078

[20] Manning G, Whyte DB, Martinez R, Hunter T, Sudarsanam S. The protein kinase complement of the human genome. Science. 2002;**298**:1912-1934. DOI: 10.1126/science.1075762

[21] Zhang YM, Cockerill S, Guntrip SB, Rusnak D, Smith K, Vanderwall D, et al. Synthesis and SAR of potent EGFR/erbB2 dual inhibitors. Bioorganic & Medicinal Chemistry Letters. 2004;**14**(1):111-114. DOI: 10.1016/j.bmcl.2003.10.010

[22] Chen YC, Tolbert R, Aronov AM, McGaughey G, Walters WP, Meireles L. Prediction of protein pairs sharing common active ligands using protein sequence, structure, and ligand similarity. Journal of Chemical Information and Modeling. 2016;**56**(9):1734-1745. DOI: 10.1021/acs.jcim.6b00118

[23] Hall DR, Kozakov D, Whitty A, Vajda S. Lessons from hot spot analysis for fragment-based drug discovery. Trends in Pharmacological Sciences. 2015;**36**(11):724-736. DOI: 10.1016/j.tips.2015.08.003

[24] Sharma PP, Bansal M, Sethi A, Poonam PL, Goel VK, Grishina M, et al. Computational methods directed towards drug repurposing for COVID-19: Advantages and limitations. RSC Advances. 2021;**11**(57):36181-36198. DOI: 10.1039/d1ra05320e

[25] Sadeghi SS, Keyvanpour MR. An analytical review of computational drug repurposing. IEEE/ACM Transactions on Computational Biology and Bioinformatics. 2021;**18**(2):472-488. DOI: 10.1109/TCBB.2019.2933825

[26] Glicksberg BS, Li L, Chen R, Dudley J, Chen B. Leveraging big data to transform drug discovery. Methods in Molecular Biology. 2019;**1939**:91-118. DOI: 10.1007/978-1-4939-9089-4_6

[27] Kleandrova VV, Scotti MT, Speck-Planche A. Computational drug repurposing for Antituberculosis therapy: Discovery of multi-strain inhibitors. Antibiotics (Basel). 2021;**10**(8):1005. DOI: 10.3390/antibiotics10081005

[28] Kadri H, Lambourne OA, Mehellou Y. Niclosamide, a drug with many (re)purposes. ChemMedChem. 2018;**13**:1088-1091. DOI: 10.1002/cmdc.201800100

[29] Chen B, Wei W, Ma L, Yang B, Gill RM, Chua MS, et al. Computational

discovery of Niclosamide ethanolamine, a repurposed drug candidate that reduces growth of hepatocellular carcinoma cells In vitro and in mice by inhibiting cell division cycle 37 Signaling. Gastroenterology. 2017;**152**(8):2022-2036. DOI: 10.1053/j.gastro.2017.02.039

[30] Zhang M, Schmitt-Ulms G, Sato C, Xi Z, Zhang Y, Zhou Y, et al. Drug repositioning for Alzheimer's disease based on systematic 'omics' data mining. PLoS One. 2016;**11**(12):e0168812. DOI: 10.1371/journal.pone.0168812

[31] Zhang M, Luo H, Xi Z, Rogaeva E. Drug repositioning for diabetes based on 'Omics' data mining. PLoS One. 2015;**10**(5):e0126082. DOI: 10.1371/journal.pone.0126082

[32] Koren G, Nordon G, Radinsky K, Shalev V. Identification of repurposable drugs with beneficial effects on glucose control in type 2 diabetes using machine learning. Pharmacology Research & Perspectives. 2019;**7**(6):e00529. DOI: 10.1002/prp2.529

[33] Khan MAB, Hashim MJ, King JK, Govender RD, Mustafa H, Al KJ. Epidemiology of type 2 diabetes - global burden of disease and forecasted trends. Journal of Epidemiology Global Health. 2020;**10**(1):107-111. DOI: 10.2991/jegh.k.191028.001

[34] Park K. A review of computational drug repurposing. Translational Clinical Pharmacology. 2019;**27**(2):59-63. DOI: 10.12793/tcp.2019.27.2.59

[35] World Health Organization. Neglected Tropical Diseases [Internet]. 2023. Available from: https://www.who.int/health-topics/neglected-tropical-diseases#tab=tab_1 [Accessed: January 24, 2023]

[36] Nigeria Centre for Disease Control and Prevention. An update of Cholera outbreak in Nigeria [Internet]. 2022. Available from: https://www.ncdc.gov.ng/diseases/sitreps [Accessed: January 24, 2023]

Chapter 11

Role of Drug Repurposing in Sustainable Drug Discovery

Shanta Bhar

Abstract

The contemporary global drug discovery scenario, in spite of several technological advances, is heavily ridden with multiple challenges of a dynamic regulatory system, escalating costs from bench to bedside investigational drugs, the increased probability of withdrawal after launch, and over-stretched timelines from discovery to approval, among others. Drug repurposing/repositioning/re-profiling/re-tasking is an effective and practical complimentary method for the selection of alternate therapies for approved, shelved, discontinued/abandoned, and investigational drugs or new chemical entities, with the parallel study of new metabolic pathways and/or protein targets. Such an approach encompasses multipronged benefits of redundant preclinical testing, toxicity evaluation, and formulation studies, based largely on serendipity. In recent years, approaches have been driven by artificial intelligence (AI) and machine learning, and bioinformatics have opened up new vistas in drug re-profiling acceleration. Increasing protocols to club the shared mechanisms among structurally diverse/dissimilar drugs include pathway analysis, phenotypic screening, signature matching, related disease genes, binding assay studies, molecular docking, and clinical data monitoring. All in all, repositioning of abandoned/investigational/existing drugs or new chemical entities for other therapeutic indications could enhance the overall productivity of the pharmaceutical industry while paradigmatically shifting the focus from new drug discovery to the optimization of available resources.

Keywords: innovation, repurposing, big data, pharmacological analysis, pathway matching

1. Introduction

The overall global population exposed to regular medicines has increased two-fold over the past few decades. To complement this, the average life expectancy has increased considerably, and newer, lesser understood diseases are on the rise. Unfortunately, the rather long timelines of drug design and approval (10-12 years), increased rates of USFDA failure/recall after launch, escalating resources for new drug discovery and development, and a paradigm shift toward green chemistry have, in totality, rendered the conventional drug discovery process largely wanting for alternative backup plans.

According to the Brundtland Commission of the United Nations: "Sustainable development is development that meets the needs of the present without compromising the ability of future generations to meet their own needs" [1]. The Sustainable Development Goals (SDGs) and the One-Health approach are analogous initiatives [2]. The various alternative ways of making drug discovery sustainable are: signature mapping, pathway matching, in silico screening and molecular docking, genetic association, retrospective analysis of clinical data, drug repurposing, high-throughput screening, and so on.

Out of all the options available for introducing sustainability in drug discovery and development, drug repositioning, also known by its alternative names of repurposing, re-profiling, or re-tasking, is the strategy of choice as the advantages far outweigh the challenges encountered in offering a drug for a new medical indication, totally distinct from its original scope.

The most important reason for the failure/withdrawal of an approved drug is addressed adequately: the potentially repurposed drug would have been in preclinical models and early-stage human clinical trials (phase I & II), thereby justifying its safety; thus, subsequent efficacy trials would be more predictable.

In addition, drug development timelines can be sufficiently squeezed, due to non-repetition of preclinical testing, safety assessment, and/or formulation development. Most significantly, it is the most economically lucrative of all the sustainable strategies employed, as mandatory investment is marginal. The regulatory and phase III costs can involve substantial savings in preclinical, phase I, and phase II expenditure.

Since the commencement of drug repurposing concept, it was rational but serendipitous; that is, an approved drug or one in clinical trials was studied for its contraindications, off-target reactions, and/or an enhanced on-target response, patented and groomed for repurposed launch. Most success stories of relaunch in a new therapeutic avatar have indeed relied hugely on serendipity, rather than on a structured and well-planned approach. Such examples include aspirin, minoxidil, sildenafil, thalidomide, celecoxib, rituximab, raloxifene, fingolimod, dapoxetine, topiramate, and ketoconazole, among others.

However, with several technological advancements, in the form of various approaches, drug repurposing in general, and specifically for rare diseases, comprising a databank of over several thousand (~7000), with 95-96% of these having no approved therapeutic agent, primarily because of unknown disease pathophysiology, contemporary drug repurposing abounds in opportunities to fill up the unmet medical space.

As we shall see further, the trade-off between challenges posed by drug repurposing and its many advantages is also laced with limitations of collation, integration, analysis, and interpretation of big data, of biomedical, clinical, pharmacological, or sequencing type.

2. Types of sustainable approaches to drug discovery

The many approaches toward sustainable drug discovery are listed below (**Figure 1**):

2.1 Signature mapping

In a broad sense, this process is based on the relative comparison of certain distinct features, thus referred to as the 'signature' of one drug against another, disease

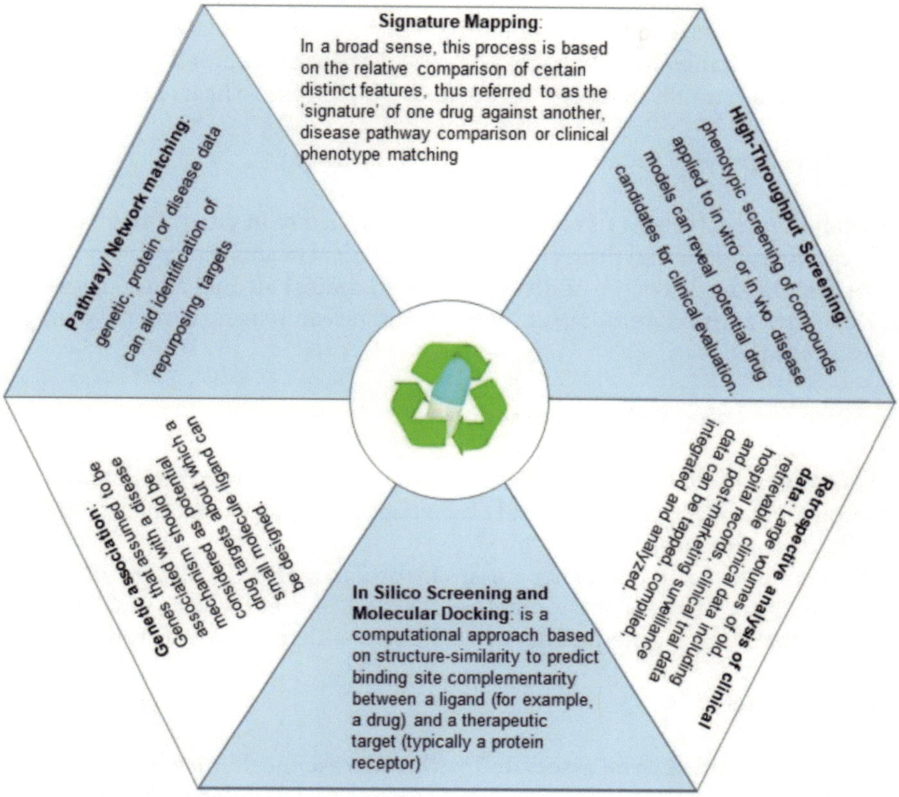

Figure 1.
Sustainable drug repurposing approaches.

pathway comparison, or clinical phenotype matching [3, 4]. This signature pattern of two comparable drugs is generally assigned from three databanks:

1. Transcriptomic (RNA), proteomic, or metabolomic data

2. Chemical structures

3. Adverse event profiles

For example, two drugs were identified using drug–disease similarity approach using the correlation between the gene expression signature of the drug and that of the disease, prednisolone, and topiramate.

2.2 Pathway/network matching

Genetic, protein, or disease data can aid the identification of repurposing targets.

In some disease pathways, the relevant genes are not druggable as targets. This is when a pathway-based comparison of genes that are either downstream or upstream or a genome-wide association studies (GWAS)-related target may be used for repurposing issues [5]. Network analysis uses available information on gene expression patterns, disease pathology, protein interactions, or GWAS data for construction of a drug or disease network to further potential repurposing candidates.

For example, pranlukast, an asthma drug/leukotriene receptor 1 antagonist, and a phosphodiesterase inhibitor amrinone are used for congestive heart failure.

2.3 High-throughput screening

Or phenotypic screening of compounds, it is applied to in vitro or in vivo disease models can reveal potential drug candidates for clinical evaluation.

For example, the discovery of disulfiram, used against alcohol abuse, turned out to be a selective antineoplastic agent, with proven research using genome-wide gene expression studies.

2.4 In Silico screening and molecular docking

It is a computational approach based on structure similarity to predict binding site complementarity between a ligand (for example, a drug) and a therapeutic target (typically, a protein receptor).

For example, molecular docking studies identified mebendazole, an anti-parasitic drug and inhibitor of vascular endothelial growth factor receptor 2 (VEGFR2), and also a mediator of angiogenesis. This was validated with experiment studies.

2.5 Genetic association

Genes that assumed to be associated with a disease mechanism should be considered as potential drug targets about which a small molecule ligand can be designed.

2.6 Retrospective analysis of clinical data

Large volumes of old, retrievable clinical data including hospital records, clinical trial data, and post-marketing surveillance data can be tapped, compiled, integrated, and analyzed. Such databases comprise both structured and unstructured data on patient response and outcomes.

For example, terbutaline sulfate, an anti-asthmatic drug candidate, was arrived at for the treatment of amyotrophic lateral sclerosis (ALS), from the retrospective clinical data analysis.

3. Drug repurposing

3.1 Challenges to overcome

3.1.1 Legal and commercial challenges

Some developing countries like India, the Philippines, Taiwan (Province of China), the Andean Pact Latin American countries (Bolivia, Colombia, Ecuador, and Peru), and Vietnam do not allow the granting of a method-of-use patent for a second or alternate medical use of an approved drug, whereas several developed nations allow second medical use patents defined as fiction of novelty. In some other cases, possible repurposing may have been discussed/covered/reported in the original literature or may be part of its non-registered uses. The international TRIPS Agreement allows flexibility to the individual signatory nations as also to their courts on the refusal/approval of second medical use patents.

The European Patent Office (EPO) does not allow a second medical use patent if it is merely noted that the drug exhibits selective binding to another receptor; yet if the claim focuses on the end result of the drug function, mentioned categorically as "any condition susceptible of being improved or prevented by inhibition or enhancement of a specific enzyme activity," the patent is granted/approved provided that it is validated/supported by experimental data, which is also disclosed in the patent application specifications. Any information related to drug re-profiling may not be controlled by intellectual property rights; however, if in the public domain, it cannot attract novelty, thus ceasing to be patentable material. Furthermore, proof-of-concept studies also need to be validated by controlled clinical trials.

Toggling the bioisosteres of existing off-patent drugs by keeping their pharmacophore intact would defeat the purpose of repurposing, as it would give rise to a new entity. Same dosage and/or formulation for off-patent drugs being re-profiled would not be legally patentable. Therefore, offering a lower dosage form than in use or an alternate formulation would be key to its re-profiling.

3.1.2 Retrieving data

With respect to shelved/abandoned/withdrawn drugs, a major hurdle is accessibility to clinical trials data that only its discovering organization may be privy to. Although a shelved drug is capable of reinventing itself as a lower dose repurposed opportunity, the pharma industry, on an average, does not resort to sharing its list/portfolio of shelved drugs, especially if the therapy area of repurposing does not cater to its organization's disease portfolio.

In another scenario, where there is a collaborative interface between industry and academia, this problem can only be facilitated by CDA (Confidentiality Disclosure Agreement) and compound sharing. Dealing with abandoned drugs, or those which have been outlived by their competitors, another challenge is posed by the availability of a suitable vendor.

3.1.3 Limited repurposing space

As more and more approved drugs are finding their way into repurposed therapeutic territories, it may seem that the druggable space for repurposing is exhausting itself out. In such a scenario, a prudent strategy would be to club drugs for combination therapy, as also to discover new pathways for their effective applications. This is visible more so in the field of infectious diseases, by employing the nifurtimox–eflornithine combination therapy for second-stage African trypanosomiasis [6]. Another avenue to expand the re-profiling horizon is personalized medicine.

4. Early examples of successful drug repositioning

The first example of drug repositioning is aspirin or acetylsalicylic acid (**Figure 2**). In 1899, Bayer marketed it as an analgesic, while at the turn of the century, in the 1980s, it was repositioned as an antiplatelet aggregation drug [7].

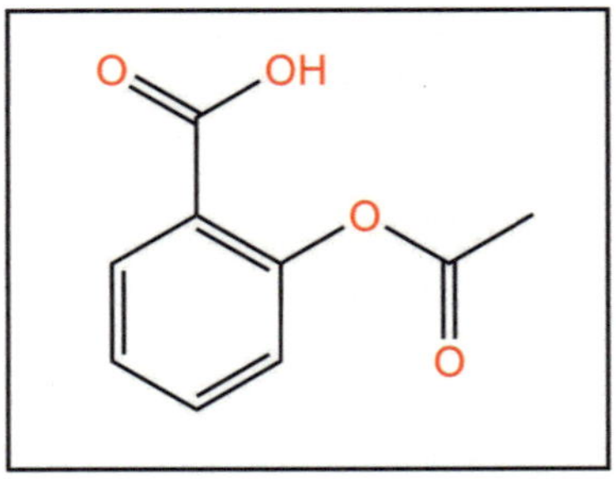

Figure 2.
Aspirin/AcetylSalicylic acid.

During the last millennium, drug repurposing successes of sildenafil, valproic acid, and minoxidil were charted by analyzing their known pharmacology in a particular domain (vis-a-vis the adverse effects) to resolve a pressing clinical problem from another therapeutic area, not relying entirely on serendipity [8].

Sildenafil (formulated as its citrate) (**Figure 3**), originally introduced by Pfizer, as an antihypertensive medication, was later repurposed for erectile dysfunction (TM Viagra) based on prior clinical experience and went on to become a blockbuster drug [9]. Moreover, as a reversible inhibitor of phosphodiesterase type 5 (PDE5), it has also been approved for pulmonary arterial hypertension (PAH) intervention under the brand name of Revatio® [10].

Valproic acid (N-dipropylacetic acid) (**Figure 4**) was discovered by Meunier and Carraz in the year 1967. On the revelation of its anticonvulsant properties, it was a popular drug widely used in epilepsy and bipolar disorder, formulated as sodium valproate. Valproic acid (VPA) has so far been the drug of choice for epilepsy and other neurological disorders since the past 66 years. Ongoing research has indicated the potential of VPA as an antineoplastic agent, partly due to its role in the inhibition of histone deacetylases, thus modulating the expression of genes and affecting changes in the cell cycle, differentiation, and subsequently apoptosis. Over and above inhibiting histone deacetylases, VPA enhances RNA interference, activating histone methyl-transferases, or suppressing the activation of transcription factors [11].

Minoxidil (**Figure 5**) was originally developed in the late 1950s, by The Upjohn Company, now Pfizer, with hopes of treating ulcers; however, it failed to treat gastric issues, and instead was shown to be a vasodilator and a potassium channel opener, hyperpolarizing the cell membranes. Two decades later, in 1979, minoxidil was repurposed for arterial hypertension [12]. During clinical trials, it was observed that unwanted hair growth was an adverse side effect, and thus, subsequently, a topical minoxidil formulation was evaluated to treat hair loss. FDA approved topical minoxidil in 1988 for androgenetic alopecia and alopecia areata, and today, generic minoxidil is sold over the counter (OTC) as Regaine Topical Solution 2%, for men and women [13].

Another drug, thalidomide, originally introduced as a sedative in the year 1957, was found to induce severe skeletal birth defects in newborn children whose mothers were administered this drug in the first pregnancy trimester; thus, after about 4 years, it was withdrawn and further repurposed for erythema nodosum leprosum (ENL) (1964), and multiple myeloma (1999) was based on serendipity [14]. The two indications were distinct of each other, and decades apart from each other. The

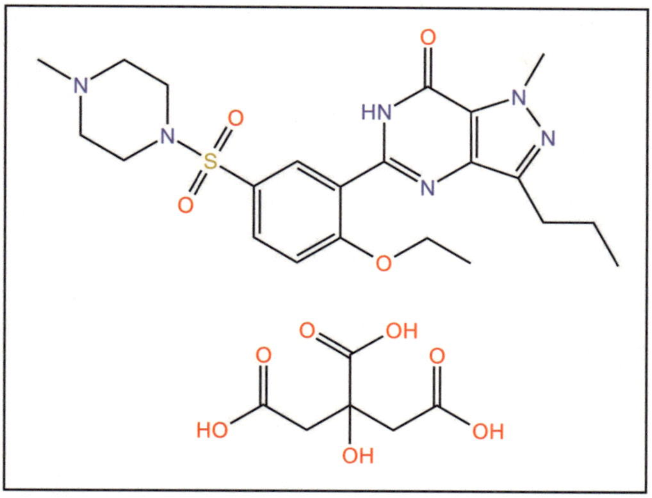

Figure 3.
Sildenafil citrate.

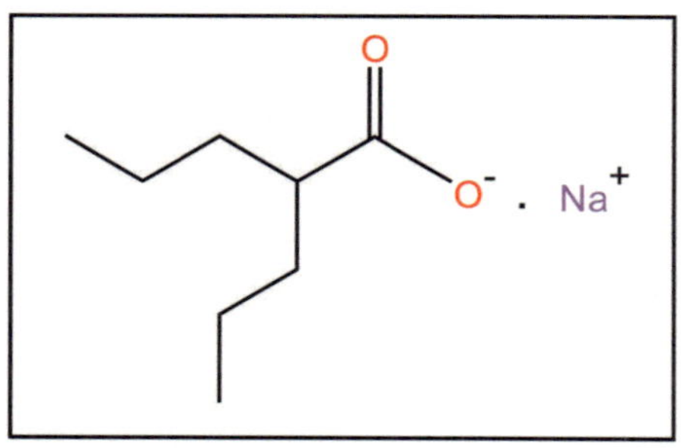

Figure 4.
Sodium valproate.

successful repurposing of thalidomide also led to the discovery, development, and approval of other highly successful derivatives, notably lenalidomide (Revlimid, Celgene) (**Figure 6**).

This strategy is especially very pertinent when applied to rare and neglected diseases and disorders, and orphan drugs, as is noticed in the drug portfolio of DNDi (Drug for Neglected Diseases initiative) repurposed NCE candidates undergoing clinical trials, including fexinidazole, fosravuconazole, Ambisome™, and miltefosine, fexinidazole being the first oral-only drug, for advanced-stage sleeping sickness [15], with a small fraction of the estimated investment for a *de novo* drug. Rare and orphan diseases often have unknown or poorly characterized metabolic pathways/ pathophysiology where computational approaches for predictive repurposing result in large-scale genome sequencing data analysis for the identification of genetic variation/s contributing to the disorder and expediting the re-profiling of existing drugs targeting the relevant protein/s [16].

During the past decade, drug repurposing as well as drug discovery is hugely complemented by artificial intelligence/machine learning methods to squeeze the drug discovery timelines while maintaining consistency in the systematic retrieval,

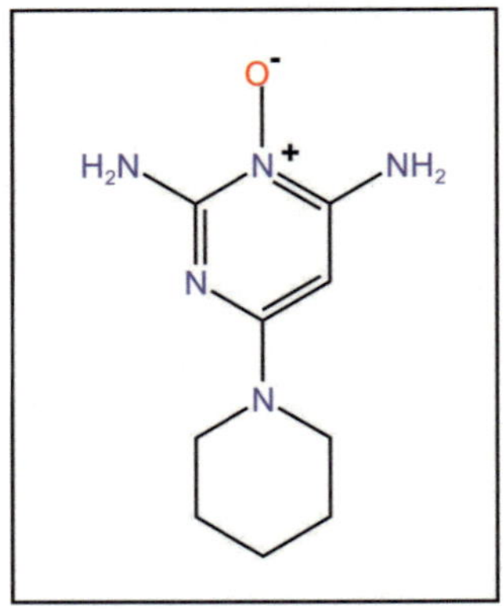

Figure 5.
Minoxidil.

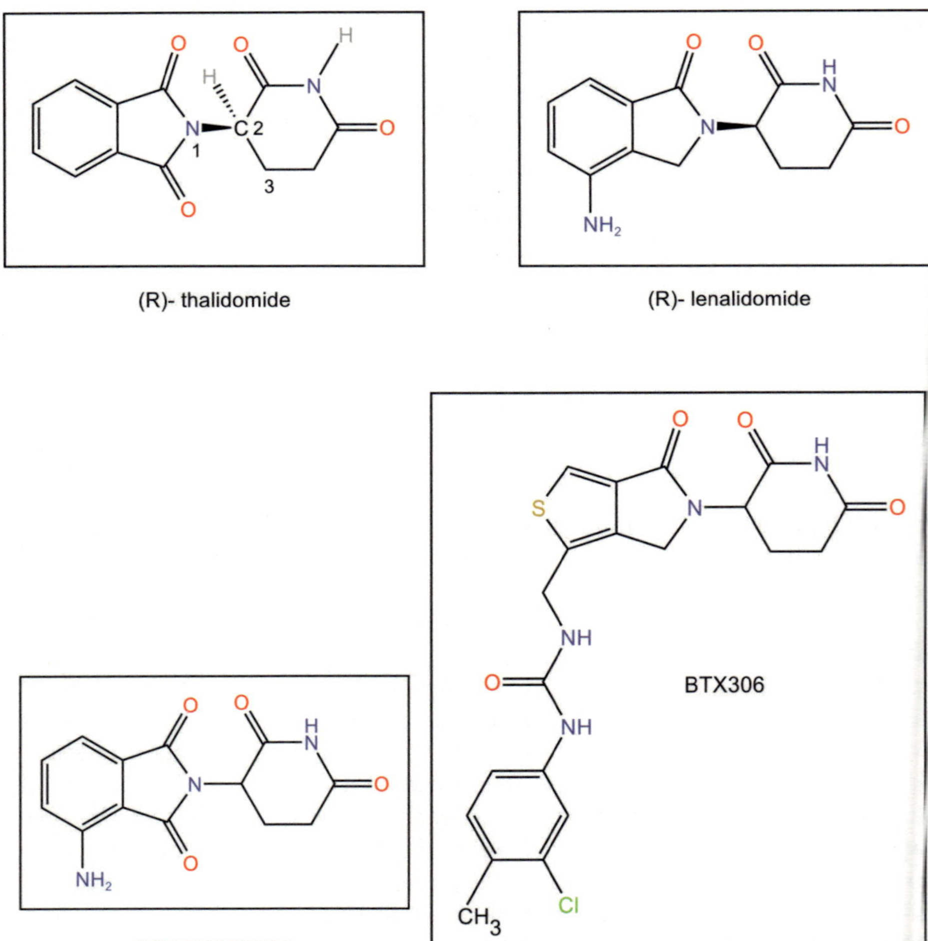

Figure 6.
Thalidomide and its derivatives, Lenalidomide, Pomalidomide, and BTX306.

analysis, and application of big data. Notable approaches in this area are systematic analysis of clinical trial data, molecular similarity approximations, signature matching of targets, transcriptomic and proteomic data, and structure-based virtual screens.

5. Unusual case studies

5.1 Dapoxetine

Dapoxetine, discovered by Eli Lilly, as a selective serotonin reuptake inhibitor (SSRI), was primarily discontinued by Eli Lilly as an adjunct therapy for analgesia. Later on, it was repurposed as an antidepressant with fluoxetine. But short half-life of the compound and the rapid onset did not permit daily dosage, an imperative criterion for any supplementary antidepressant, and thus, it fizzled out.

Finally, dapoxetine's rapid onset and short half-life were considered to be a pharmacokinetic advantage for the therapy of premature ejaculation, which prompted patenting the findings and validating with phase II proof-of-concept studies, and after changing hands, with a new method-of-use patent, dapoxetine (now a part of Johnson & Johnson portfolio) is now in phase III clinical development for premature ejaculation.

5.2 Thalidomide

As noted previously, after severely unfortunate fallouts, thalidomide made a grand role reversal. Originally marketed as a sedative in 1957 in Germany and England, Thalidomide created unforeseen complications in pregnant women facing morning sickness. It was subsequently repurposed as a drug of choice to treat the erythema nodosum laprosum (ENL), an agonizing inflammation caused due to leprosy whereby painfully large boils often lead to blindness.

6. Future outlook

Currently, almost a third of approvals are repurposed drugs. This clearly indicates the success of several repurposed drugs. New avenues for repositioning can emerge from increased collaboration between pharmaceutical industry and allied sectors of academia, with priority awarded to orphan diseases, rare and neglected disorders, and synergistic drug combinations of repurposed drugs, in such cases as metformin, where the efficacy of the original drug continues unabated. Rare and neglected diseases are not usually profitable for pharmaceutical giants, and their involvement in terms of corporate social responsibility, which endeavors to bridge the gap between profit margins and overall societal welfare, can also add up to generate awareness about several lesser-known disorders. These can be heavily incentivized, parallelly by governmental agencies/organizations, to sustain the equilibrium between commercial viability and redressal of new therapeutic solutions for marginalized diseases.

To supplement this, personalized/precision medicine will add to newer information regarding the characterization and classification of disease pathways, leading to a better understanding of repositioning old/abandoned drugs for diverse therapeutic areas, revitalizing drug re-profiling even further. Contraindications/adverse reactions relating to a prior allotted pharmacokinetic metabolism can assist and enhance our knowledge of expected drug reactions. Sustainable drug re-profiling is also complimented by advances in technology such as artificial intelligence and machine learning, which are instrumental in the expedition of large-scale extraction and integration of heterogeneous data, comprising a mixed bag of imaging, HTS data, DMPK profiles, clinical trials records, and electronic health reports and records, to name a few.

Thus, *de novo* drug discovery and drug repositioning can support each other to make pharmaceutical innovation more sustainable in terms of resources, time, and setbacks.

Author details

Shanta Bhar
Indian Institute of Information Technology, Guwahati, India

*Address all correspondence to: shanta.bhar@gmail.com

References

[1] Brundtland GH. Our common future: Report of the world commission on environment and development. In: UN Document; 1987. Geneva: A/42/427; 1987

[2] Dye C. One health as a catalyst for sustainable development. Nature Microbiology. 2022;**7**:467-468. DOI: 10.1038/s41564-022-01076-1

[3] Keiser MJ, Setola V, Irwin JJ, Laggner C, Abbas AI, Hufeisen SJ, et al. Predicting new molecular targets for known drugs. Nature. 2009;**462**:175-181. DOI: 10.1038/nature08506

[4] Hieronymus H, Lamb J, Ross KN, Peng XP, Clement C, Rodina A, et al. Gene expression signature-based chemical genomic prediction identifies a novel class of HSP90 pathway modulators. Cancer Cell. 2006;**10**(4):321-330. DOI: 10.1016/j.ccr.2006.09.005

[5] Greene CS, Voight BF. Pathway and network-based strategies to translate genetic discoveries into effective therapies. Human Molecular Genetics. 2016;**25**(R2):R94-R98. DOI: 10.1093/hmg/ddw160

[6] Alirol E, Schrumpf D, Amici HJ. Nifurtimox-eflornithine combination therapy for second-stage gambiense human African trypanosomiasis: Médecins Sans Frontières experience in the Democratic Republic of the Congo. Clinical Infectious Diseases. 2013;**56**(2):195-203. DOI: 10.1093/cid/cis886

[7] Monneret C, Bohuon C. Fabuleux hasards: histoire de la découverte de médicaments. Paris: EDP; 2009. p. 22. DOI: 10.1016/j.pharma.2009.09.002

[8] Thor KB. Drug repositioning: Identifying and developing new uses for existing drugs. Nature Review. 2004;**3**:673-683. DOI: 10.1038/nrd1468

[9] Jackson G, Gillies H, Osterloh I. Past, present, and future: A 7-year update of Viagra® (sildenafil citrate). The International Journal of Clinical Practice. 2005;**59**(6):680-691. DOI: 10.1111/j.1368-5031.2005.00578.x

[10] Corbin JD, Beasley A, Blount MA, Francis SH. High lung PDE5: A strong basis for treating pulmonary hypertension with PDE5 inhibitors. Biochemical and Biophysical Research Communications. 2005;**334**(3):930-938. DOI: 10.1016/j.bbrc.2005.06.183

[11] Soria-Castro R, Schcolnik-Cabrera A, Rodríguez-López G, Campillo-Navarro M, Puebla-Osorio N, Estrada-Parra S, et al. Exploring the drug repurposing versatility of Valproic acid as a multifunctional regulator of innate and adaptive immune cells. Journal of Immunology Research. 2019;**96**:1-24. DOI: 10.1155/2019/9678098

[12] Gottlieb TB, Katz FH, Chidsey CA. Combined therapy with vasodilator drugs and beta-adrenergic blockade in hypertension. A comparative study of minoxidil and hydralazine. Circulation. 1972;**45**(3):571-582. DOI: 10.1161/01.cir.45.3.571

[13] Clissold SP, Heel RC. Topical minoxidil. A preliminary review of its pharmacodynamic properties and therapeutic efficacy in alopecia areata and alopecia androgenetica. Drugs. 1987;**33**:107-122. DOI: 10.2165/00003495-198733020-00002

[14] Brynner R, Stephens T. Dark Remedy: The Impact of Thalidomide and its Revival as a Vital Medicine.

Cambridge: Perseus Publishing; 2001. p. 240. DOI: 10.1136/bmj.322.7302.1608

[15] Pollastri MP. Fexinidazole: A new drug for african sleeping sickness on the horizon. Trends in Parasitology. 2018;**34**(3):178-179. DOI: 10.1016/j.pt.2017.12.002

[16] Pushpakom S, Iorio F, Eyers PA, Escott JK, Hopper S, Wells A, et al. Drug repurposing: Progress, challenges and recommendations. Nature Reviews Drug Discovery. 2019;**18**:41-58. DOI: 10.1038/nrd.2018.168

Section 3

Natural Products and Drug Discovery

Chapter 12

Development of Phytomedicines as Novel Antimalarial Lead Molecules: Progress towards Successful Antimalarial Drug Discovery

Mithun Rudrapal, Dipak Chetia and Soumya Bhattacharya

Abstract

Among numerous life-threatening infectious diseases (HIV/AIDS, TB, NTDs and EIDs), malaria continues to be the deadliest parasitic disease caused by *Plasmodium* protozoa transmitted by an infective female *Anopheles* mosquito. *Plasmodium falciparum*, the potentially fatal malaria parasite, is believed to be responsible for most of the morbidities and mortalities associated with malaria infections. Artemisinin-based Combination Therapies (ACTs) are currently considered to be the frontline therapy against malaria caused by *P. falciparum*. Despite significant progresses in antimalarial drug discovery, the control and prevention of malaria is still a challenging task. It is primarily because of the reduced clinical efficacy of existing antimalarial therapies including ACTs due to the widespread emergence of drug-resistant strains of malaria parasites, especially *P. falciparum*. It is, therefore, necessary to discover and develop novel drug candidates and/or alternative therapies for the treatment as well as prevention of resistant malaria. In this chapter, the potential of phytomedicines as natural sources of novel antimalarial lead molecules/ drugs with recent advances in phytomedicine-based antimalarial drug discovery has been reviewed.

Keywords: antimalarials, phytomedicines, *P. falciparum*, lead molecules, drug discovery

1. Introduction

Malaria is a potentially life-threatening parasitic disease caused by *Plasmodium* protozoa transmitted by an infective female *Anopheles* mosquito. Along with human immunodeficiency virus/ acquired immunodeficiency syndrome (HIV/AIDS), tuberculosis (TB), neglected tropical diseases (NTDs) and viral hepatitis (hepatitis B), malaria affects billions of people, and causes more than 4 million deaths every year globally [1]. Apart from these infectious diseases, emerging infectious diseases (EIDs) are serious public health threats in the twenty-first century. Some deadly EIDs include severe acute respiratory syndrome (SARS), Ebola virus disease (EVD), Zika virus disease (ZVD), swine flu (H1N1 influenza), bird flu (avian influenza), chikungunya

IntechOpen

(CHIKV), dengue fever (DENV), hanta pulmonary syndrome (HPS, hanta virus), antibiotic-resistant infections (superbugs) and coronavirus disease (COVID-19, SARS-CoV-2) [2, 3].

According to the latest report by World Health Organization (WHO), about 229 million clinical cases of malaria with a death toll of 409,000 have been documented for the year 2019. In the same year, 94% of all malaria cases and deaths were found in the WHO African region. In the Southeast Asian region of WHO, there were an estimated 7.9 million cases of malaria in 2018. Children under 5 years of age are considerably at higher risk of malaria. They have been accounted for 67% of all malaria deaths worldwide in 2019 [4–6]. However, *Plasmodium falciparum*, the deadliest malaria parasite, is attributed to be responsible for most of the morbidity and mortality associated with malaria [7, 8]. Artemisinin-based Combination Therapies (ACTs) are currently considered as the frontline therapy against malaria caused by *P. falciparum* [9, 10]. Due to the widespread emergence and spread of drug resistant strains of *P. falciparum*, the clinical utility of existing antimalarial therapies including ACTs has been drastically declined [11, 12]. It has, therefore, become a serious health concern, which urgently necessities the discovery and development of novel drug candidates and/or alternative therapies for the treatment as well as prevention of resistant malaria. In this chapter, the potential of phytomedicines as natural sources of novel antimalarial lead molecules/ drugs with recent advances in phytomedicine-based antimalarial drug discovery has been briefly summarized.

2. Phytomedicines and antimalarial drugs

The discovery of antimalarial drugs from plant sources was started in 200 years back when quinine (QN), a cinchona alkaloid, was isolated from *Cinchona* bark in the year 1820. Earlier, the extract of *Cinchona* bark (also known as Peruvian Bark) was traditionally used for the treatment of fever by native Peruvian Indians in 1600s [13]. QN was the only known antimalarial drug for more than three centuries, and until the 1930s was the only effective therapeutic agent for the treatment of malaria. Later, the structure of quinine served as a template for the development of several synthetic congeners as potent antimalarial agents [13, 14]. The introduction of CQ, a 4-aminoquinoline derivative of QN, in the mid-twentieth century (1940) ceased the wide spread use of QN. Soon after its introduction, CQ became the mainstay of malaria chemotherapy, since it was clinically effective, less toxic and cheaper drug [15]. Another synthetic antimalarial, primaquine (PQ, 1950) was also developed thereafter based on the

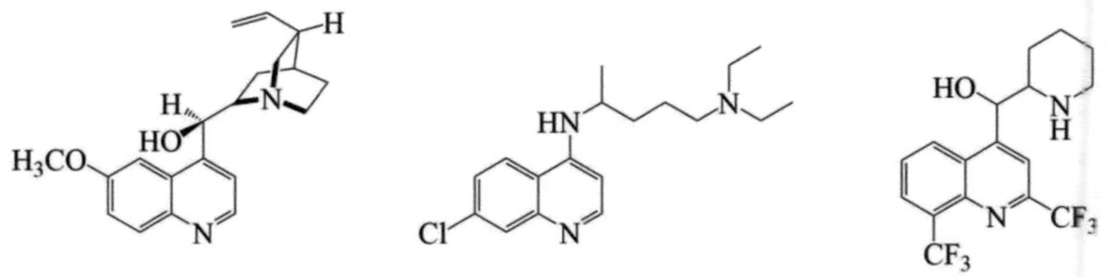

QN **CQ** **MQ**

Figure 1.
Some QN-based antimalarial drugs.

structure of lead QN molecule. PQ is a 8-aminoquinoline analogue of QN. Mefloquine (MQ), a synthetic quinoline methanol derivative of QN, was developed (1975) after CQ to treat resistant cases of malaria. Malaria parasites resistance to CQ and MQ began to appear within a few decades of introduction [16]. Later, several quinoline derivatives related to CQ (amodiaquine, AQ and isoquine, IQ) and MQ [halofantrine (HL), lumefantrine (LUM) and pyronaridine (PYN)] were developed and found effective (in combination with ART-based drugs such as dihydroartemisinin, artemether and artesunate) against CQ-resistant and/or multi-drug resistant (MDR) *P. falciparum* infections. Hepatotoxicity and cardiotoxicity are some serious toxic effects associated with these drugs [17]. Moreover, rapid development of resistance has severely limited the use of QN-based drugs alone, and therefore, they are used in combination with other drugs in the treatment of resistant malaria. The increasing prevalence of MDR strains of malaria parasites, particularly *P. falciparum* in most malaria endemic areas (Southeast Asia including Myanmar, Thailand, Vietnam and India, African continent and Eastern Mediterranean region) has significantly reduced the efficacy of CQ and other potent QN-based antimalarials in the treatment of malaria [8]. **Figure 1** depicts structures of some QN-based antimalarial drugs.

QN-based antimalarials are used widely in the treatment and prophylaxis of malaria. QN still remains an important antimalarial drug due to the emergence of CQ-resistant and MDR strains of malaria parasites, especially *P. falciparum*. Due to its undesirable side effects, it is now only used as an intravenous injection (as sulphate salt) to treat severe malaria. CQ (as phosphate salt) still remains the first-line drug in the treatment of uncomplicated sensitive *P. falciparum* malaria, despite its increasing resistance to parasites, due to its easy availability, low cost and good tolerability. In CQ-resistant malaria, the next drug of choice is MQ, followed by QN in combination with tetracycline, doxycycline or sulphadoxine-pyrimethamine (SP). MQ and AQ are widely available and are used to treat cases of uncomplicated malaria in areas where CQ resistance is prevalent [18, 19].

QN-based drugs are blood stage schizonticidal. CQ/MQ is selectively active against the intra-erythrocytic mature forms (trophozoites) and also younger ring forms of malaria parasites, without any activity against gametocytes. QN-based drugs inhibit the heme polymerase enzyme resulting in specific toxicity during the developmental stage of the parasite. CQ accumulates by a weak base mechanism in the acidic food vacuole of trophozoite-infected cells and act by forming a complex with heme in the parasite food vacuole, which prevents heme polymerization and consequently, hemozoin formation. Simply, they these drugs block the polymerisation of heme to haemozoin (malaria pigment). As a result, the heme which is released during haemoglobin degradation builds up toxic accumulation of heme (haematin), thereby kills the parasite with its own toxic effects. The mode of action of QN is similar to CQ. QN binds strongly to heme protein and forms complexes that are toxic to the malaria parasite, as already delineated above. MQ also acts by inhibiting the heme polymerase, similar to CQ [8, 18–20].

ART, an active constituent of *Artemisia annua* L. (Sweet wormwood) and related compounds (semi-synthetic derivatives) showed promising antimalarial efficacy in clinical trials in 1970s (1972) and till date they are considered as the most effective and potent antimalarial agents [21]. Since ART is not soluble in water or oil, it has several limitations such as poor aqueous solubility, oral absorption and bioavailability. Reduction of ART (sesquiterpene lactones or cyclic endoperoxide) produced dihydroartemisinin (DHA), a sesquiterpene lactol, which served later as a template for the synthesis of a series of semi-synthetic analogues such as artemether (AM), arteether

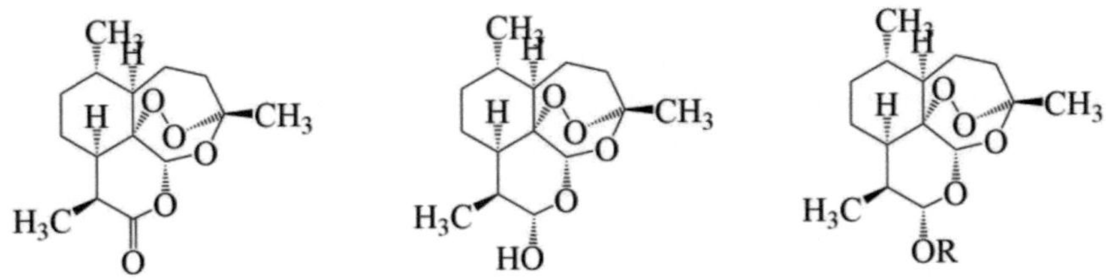

ART **DHA** R=Me, **AM**
R=Et, **AE**
R=$CO(CH_2)_2COONa$, **AS**

Figure 2.
ART and some ART-based antimalarials.

(AE) and artesunate (AS). They are collectively termed as the first-generation derivatives of ART [22, 23]. First-generation ART derivatives can be further grouped into oil soluble C(10) β-alkyl ethers (AM and AE) and water soluble C(10) β-(substituted) esters (sodium artesunate and sodium artelinate). These drugs possess better oil/water solubility, and therefore, have superior pharmacokinetics properties with increased antimalarial efficacies over the parent compound, ART [8]. **Figure 2** represents the structures of ART and some ART-based antimalarial drugs.

Because of having excellent antiparasitic efficacy against resistant parasites, ART-based drugs mostly replaced the use of QN- and antifolate-based drugs. ART derivatives are fast-acting antimalarials effective against MDR strains of *P. falciparum* and are used for the treatment of severe and complicated malaria. ART-based drugs showed very rapid clearance of parasites and faster resolution of fever as compared to QN. In some areas of Southeast Asia, combinations of ART-based drug and MQ offer the only reliable treatment for uncomplicated MDR *P. falciparum* malaria [24, 25].

ART and its analogues are active against all blood stages, particularly against younger ring forms and gametocytes. They have no activity on hepatic stages of parasites. They reduce parasitemia very rapidly and are well tolerated in both adults and children. ART and related compounds are concentrated in parasite-infected erythrocytes and exert their parasiticidal activity subsequent to reductive activation by heme in an irreversible redox reaction, which produces toxic carbon-centred free radicals. Toxic free radicals may lead to alkylation of heme or bring about oxidative damage to parasite proteins/lipids. The endoperoxide group, therefore, appears to be crucial for the antimalarial activity. The antimalarial activity of ART may also result from the inhibition of a parasitic calcium ATPase enzyme [8, 24–26].

The development of atovaquone (ATO), a 2-hydroxy-1,4-napthoquinone antimalarial, began more than 50 years ago when the outbreak of World War II caused substantial shortages in the supply of QN. ATO is an analogue of lapachol (a prenylnaphthoquinone isolated from *Tabebuia* species, Lapacho tree, 1892). Lapachol was used as an antimalarial lead molecule for the development of ATO. It is effective against CQ-resistant *P. falciparum*, but because, when used alone, resistance develops rapidly, ATO is often given in combination with proguanil (PG). A new fixed-dose antimalarial combination of ATO and PG (Malarone, 1998) is available in the market worldwide. Malarone shows good tolerability with minimal side effects in children and adults with uncomplicated malaria. It is used as chemoprophylaxis for the prevention of malaria in travellers. ATO represents a novel class of expensive antimalarial drug.

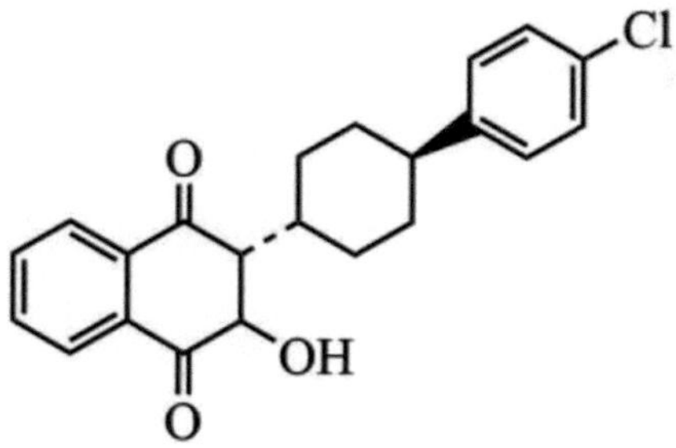

ATO

Figure 3.
Structure of ATO.

ATO is used in combination with PG (a selective inhibitor of dihydrofolate reductase, DHFR) or tetracycline for the prevention as well as treatment of CQ-resistant malaria, including cerebral malaria caused by *P. falciparum*. It is as effective as MQ or doxycycline. ATO acts through the inhibition of electron transport at the *Plasmodium* mitochondrial cytochrome bc1 complex and depolarizes the membranes of *Plasmodial* mitochondria[15, 16]. The structure of ATO is given in **Figure 3.**

3. Approaches to antimalarial drug discovery

The objective of antimalarial drug discovery is to find out new and potent drug candidates based on the knowledge of existing and/or novel drug targets. It is necessary to develop affordable and safe drugs that would be reasonably cheaper, non-toxic to host tissues, and clinically effective against resistant malaria parasites. Suitable *in vitro* and *in vivo* experimental methods are, therefore, used for the evaluation of efficacy as well as toxicity of newer antimalarial agents. However, there are several traditional and modern approaches to antimalarial drug discovery programme, which include traditional evaluation of bioactive natural products/phytomedicines, molecular modifications of existing lead molecules, reverse pharmacological or drug repurposing approach and drug discovery based on CADD/SBDD approach [8]. Brief explanations of these approaches are given here under (**Figure 4**).

3.1 Ethnomedicinal evaluation based approach

The investigation of medicinal plants having traditional/ folkloric uses as antimalarial medicine may be potential sources of novel bioactive compounds that can be further developed into potent antimalarial drugs and/or lead molecules. Several tribes and aboriginals of Asian, African and South American continents still rely on plant-based ethnomedicines for the management of fever and malaria-like illness. QN and ART were discovered from the ethnomedicinal use of *Cinchona* and *Artemisia* plants, respectively. They served as lead structures in the development of many more potent antimalarial drugs of current use. Considering the above fact, thousands of medicinal plants and traditional formulations have been screened (*in vitro* and *in vivo*) to aid bioactive fraction guided discovery of antimalarial lead molecules [27].

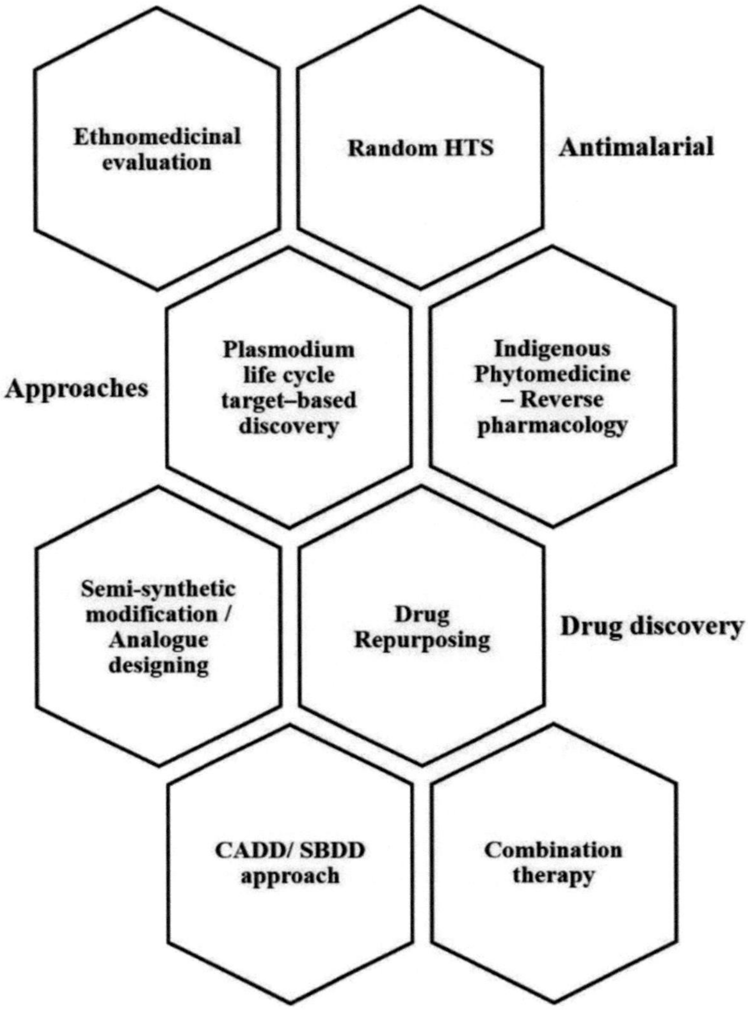

Figure 4.
Approaches to antimalarial drug discovery.

3.2 Random high-throughput screening

Random high-throughput screening of plant extracts is one of the common approaches for antimalarial drug discovery. Scientists and researchers perform random screening of plant extracts against *Plasmodium* strains by various *in vitro* methods in search for novel antimalarial compounds. Depending upon preliminary antimalarial efficacy (IC_{50}) and cytotoxicity profile (CC_{50}) obtained *in vitro*, plant extracts and/or isolated pure compounds can be further subjected to *in vivo* experimental (ED_{50} and Pharmacokinetics) studies [28].

3.3 *Plasmodium* life cycle targeted drug discovery

This is believed to be the most potential approach in antimalarial drug discovery programme. Specific proteins or enzymes that are essential biological components in the life cycle of *Plasmodium* parasite may provide novel targets for the discovery of drug molecules. For instance, falcipains (FP), plasmepsins (PM), dihydrooroate dehydrogenase (DHOH), phosphatidylisositol-4-kinase (PI4K), cytochrome *bc1* (Cyt *bc1*) and Na^+-ATPase 4 are some novel drug targets discovered from the biology of *P. falciparum* [8].

3.4 Indigenous phytomedicine-based reverse pharmacological approach

Reverse Pharmacology deals with the precisely designed preclinical and clinical research of age old herbal medicine used in well documented indigenous system of medicine (*Ayurvedic* medicine, Chinese medicine etc.) with a view of better understanding of the mechanism of action (even at molecular level) followed by the isolation of bioactive molecule(s) and finally the development of lead molecule(s). In fact, the discovery and development of ART (from *A. annua*) and its derivatives are the result of reverse pharmacological approach. Another interesting example is the discovery of antiplasmodial protoberberine type alkaloids allocryptopine and protopine from *A. mexicana*. This approach is considered to be quite reliable and faster technique due to the availability of prior information about therapeutic and toxic properties of the plant species under investigation. However, the discovery of potent lead molecule(s) with desired pharmacological/toxicity profile may sometimes be difficult because herbal medicine/ plant extracts possess therapeutic efficacy due to the synergistic activity of multiple ingredients in the crude mixture [26, 29].

3.5 Drug repurposing approach

Repurposing of existing drugs with new therapeutic indications is also considered as one of the effective alternatives for the discovery of antimalarial drugs. The notable advantage of this approach is that the mechanism of action and toxicity of drugs have already been established in clinical trials for other diseases. Folate antagonists (sulphonamides, sulphones, biguanides, pyrimethamine, triazines, etc.) and several antibacterials/ antibiotics (tetracycline, doxycycline, clindamycin etc.) have been reported to exhibit promising antiplasmodial efficacy against malaria parasites. In recent days, drug repurposing involves the combined efforts of *in silico* and *in vitro* methods to identify new therapeutic uses of existing drug molecules on a rational basis. Using the same strategy, researchers have been working on existing drugs in search for new antimalarial drug candidates. Repurposing of azithromycin, auranofin, loperamide hydrochloride, amlodipine besylate, cyclosporin A, esomeprazole magnesium, omeprazole etc. with antimalarial activity have been reported in literature [30, 31].

3.6 Semi-synthetic modifications or designing of analogues

Novel antimalarial drugs can be developed from the semi-synthetic modification of naturally derived lead molecules and/or by designing of newer synthetic analogues/ derivatives of existing drugs based on the structure-activity relationship (SAR) approach. This approach mainly emphasizes on reducing the toxicity with retaining and/or enhancing the therapeutic efficacy of the basic template structure/ lead molecule. Synthetic quinolines like CQ, AQ, IQ (4-aminoquinolines), PQ (8-aminoquinolines) MQ, HL, LUM (quinoline amino alcohols), piperaquine (PIP, bisquinoline analogue) and PYN (benzonaphthyridine derivative) were developed based upon the structural template of QN. Several chemical strategies were involved in structural modification of QN or other lead molecules in order to improve the therapeutic efficacy as well as toxicity of the parent molecule. Tebuquine (4-aminoquinoline derivative, a CQ analogue) and tafenoquine (8-aminoquinoline derivative, a derivative of PQ), are two newer drugs developed recently. Ferroquine (4-aminoquinoline derivative, a CQ analogue, Phase II terminated), AQ-13 (4-aminoquinoline analogue, Phase II) are presently under development. Following similar approach, DHA, AM and AS were also developed from ART. Some newer drugs (belonging to different classes) that are under development include DSM265 [Pf dihydrooroate dehydrogenase (DHOH) inhibitor, a triazolopyrimidine-based drug, Phase II], MMV390048 [Pf phosphatidylisositol-4-kinase (PI4K) inhibitor, Phase I] and KAE609 or cipargamin (Na+-ATPase 4 inhibitor) [8, 32–38].

3.7 Combination therapy approach

The concept of combination therapy (CT) is based on the synergistic or additive activity of two or more drugs, which improves therapeutic efficacy and also delays the development of resistance to the individual drugs of the combination. In antimalarial combination therapy, two or more drugs are used together that act with independent mode of action probably at different biochemical targets in the life cycle of *Plasmodium* parasite. WHO recommended combining the rapid schizonticidal ART derivative (DHA, AM or AS) with one or more partner drugs (from different class of antimalarials having longer biological half-lives) for the treatment of resistant *P. falciparum* malaria. Such combined antimalarial drug regimens (for examples, AM + LUM (Co-Artem, fixed dose, AL), AS + MQ (AM), AS + CQ, AS + SP, AS + DOX, AS + DOX + CQ etc.) are known as ACTs. Some ACTs which are in pipeline include AS + PYN, DHA + PIP (Artekin), DHA-PIP- Trimethoprim and DHA + PIP + MQ [8, 25].

3.8 Drug discovery by CADD/SBDD approach

Traditionally, drugs are discovered by testing naturally derived or synthetically obtained compounds in time-consuming multi-step processes against a battery of *in vitro* and *in vivo* screening methods. Compounds having promising therapeutic potential are further investigated for their development as drug candidates after pharmacokinetic, metabolism and toxicity studies. Today's modern drug discovery process involves rational design and development of novel drug molecules based on a particular disease target using modern tools and techniques of virtual and experimental screening techniques. In virtual screening, computational methods screen large chemical libraries targeted towards a specific biological receptor, using advanced high performance computing environments, data management software and internet. It delivers new drug candidates quickly and at lower costs. Virtual screening is an approach of structure-based drug design (SBDD) that uses computer-based (*in silico*) methods to discover and develop new drug molecules on the basis of biological structures of particular disease of interest. SBDD methods mainly focus on the design of molecules for a disease target with known three dimensional structures followed by the determination of their binding affinity for the target by molecular docking along with other *in silico* screening methods (ADMET and toxicity screening) for optimization of molecules during development. The process of SBDD proceeds through design and development of a series of consecutive steps from hit identification to lead optimization followed by preclinical and clinical development of drug candidates [38, 39]. Antimalarial drug

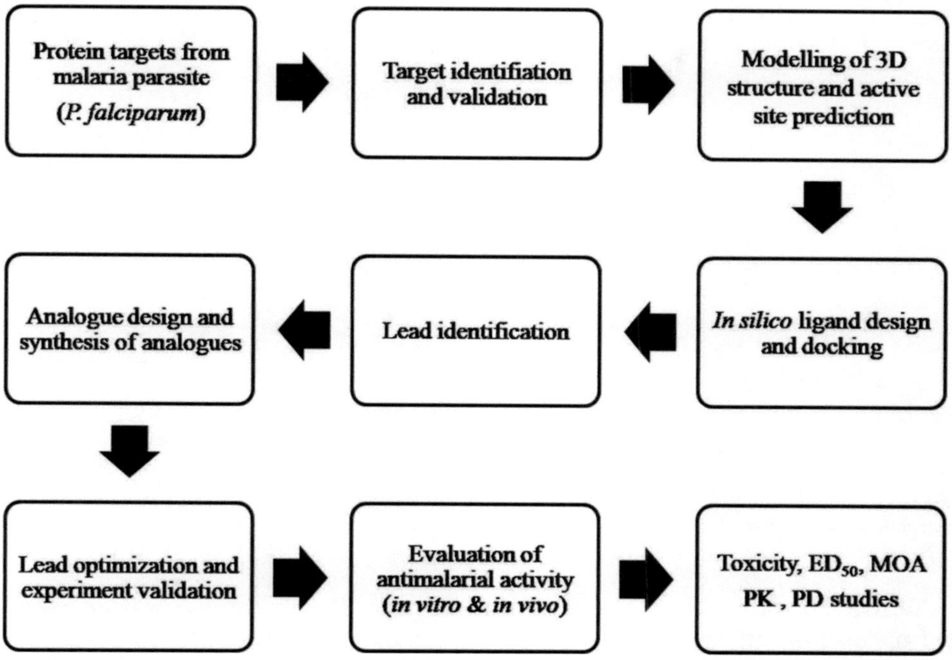

Figure 5.
Antimalarial drug discovery based on SBDD approach.

discovery based on SBDD approach involves the application of modern tools of molecular modelling and other *in silico* techniques in the development of novel antimalarial drug candidates (**Figure 5**).

4. Phytomedicines and antimalarial lead molecules: recent developments

Phytomedicines (i.e., plant-based/ herbal traditional medicine systems) served as potential sources of lead molecules for the development of several clinically useful antimalarial drug candidates. For example, QN isolated from *Cinchona* bark was used as a template for the development of CQ and MQ. ART isolated from *Artemisia annua* has been utilized for the successful development of various semi-synthetic derivatives (DHA, AM and AS) which are currently used in the treatment of CQ-resistant *P. falciparum* malaria [40, 41]. Apart from QN and ART, some examples of antimalarial natural products that were developed from plants include yingzhausu A, febrifugine, sergeolide, chaparrin, glaucarubin, tehranholide and brusatol [42].

During the last few decades, a large number of plant species have been identified to be effective as antimalarial agents. Pure phytochemicals isolated from these plants have been reported to exhibit antimalarial effectiveness, particularly, against CQ-sensitive and CQ-resistant strains of *P. falciparum*. It is, therefore, imperative that antimalarial phytochemicals reported with promising *in vitro* and *in vivo* activities can be further subjected to preclinical and clinical confirmation for their development as novel antimalarial lead molecules and/ drug candidates. Plant-derived antimalarial compounds belong to several phytochemical classes of natural products such as alkaloids, terpenoids, quassinoids, limonoids, Polyphenols and flavonoids, coumarins, steroids, anthraquinones, naphthoquinones etc.

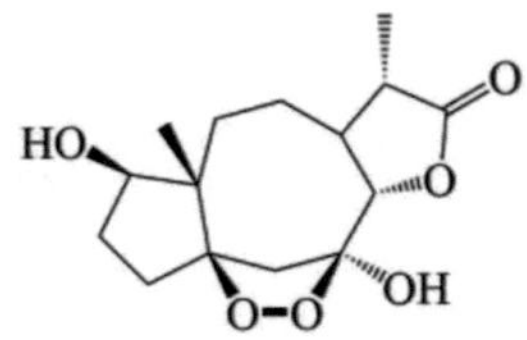

Artediffusin

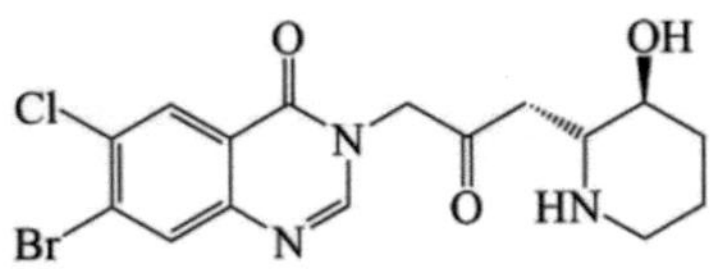

Halofuginone

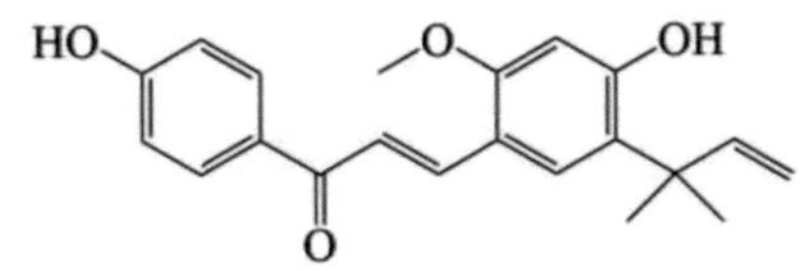

Licochalcone A

Figure 6.
Structures of some recently developed plant-derived antimalarial compounds.

Terhanolide (artediffusin), a sequiterpene lactone isolated from *A. diffusa* exhibited antimalarial efficacy against *P. falciparum* (*in vitro*) and *P. berghei* (*in vivo*) [43]. Halofuginone, an analogue of febrifugine (an alkaloid originally isolated from the plant *Dichroa febrifuga*) exhibited antiplasmodial effects against CQ-sensitive and CQ-resistant *P. falciparum (in vitro)* with curative effects in *P. berghei*-infected mice [44]. Sergeolide, a quassinoid from *Picrolemma pseudocoffa* showed antimalarial activities *in vitro* against *P. falciparum* and *in vivo* against *P. berghei* in mice [45]. Further, the antimalarial property licochalcone A (oxygenated chalcone) obtained from Chinese licorice has been reported to exhibit antimalarial activity against CQ-sensitive and CQ-resistant *Plasmodium* strain. Lichochalcone-A was the first natural

Name of specific phytochemical(s)	Type of compound(s)	Plant source (Family)	Antimalarial/ Antiplasmodial activity
Alkaloids			
Strychnogucine B Strychnobaillonine	Bisindole alkaloid	*Strychnos icaja* Baill. (Loganiaceae)	*In vivo* antimalarial activity (30 mg/kg/d dose) against *P. berghei* in murine model Potent *in vitro* antimalarial activity against CQ-sensitive 3D7 strain of *P. falciparum* with IC_{50} value of 1.1 μM
Lycorine	Indolizidine alkaloid	Plants from Amaryllidaceae family	*In vitro* antimalarial activity with IC_{50} value of 0.029 μg/mL against FCR-3 African strain of *P. falciparum*
Caesalminines A & B	Tetracyclic cassane-type diterpenoids alkaloids	*Caesalpinia minax* Hance (fabaceae)	Antiplasmodial activity with IC_{50} values between 0.42 and 0.79 μM

Name of specific phytochemical(s)	Type of compound(s)	Plant source (Family)	Antimalarial/ Antiplasmodial activity
8α-Polyeolinone, polyalthenol, *N*-acetyl-8α-polyeolinone and *N*-acetyl-polyveoine	Indolosesquiterpene alkaloid	*Polyalthia oliveri Pellegr. (Annonaceae) Polyalthia suaveolens* Engl. & Diels. (Annonaceae) (syn.*Greenwayodendron suaveolens* Engl. & Diels. Verdc. (Annonaceae)	Antiplasmodial activity against NF54 strain of *P. falciparum* with IC_{50} of 2.8 μM
Strychnochrysine	Bisindolomonoter penoid alkaloid	Strychnos nux-vomica Linn. (Loganiaceae)	Antiplasmodial activity against CQ-sensitive and CQ-resistant strains of *P. falcipaum*
Conessine	Steroidal alkaloid	*Holarrhena antidysenterica* (L.) Wall. Ex A. DC. (Apocynaceae)	Antimalarial activity against CQ-sensitive *P. berghei* NK65 strain in BALB/c mice
Conessine	Steroidal alkaloid	*Holarrhena antidysenterica* (L.) Wall. Ex A. DC. (Apocynaceae)	IC_{50} values of 1.9 μg/ml and 1.3 μg/ml in the schizont maturation and pLDH assays,
Mokluangin D irehline and mokluangin A	Pregnene-type alkaloid	*Holarrhena pubescens* (Buch.-Ham.) Wall. Ex G. Don. (Apocynaceae)	Antimalarial activity against MDR *P. falciparum* K1 strain with IC_{50} values between 1.2 and 2.0 μM
N-3-benzoyldihydrocyclo microphylline F	Steroidal alkaloid	*Buxus cochinchinensis* Pierre ex Gagnep. (Buxaceae)	Antimalarial activity against DR Dd2 strain of *P. falciparum* with IC_{50} value of 2.07 μM
Alstonisine	Indole alkaloid	*Alstonia macrophylla* Wall. ex G.Don (Apocynaceae)	Antiplasmodial activity against *P. falciparum* with IC_{50} value of 7.6 μM
20-Epi-dasycarpidone	Indole alkaloid	*Aspidosperma ulei* Markgr. (Apocynaceae).	Active against MDR K1 strain of *P. falciparum* with IC_{50} value of 16.7 μM
16-demethoxycar bonylvoacamine	Sarpagine-type indole alkaloids	*Tabernaemontana macrocarpa* Jack. (Apocynaceae)	Antiplasmodial activity against 3D7 strain of *P. falciparum*
Dehydrotylophorine, dehydroantofine and tylophoridicine D	Phenanthroindolizine alkaloids	*Ficus septica* Burm.f. (Moraceae)	Antimalarial activity against 3D7 strain of *P. falciparum* with IC_{50} values of 0.42, 0.028, 0.058 μM
10-Demethylxylopinine	Isoquinoline alkaloids	*Actinodaphne macrophylla* (Blume)Nees (Lauraceae)	*In vitro* antiplasmodial activity against 3D7 strain of *P. falciparum*
(+)-*N*-methylisococlaurine, atherosperminine, 2-hydroxyathersperminine	Isoquinoline	*Cryptocarya nigra* R.Br. (Lauraceae)	Antiplasmodial activity against CQ-resistant strain of *P. falciparum* (K1 strain) with IC_{50} values of 5.40, 5.80, and 0.75 μM

Name of specific phytochemical(s)	Type of compound(s)	Plant source (Family)	Antimalarial/ Antiplasmodial activity
Dihydronitidine	dihydronitidine	*Zanthoxylum heitzii* (Aubrey. & Pellegr.) P.G. Waterm. (Rutaceae)	Potent against *P. falciparum* with IC_{50} value of 25 nM
(−)-Pseudocurine	Bisbenzylisoquinoline	*Stephania abyssinica* Oliv. (Menispermaceae)	Antiplasmodial activity against both CQ-susceptible D6 and CQ-resistant W2 strains of *P. falciparum* (IC_{50} = 0.29±0.00 and 0.31±0.01 μg/ml, respectively)
(+)-laurotetanine, (+)-norstephasubine	Bisbenzylisoquinoline	*Alseodaphne corneri* Kosterm. (Lauraceae)	*In vitro* antiplasmodial efficacy with IC_{50} values of 0.189 and 0.116 μM
Dioncophylline F	Naphthylisoquinoline alkaloid	*Ancistrocladus ileboensis* Heubl, Mudogo & G. Bringmann. (Ancistrocladaceae)	Highly effective and specifically active against *P. falciparum*
Pseudopalmatine Obtusipetadione Anonaine Tavoyanine A, roemerine, Laurolitsine and boldine	Aporphine alkaloid	*Stephania rotunda* Lour. (Menispermaceae) *Dasymaschalon obtusipetalum* Jing Wang & R.M.K. Saunders. (Annonaceae) *Xylopia sericea* A.St.-Hil. (Annonaceae) *Phoebe tavoyana* (Meissn.) Hook f. (Lauraceae)	Effective against W2 strain of *P. falciparum* with IC_{50} value of 2.8 μM *In vitro* antiplasmodial activity against MDR *P. falciparum* strains (TM4 and K1) with IC_{50} values of 2.46 ± 0.12 and 1.38 ± 0.99 μg/mL Antiplasmodial activity against CQ-resistant W2 strain of *P. falciparum* With IC_{50} value of 23.2 ± 2.7 μg/ml Potent inhibitory activity against 3D7 strain of *P. falciparum* 3D7 with IC_{50} values of 0.89, 1.49 and 1.65 μg/ml
Sebiferine	Morphinandienone type alkaloid	*Phoebe tavoyana* (Meissn.) Hook f. (Lauraceae)	Potent inhibitoryactivity against the growth of *P. falciparum* 3D7 clone, with IC_{50} values of 2.76 μg/ml
Simplicifolianine	Protoberberine	*Meconopsis simplicifolia* (D. Don) Walpers (Papaveraceae)	Antiplasmodial activity against *P. falciparum* strains, TM4/8.2 (CQ-antifolate-sensitive strain) and K1CB1 (MDR) with IC_{50} values of 0.78 μg/mL and 1.29 μg/mL, respectively
Coptisine	Protoberberine-type alkaloid	*Coptis chinesis* Franch. (Ranunculaceae)	Potent inhibitory activity against *P. falciparum* dihydroorotate dehydrogenase (Pf DHODH) with IC_{50} value of 1.83 ± 0.08 μM

Name of specific phytochemical(s)	Type of compound(s)	Plant source (Family)	Antimalarial/ Antiplasmodial activity
Miliusacunines A	Oxoprotoberberine	*Miliusa cuneata* (Graib). (Annonaceae)	*In vitro* antimalarial activity against TM4 strain of *P. falciparum* with IC_{50} value of 19.3 ± 3.4 μM
Hymenocardine *N*-oxide	Cyclopeptide alkaloids	*Hymenocardia acida* Tul. (Phyllanthaceae)	Antiplasmodial activity against *P. falciparum* with IC_{50} value of 12.2 ± 6.6 μM
Microthecaline A	Quinoline alkaloid	*Eremophila microtheca* F.Muell. (Scrophulariaceae)	Moderate antimalarial activity against *P. falciparum* (3D7 strain) with IC_{50} value of 7.7 *μM*
Sauristolactam	Pyridocoumarin alkaloid	*Goniothalamus australis* Jessup. (Annonaceae)	Potent antimalarila activity against CQ-sensitive *P. falciparum* (3D7 strain) with IC_{50} value of 9.0 μM
Normelicopidine	*Acridone Alkaloid*	*Zanthoxylum simullans* Hance (Rutaceae)	Active against drug resistant Dd2 strain of *P. falciparum* with IC_{50} value of 18.9 ug/mL
Carpaine	Macrocyclic dilactone	*Carica papaya* L. (Caricaeae)	Potent antimalarial activity activity against 3D7 (sensitive) and Dd2 (resistant) strains of *P. falciparum* with IC_{50} values of 4.21 μM and 4.57 μM, respectively
Palmitine and jatrorrhizine	Indole alkaloid	*Penianthus longifolius* Miers. (Menispermaceae)	In vitro antimalarial activity against *P. falciparum* with IC_{50} values ranging from 0.28 to 0.35 μg mL^{-1}
Liriodenine	Indole alkaloid	*Glossocalyx brevipes* Benth. (Siparunaceae)	Antimalarial activity against drug sensitive D-6 strain and NF54 strains of *P. falciparum* with IC_{50} values of 2.37 μM and 1.32 μM, respectively
Fagaronine	Indole alkaloid	*Fagara zanthoxyloides* (Lam). (Rutaceae)	Antimalarial activity *in vitro* against *P. falciparum* with IC_{50} value of 0.018 μg mL^{-1}
Strychnopentamine chrysopentamine	Indole alkaloid	*Strychnos usambarensis* Glig ex Engl. (Loganiaceae)	Antimalarial activity against CQ-sensitive (FCA 20) (IC_{50} = 117 to 579 nM), moderately CQ-resistant (FCB1-R) (IC_{50} = 107–550 nM) and CQ-resistant (W2) (IC_{50} = 145–507 nM) strains of *P. falciparum*

Name of specific phytochemical(s)	**Type of compound(s)**	**Plant source (Family)**	**Antimalarial/ Antiplasmodial activity**
Ancistrobrevine; Ancistrobertsonine A, Ancistrobertsonine B, Ancistrobertsonine C, Ancistrobertsonine D	Naphthoisoquinolines	*Ancistrocladus robertsoniorum* J. Leonard. (Ancistrocladace)	Moderate antimalarial activity against K-1 and NF54 strains of *P. falciparum* (IC_{50} values ranges from 2.0 to 15.9 µM)
Habropetaline A, 5′-Odemethyl-dioncohylline A	Naphthoisoquinolines	*Triphyophyllum peltatum* (Hutch. & Dalz.) Airy Shaw (Dioncophyllaceae)	Antiplasmodial activities against K1 (CQ and pyrimethamine resistant) and NF54 (sensitive to all known drugs) strains of *P. falciparum* with IC_{50} values of 5.0 and 2.3 ng mL^{-1}, respectively
Nitidine	Furoquinolines alkaloid	*Toddalia asiatica* (L.) Lam. (Rutaceae)	*In vitro* antiplasmodial activity against K39 strain of *P. falciparum* with IC_{50} value of 0.0[illegible]5 µg mL^{-1}
β-hydroxydihydrochalcone Deguelin, obovatin	Flavonoids	*Tephrosia elata* Deflers . (Fabaceae)	Antiplasmodial activity against D6 and W2 strains of *P. falciparum* with IC_{50} values of 8.2 ± 0.8 and 16.3 ± 0.9 µM, respectively Antimalarial activity against D6 and W2 strains of *P. falciparum* with IC_{50} values ranging from 12.4 to 27.6 µM
Chrobisiamone A	Bischromone	*Cassia siamea* (Lam). (Fabaceae)	*In vitro* antiplasmodial activity against 3D7 strain of *P. falciparum* 3D7 (IC_{50} = 5.6 µM)
Series of twelve biflavonoids (amentoflavone and hinokiflavone derivatives)	Flavonoids	*Selaginella bryopteris* L. (Selaginellaceae)	Antiplasmodial activity against *P. falciparum* strains with IC_{50} value between 0.30 and 0.26 µM
Citflavanone lonchocarpol A 8-prenyldaidzein	Flavonoids	*Erythrina fusca* Lour. (Fabaceae)	*In vitro* antiplasmodial activity against *P. falciparum* at 12.[illegible] µg/mL
Butyraxanthones A-D	Xanthone	*Pentadesma butyracea* Sabine (Clusiaceae)	Antiplasmodial activity against *P. falciparum* with IC_{50} values ranging from 4.4 to 8.0 µM

Name of specific phytochemical(s)	Type of compound(s)	Plant source (Family)	Antimalarial/ Antiplasmodial activity
Kaempferol	Flavonols	Onions, kale, broccoli, apples, cherries, fennel, sorrel, berries, tea	*In vitro* antiplasmodial activity against *P. falciparum* with IC_{50} values 33 ± 7 μM(3D7 strain) and 25 ± 2 μM (7G8 strain)
Myricetin	Flavonols	Onions, kale, broccoli, apples, cherries, fennel, sorrel, berries, tea	*In vitro* antiplasmodial activity against *P. falciparum* with IC_{50} values 40 ± 10 μM (3D7) and 76 ± 2 μM (7G8)
Quercetin	Flavonols	Onions, kale, broccoli, apples, cherries, fennel, sorrel, berries, tea	*In vitro* antiplasmodial activity against *P. falciparum* with IC_{50} values 15± 5μM μM (3D7) and 14 ± 1 μM (7G8)
Isoquercitrin	Flavonols	Onions, kale, broccoli, apples, cherries, fennel, sorrel, berries, tea	*In vitro* antiplasmodial activity against *P. falciparum* with IC_{50} values 66± 10μM (3D7) and 66± 10μM (7G8)
Luteolin	Flavones	Parsley, thyme, celery, sweet red pepper	*In vitro* antiplasmodial activity against *P. falciparum* with IC_{50} values 11± 1μM (3D7) and 12 ± 1 μM (7G8)
Chrysin	Flavones	Parsley, thyme, celery, sweet red pepper	*In vitro* antiplasmodial activity against *P. falciparum* with IC_{50} values 18± 3μM (3D7) and 22 ± 4 μM (7G8)
Okundoperoxide	bicyclofarnesyl sesquiterpene endoperoxide	*Scleria striatinux* de Wild (syn. *S. striatonux*) (Cyperaceae)	Antiplasmodial activity against CQ-sensitive (D6) and CQ-resistant (W2) strains of *P. falciparum* with IC_{50} values ranging from 176 to 180 μM
Fagraldehyde	Secoiridoid aglycone	*Fagraea fragrans* (Roxb.) DC. (Gentianaceae)	Effective *in vitro* against *P. falciparum*, exhibiting an IC_{50} value of 116.6 ± 9.4 μM (W2 strain)
6α,7β-Diacetoxyvouacapane	Diterpene	*Bowdichia nitida* Benth. (Fabaceae)	*In vitro* antiplasmodial activity against 3D7 strain of *P. falciparum* (IC_{50} = 1 μM)

Name of specific phytochemical(s)	Type of compound(s)	Plant source (Family)	Antimalarial/ Antiplasmodial activity
Geraniol	Monoterpene	Pure isolated compound	Antiplasmodial activities against CQ-resistant FcM29-Cameroon strain of *P. falciparum* (IC_{50} = 52 μM)
Limonene	Monoterpene	Pure isolated compound	IC50 = 66 μ Mantiplasmodial activities against the chloroquine-resistant FcM29-Cameroon strain of *P. falciparum*
Ineupatorolide A	Sesquiterpene lactone	*Carpesium rosulatum* (Asteraceae)	*In vitro* antiplasmodial activity against CQ-resistant D10 strain of *P. falciparum* (IC_{50} = 0.019 μM) *In vivo* antimalarial activity against *P. berghei* in mice at doses of 2, 5 and 10 $mg.kg^{-1}.day^{-1}$

Table 1.
Phytomedicines as potential sources of antimalarial compounds [41, 47, 48, 52–58].

derivative of chalcones with antimalarial effectiveness against CQ-resistant strain of *P. falciparum* [43]. **Figure 6** displays structures of some recently developed plant-derived antimalarial compounds.

Herein, phytomedicine-derived antimalarial compounds are categorized into two broad groups, viz. alkaloids and non-alkaloids [46]. Different alkaloids such as indoles, bisindols, isoquinolines (naphthyl and benzyl), piperidines, pyrroles, quinolones, steroidal alkaloids have been reported to possess antimalarial effectiveness. Polyphenolic compounds and bioflavonoids including dietary flavonoids such as kaempferol, myricetin, quercetin and isoquercitrin possess *in vitro* antimalarial activities. Different terpenenoids (farnesol, nerolidol, limonene, and linalool), quassinoids, coumarins and limonoids also exhibited antiplasmodial activity when tested *in vitro* against *P. falciparum* strains [47, 48]. Semi-synthetic triterpenes such as balsaminoside B, karavilagenin C, *S*-farnesylthiosalicylic acid, and karavoates B and D have been reported to exhibit *in vitro* and *in vivo* antimalarial activity [49–51]. **Table 1** describes phytomedicines as potential sources of novel antimalarial compounds.

5. Challenges in antimalarial drug discovery

There are several challenges that exist in the domain of antimalarial drug discovery from plant sources. Some major challenges are low natural abundance of phytoconstituents, difficulty in isolation of the specific active compound in pure form, safety/toxicity and ADMET/pharmacokinetics issues, and high cost of production. Due to synergistic nature of crude plant extracts, it is also difficult to select the specific phytochemical responsible for the antimalarial action for isolation. Other issues include limited oral bioavailability and target specificity of natural molecules isolated from plants [59, 60]. Natural products with high degree of structural complexity and chemical instability are the other notable hindrances in the drug discovery pipeline of antimalarial drugs from plants. *In vitro* screening using parasitic cell cultures is a tedious work protocol which requires an expensive experimental set up and skilled laboratory personnel for the successful evaluation of antiparasitic activity. Similarly, the *in vitro* toxicity evaluation on normal cell lines requires extensive efforts, skills and labours. Compounds having high *in vitro* efficacy ($IC_{50} \leq 1\mu M$) and sufficient oral bioavailability can be considered for further *in vivo* testing. Compounds with ED_{90} values of less than 10 mg/kg per os in *in vivo* murine model is essential for further development [12, 17]. An important challenge is the lacking of efficacy in preclinical trials after the successful *in vitro* and *in vivo* studies. Further, development of semi-synthetic derivatives from the natural lead(s) is a challenging task in context of designing scheme of synthesis, synthetic modification, purification of compounds and finally chemical characterization of pure compounds. High-throughput experimental assays eliminate potent antimalarial compounds due to toxicity issues and lack of pharmacokinetic properties [42]. Another challenge is the geochemical and climatic variation of plants. One more important challenge is that since no molecular mechanism and target specificity is known, it is very difficult to choose the *in vitro* or *in vivo* models for preliminary screening, and final confirmation of antimalarial efficacy with the exploration of mode(s) of action [59, 60]. Recently, *in silico* techniques based discovery of antimalarial drugs could reduce the chances of failure in the discovery pipeline. However, newer assays and target based approaches are required to be developed for discovery of newer congeners/ derivatives of naturally occurring potent molecules with desired antimalarial potency and less toxicity.

6. Conclusion

Re-emergence of resistance of existing drugs against *P. falciparum*, toxicity and unsatisfactory pharmacokinetics and less cost-effectiveness and poor patient compliance, particularly in South-east Asian and African regions are some major concerns in the malaria control and prevention programme worldwide. Although QN- and ART-based existing drugs/ therapies are considered as gold standards in malaria chemotherapy, the clinical utility of these drugs is challenging. Potent antimalarial compounds derived from phytomedicines could serve as potential sources of future antimalarial leads/ agents after a plethora of drug development (pre-clinical and clinical studies) processes. Target-based discovery of bioactive phytochemical entities is required for their successful development as effective and safe antimalarial drug molecules.

Conflict of interest

Authors declare that there is no conflict of interest.

Author details

Mithun Rudrapal[1*], Dipak Chetia[2] and Soumya Bhattacharya[3]

1 Rasiklal M. Dhariwal Institute of Pharmaceutical Education and Research, Pune, Maharashtra, India

2 Department of Pharmaceutical Sciences, Dibrugarh University, Dibrugarh, Assam, India

3 Guru Nanak Institute of Pharmaceutical Science and Technology, Kolkata, India

*Address all correspondence to: rsmrpal@gmail.com

References

[1] Communicable Diseases (CDS) ((World Health Organization). Available from URL: https://www.who.int/about/structure/organigram/htm/en/ [Accessed: 18 February 2021]

[2] McArthur DB. Emerging infectious diseases. The Nursing Clinics of North America. 2019;**54**(2):297-311

[3] World Malaria Report 2020 (World Health Organization). Available from URL: https://www.who.int/teams/global-malaria-programme/reports/world-malaria-report-2020 [Accessed: 15 February 2021]

[4] Kalita J, Chetia D, Rudrapal M. Design, synthesis, antimalarial activity and docking study of 7-Chloro-4-(2-(substituted benzylidene)hydrazineyl) quinolines. Medicinal Chemistry. 2020;**16**(7):928-937

[5] Rudrapal M, Khairnar SJ, Borse LB, Jadhav AG. Coronavirus disease-2019 (COVID-19): An updated review. Drug Reseaarch. 2020;**70**:389-400

[6] Rudrapal M, Banu ZW, Chetia D. Newer series of trioxane derivatives as potent antimalarial agents. Medicinal Chemistry Research. 2018;**27**(2):653-668

[7] Rudrapal M, Chetia D, Singh V. Novel series of 1,2,4-trioxane derivatives as antimalarial agents. Journal of Enzyme Inhibition and Medicinal Chemistry. 2017;**32**(1):1159-1173

[8] Rudrapal M, Chetia D. Endoperoxide antimalarials: Development, structural diversity and pharmacodynamic aspects with reference to 1,2,4-trioxane-based structural scaffold. Drug Design Devlopmental Therapy. 2016;**10**:3575-3590

[9] Kalita J, Chetia D, Rudrapal M. Molecular docking, drug-likeness studies and ADMET prediction of quinoline imines for antimalarial activity. Journal of Medical and Chemical Drugs Design. 2019;**2**(1):1-7

[10] Medhi A. Synthesis and antimalarial activity of lawsone mannich base derivatives. Indian Journal of Pharmaceutical Education and Research. 2018;**52**(3):472-479

[11] Patowary P, Chetia D, Kalita J, Rudrapal M. Design, synthesis and antimalarial activity of flavonoid derivatives. Indian Journal of Heterocyclic Chemistry. 2019;**29**(1):53-58

[12] Rudrapal M, Chetia D. *In vitro* and *in vivo* models used for antimalarial activity: A brief review. Asian Journal of Pharmaceutical and Pharmacology. 2019;**5**(6):1251-1255

[13] Biamonte MA, Wanner J, Le Roch KG. Recent advances in malaria drug discovery. Bioorganic & Medicinal Chemistry Letters. 2013;**23**:2829-2843

[14] Rudrapal M, Chetia D. Malaria: Chemotherapy and Development of Novel Antimalarial Agents. Germany: LAP LAMBERT Academic Publishing; 2014

[15] Bhagavathula AS, Elnour AH, Shehab A. Alternatives to currently used antimalarial drugs: In search of a magic bullet. Infectious Diseases of Poverty. 2016;**5**:103

[16] Robert A, Benoit-Vical F, Dechy-Cabaret O, Meunier B. From classical antimalarial drugs to new compounds based on the mechanism of action of artemisinin. Pure and Applied Chemistry. 2001;**73**:1173-1180

[17] Meshnick SR, Dobson MJ. History of antimalarial drugs. In: Rosenthal PJ, editor. Antimalarial Chemotherapy: Mechanisms of Action, Resistance, and New Directions in Drug Discovery. New Jersey: Humana Press; 2001. pp. 2-25

[18] Rudrapal M, Chetia D. Novel 4-aminoquinoline analogues as antimalarial agents: A review. Der Pharmacia Letter. 2011;**3**(3):29-36

[19] Rudrapal M. A brief review on malaria and current antimalarial drugs. Current Pharmaceutical Research. 2011;**1**(3):286-292

[20] Dinio T, Gorka AP, McGinniss A, Roepe PD, Morgan JB. Investigating the activity of quinine analogues versus chloroquine resistant *Plasmodium falciparum*. Bioorganic & Medicinal Chemistry. 2012;**20**:3292-3297

[21] Bray PG, Ward SA, O'Neill PM. Quinolines and artemisinin: Chemistry, biology and history. Current Topics in Microbiology and Immunology. 2005;**295**:3-38

[22] Luo XD, Shen CC. The chemistry, pharmacology, and clinical applications of Qinghaosu (Artemisinin) and its derivatives. Medicinal Research Reviews. 1987;**7**:29-52

[23] Balint GA. Artemisinin and its derivatives: An important new class of antimalarial agents. Pharmacology & Therapeutics. 2001;**90**:261-265

[24] Meshnick SR. Artemisinin: Mechanisms of action, resistance and toxicity. International Journal for Parasitology. 2002;**32**:1655-1660

[25] Garner P, Graves PM. The benefits of artemisinin combination therapy for malaria extend beyond the individual patient. PLoS Medicine. 2005;**2**:e105

[26] Borstnik K, Paik IH, Shapiro TA, PosnerGH. Antimalarialchemotherapeutic peroxides: Artemisinin, yingzhaosu A and related compounds. International Journal for Parasitology. 2002;**32**(4):1661-1667

[27] Liu C. Discovery and development of artemisinin and related compounds. China Herbal Medicine. 2017;**9**:101-114

[28] Achan J et al. Quinine, an old anti-malarial drug in a modern world: Role in the treatment of malaria. Malaria Journal. 2011;**10**:144

[29] Rosenthal PJ. Antimalarial drug discovery: Old and new approaches. The Journal of Experimental Biology. 2003;**206**:3735-3744

[30] Flannery EL, Chatterjee AK, Winzeler EA. Antimalarial drug discovery-approaches and progress towards new medicines. Nature Reviews. Microbiology. 2013;**11**:849-862

[31] Rudrapal M, Khairnar SJ. Drug repurposing: An emerging approach in drug discovery. In: Dekebo A, editor. Drug Repurposing: Hypothesis, Molecular Aspects and Therapeutic Applications. London: IntechOpen; 2020, 2020

[32] Roy S, Chetia D, Rudrapal M, Prakash A. Synthesis and antimalarial activity study of some new Mannich bases of 7-Chloro-4-Aminoquinoline. Medicinal Chemistry. 2013;**9**(3):379-383

[33] Rudrapal M, Chetia D, Prakash A. Synthesis, antimalarial and antibacterial activity evaluation of some new 4-aminoquinoline derivatives. Medicinal Chemistry Research. 2013;**22**:3703-3711

[34] Sharma D, Chetia D, Rudrapal M. Design, synthesis and antimalarial activity of new 2-hydroxy-1,4-naphthoquinone-4-hydroxyanilino

hybrid Mannich bases. Asian Journal of Chemistry. 2016;**28**(4):782-788

[35] Gogoi J, Chetia D, Kumawat MK, Rudrapal M. Synthesis and antimalarial activity evaluation of some mannich bases of tetraoxane-phenol conjugate. Indian Journal of Pharmaceutical Education and Research. 2016;**50**(4):591-597

[36] Kashyap A, Chetia D, Rudrapal M. Synthesis, antimalarial activity evaluation and drug-likeness study of some new Quinoline-Lawsone hybrids. Indian Journal of Pharmaceutical Sciences. 2016;**78**(6):892-911

[37] Rudrapal M, Chetia D. QSAR analysis of 7-chloro-4-aminoquinoline derivatives as antimalarial agents. Asian Journal of Organic Medical Chemistry. 2013;**1**:51-54

[38] Bhagat S, Gahlawat A, Bharatnam PV. Structure-based drug design PfDHODH inhibitors as antimalarial agents. In: Mohan C, editor. Structural Biinformatics: Applications in Preclinical Drug Discovery Process. Challenges and Advances in Computational Chemistry and Physics. Cham: Springer; 2019

[39] Rudrapal M, Chetia D. Virtual screening, molecular docking and f QSAR studies in drug discovery and development programme. Journal of Drug Delivery Therapy. 2020;**1094**:225-233

[40] Ashley EA, Phyo AP. Drugs in development for malaria. Drugs. 2018;**78**:861-879

[41] Rudrapal M, Chetia D. Plant flavonoids as potential source of future antimalarial leads. Systematic Review in Pharmacology. 2017;**8**:13-18

[42] Mojab F. Antimalarial natural products: A review. Avicenna Journal of Phytomedicine. 2011;**2**:52-62

[43] Mishra LC, Bhattacharya A, Bhasin VK. Phytochemical licochalcone A enhances antimalarial activity of artemisinin in vitro. Acta Tropical. 2009;**109**:194-198

[44] Pines M, Spector I. Halofuginone-The multifaceted molecule. Molecules. 2015;**20**(1):573-594

[45] Fandeur T, Moretti C, Polonsky J. *In vitro* and *in vivo* assessment of the antiomalarial activity of sergeolide. Planta Medica. 1985;**51**:20-23

[46] Oliveira BA, Dolabela MF, Braga FC, Jácome RLRP, Varotti FP, Póvoa MM. Plant-derived antimalarial agents: New leads and efficient phythomedicines. Part I. Alkaloids. Anais da Academia Brasileira de Ciencias. 2009;**81**:715-740

[47] Amoa Ntie-Kang F, Lifongo LL, Ndom JC, Sippl W, Mbaze LM. The potential of anti-malarial compounds derived from African medicinal plants, part I: A pharmacological evaluation of alkaloids and terpenoids. Malaria Journal. 2013;**12**:449

[48] Batista R, Silva Ade J Jr, de Oliveira AB. Plant-derived antimalarial agents: New leads and efficient phytomedicines. Part II. Non-alkaloidal natural products. Molecules. 2009;**14**:3037-3072

[49] Tse EG, Korsik M, Todd MH. The past, present and future of anti-malarial medicines. Malaria Journal. 2019;**18**:93

[50] Tajuddeen N, Van Heerden FR. Antiplasmodial natural products: An update. Malaria Journal. 2019;**18**:404

[51] Pawar HA. Natural product as a source of lead to the design of new drugs. Natural Products in Chemical Research. 2014;**2**:156

[52] Rustaiyan A, Nahrevanian H. An investigation on Anti-malarial Effects of Tehranolide Isolated from Artemisia diffusa against Human Malaria Parasite *Plasmodium falciparum in vitro*. Research Journal of Parasitology. 2015;**10**(2):73-78

[53] Beaufay C, Ledoux A, Jansen O, Bordignon A, Zhao S, Teijaro CN, et al. *In vivo* antimalarial and antitrypanosomal activity of Strychnogucine B, a Bisindole Alkaloid from *Strychnos icaja*. Planta Medica. 2018;**84**:881-885

[54] Dua VK, Verma G, Singh B, Rajan A, Bagai U, Agarwal DD, et al. Anti-malarial property of steroidal alkaloid conessine isolated from the bark of *Holarrhena antidysenterica*. Malaria Journal. 2013;**12**:194

[55] Nair JJ, van Staden J. Antiplasmodial lycorane alkaloid principles of the plant family amaryllidaceae. Planta Medica. 2019;**85**(8):637-647

[56] Qidwai T, Jamal F, Khan MY, Sharma B. Exploring drug targets in isoprenoid biosynthetic pathway for *Plasmodium falciparum*. Biochemistry Research International. 2014;**2014**: 657189

[57] Gabriel HB, Sussmann RAC, Kimura EA, Rodriguez AAM, Verdaguer IB, Leite GCF. Terpenes as potential antimalarial drugs. In: Perveen S, Al-Taweel A, editors. Terpenes and Terpenoids. London: IntechOpen; 2018

[58] Lehane AM, Saliba KJ. Common dietary flavonoids inhibit the growth of the intraerythrocytic malaria parasite. BMC Research Notes. 2008;**1**:26

[59] Burrows JN, Leroy D, Lotharius J, Waterson D. Challenges in antimalarial drug discovery. Future Medicinal Chemistry. 2011:31401-31412

[60] Uzor PF. Alkaloids from plants with antimalarial activity: A review of recent studies. Evidence-based Complementary and Alternative Medicine. 2020;**2020**:8749083

Chapter 13

Effects and Pharmacological Use of Alkaloids on the Eyes

Jin-Ho Joo

Abstract

Alkaloids can have a variety of effects on the eyes. Some alkaloids are used as a treatment for eye diseases, such as keratoconjunctivitis, but they are also toxic to the retina. Other alkaloids are known to protect neuroretina from damage caused by oxidative stress. Numerous ophthalmic drugs, such as glaucoma and antibiotic eye drops, have long been developed through alkaloids. In this chapter, we will introduce the beneficial and detrimental effects of alkaloids on the eye. In addition, the action of alkaloids as existing eye drops and the possibility of developing them as drugs in the future will be discussed.

Keywords: alkaloid, eye, mydriasis, miosis, repurposing, myopia, presbyopia, intraocular pressure, retina, cataract, glaucoma, optic neuropathy, angiogenesis

1. Introduction

Alkaloid is a generic term for compounds derived from natural substances and having a nitrogen atom as a base. Alkaloids can be obtained from a variety of organisms, including bacteria, fungi, plants, and animals. The first alkaloid to be isolated was morphine from opium in 1804 by Friedrich Sertürner, a German pharmacist [1, 2]. Alkaloids with pharmacological effects are often known to be used as medicines, for example, physostigmine and pilocarpine as a treatment for glaucoma, and cocaine as a topical ocular anesthetic. However, in some cases, they are toxic, just as cocaine is highly toxic to corneal epithelial cells. Sometimes alkaloids cause undesirable constriction or dilation of the pupil, making us uncomfortable.

Recently, several studies have shown the potential of alkaloids as new drugs in the field of ophthalmology. Previously used, atropine plays a role in inhibiting the progression of myopia, and pilocarpine is attracting attention as a new treatment for presbyopia. In addition, some alkaloids are known to have antioxidant effects to prevent the progression of cataracts, protect the optic nerve through various mechanisms, and protect the retina by inhibiting angiogenesis.

Therefore, in this chapter, we would like to introduce the positive effects of using alkaloids as medicines and the various effects of alkaloids on the eyes. And among the recent studies, alkaloids would like to introduce the possibility of novel treatment in the field of ophthalmology.

2. Medicinal use of alkaloids in the field of ophthalmology

2.1 Atropine

Atropine ($C_{17}H_{23}NO_3$) is a drug widely used by ophthalmologists for ophthalmic diagnosis and treatment since the 1800s and not only derived from the leaves of *Atropa belladonna* but is also found in other plants mainly from the Solanaceae family, such as *Datura stramonium, A. belladonna, Hyoscyamus niger*, and *Mandragora officinarum* [3]. It is an anticholinergic drug that causes powerful and long-lasting mydriasis and paralyzes the ciliary body, causing cycloplegia. For muscarinic receptors, it competes with acetylcholine or muscarine to inhibit parasympathetic nerves and selectively block the action of acetylcholine or muscarine. Acetylcholine secreted by stimulation binds to muscarinic receptors to continue signal transmission, and then, acetylcholine must be degraded by an enzyme called "acetylcholinesterase" to continue normal signal transmission. Atropine binds to muscarinic receptors but does not cause signal transduction, and since atropine and acetylcholine competitively bind to muscarinic receptors, atropine acts to inhibit the action of acetylcholine [4].

Until now, atropine eye drops have been used in ophthalmology to make mydriasis for diagnosis and surgical treatment, to help reduce intraocular inflammation and control the spasm of the near reflex. Recently, low concentrations of atropine have been found to be effective in controlling myopia. In a randomized clinical trials study, it was known that 0.05% atropine was less effective at the optimal concentration and minimized the side effects of near blurry and photophobia [5, 6].

Although the mechanism by which atropine suppresses the progression of myopia is not known, the following hypotheses are known to be highly likely through several studies. First, atropine affects the sclera, which is a fibrous connective tissue that protects the eye. It has been reported that atropine reduces the activity of the epidermal growth factor receptor in sclera fibroblasts, thereby reducing the proliferation of these cells, increasing the thickness of the scleral fibrous layer in the myopic eye, and reducing extracellular matrix production by reducing glycosaminoglycan synthesis. This can explain that myopia is prevented by suppressing the increase in the axial length of the eye. Second, atropine may affect the choroid, a layer of blood vessels that supply oxygen and nutrients to the outer retina. Originally, the choroid responds to optic defocus and controls the choroid thickness to focus. Atropine blocks the muscarine receptors of the choroid retinal pigment epithelium (RPE), modulates the transforming growth factor and basal fibroblast growth factor, and eventually suppresses choroid thinning, which is known to prevent the progression of myopia [7].

2.2 Physostigmine

In 1862, Thomas Fraser discovered the first intraocular pressure (IOP) lowering medication, physostigmine ($C_{15}H_{21}N_3O_2$), from the Calabar beans [8]. Physostigmine is a highly toxic parasympathomimetic alkaloid and a reversible cholinesterase inhibitor. After instillation into the eye, it increases the activity of free acetylcholine in the pupil sphincter, causing miosis leading to contraction of the ciliary muscle. Contraction of the ciliary muscle has been shown to decrease IOP by increasing the drainage of aqueous humor into the trabecular pathway. However, physostigmine has been replaced with safer drugs, which will be introduced below, due to side effects, such as headache, spasm of accommodation, blurred vision due to miosis, increased risk of retinal detachment, and inflammation of the conjunctiva, cornea, and iris [9].

2.3 Pilocarpine

Pilocarpine ($C_{11}H_{16}N_2O_2$) is a cholinergic agent that was isolated by Hardy and Gerrard from *Pilocarpus* in 1875 and used as an eye drops for the treatment of glaucoma. Installation of pilocarpine reduces the size of the pupil, which can help reduce glare.

Pilocarpine is a cholinergic parasympathomimetic agent that acts through direct stimulation of muscarinic receptors and smooth muscles, such as the iris [10]. Aqueous humor is secreted from the ciliary body, travels through the pupil to the anterior chamber, and exits through the trabecular meshwork into Schlemm's canal. In angle closure glaucoma, IOP rises because aqueous flow obstruction occurs by the pupillary block. This can cause vision loss and pain in the eyeball. The therapeutic principle in angle closure is by removing the pupillary block. Pilocarpine contracts the iris sphincter muscle and pulls it away from the trabecular meshwork, widening the anterior chamber angle. As a result, it is used as an important treatment for angle closure glaucoma by resolving a pupillary block [11, 12].

Pilocarpine is also used for diagnostic purposes. Dilated pupils can appear for a variety of reasons. Among them, Adie's tonic pupil is caused by damage to the post-ganglionic parasympathetic nerve of the iris sphincter muscle. Denervation supersensitivity is a characteristic sign in Adie's tonic pupil that is confirmed by pharmacologic testing with a direct-acting weak muscarinic agonist, dilute pilocarpine [13].

Recently, pilocarpine 1.25% eye drops have been approved by the FDA for the treatment of presbyopia. Presbyopia is a condition in which near vision loss occurs due to a progressive physiological loss of accommodation. Accommodation is adjusting refraction to make focus on a near object. This can be achieved by increasing lens thickness by reducing zonular tension with ciliary muscle contraction, pupillary constriction, and convergence of both eyes. Presbyopia is known to occur due to the stiffening of the lens due to aging. About 1.25% pilocarpine is a muscarinic agent that induces miosis and ciliary body contraction and has been demonstrated to improve near vision without significantly impairing distance vision [14, 15].

2.4 Cocaine

It was first used in 1884 by Karl Köller as cocaine ($C_{17}H_{21}NO_4$) for topical ocular anesthesia. As a local anesthetic, cocaine reduces pain by blocking sodium channels in the membranes of sensory nerve endings. However, cocaine is highly toxic to corneal epithelial cells and is no longer used for anesthesia. Since then, local anesthetics for ophthalmic use have changed to tetracaine, proparacaine, and lidocaine [16, 17].

Cocaine inhibits norepinephrine reuptake and causes pupillary dilation. High concentrations can cause cycloplegia, and chronic users can cause exophthalmos and retraction of the upper eyelid [18]. Cocaine users may develop superficial punctate keratitis, epithelial defects, and ulcers through eye rubbing or retrograde passage through the nasolacrimal duct [19]. Although not directly affected by drugs, unilateral vision loss along with proptosis and ophthalmoplegia may occur due to orbital congestion and ophthalmic/central retinal artery occlusion due to continuous pressure on the orbital socket while sleeping in an abnormal posture due to unconsciousness after excessive drug abuse. Orbital congestion and proptosis improved with time, but the visual prognosis was poor [20].

2.5 Pyrrolizidine alkaloid

Heliotropium Indicum is used traditionally as a remedy for conjunctivitis. This plant is an annual, hirsute plant that is a common weed in waste places and settled areas. It is native to Asia. It is widely used in native medicine in India. The extract from the pounded leaves of this plant contains several pharmacologically active alkaloids, such as indicine ($C_{15}H_{25}NO_5$), acetyl-indicine ($C_{17}H_{27}NO_6$), indicinine-N-oxide ($C_{15}H_{25}NO_6$), heleurine ($C_{16}H_{27}NO_4$), heliotrine ($C_{16}H_{27}NO_5$), supinidine ($C_8H_{13}NO$), and lindelofidine ($C_8H_{15}NO$). These alkaloids have anti-allergic effects, possibly by immunomodulation or immunosuppression in allergic conjunctivitis. Also, this extraction exhibits an anti-inflammatory effect on uveitis, possibly by reducing the production of pro-inflammatory mediators. It was confirmed that this extract significantly reduced the concentrations of tumor necrosis factor-α (TNF-α), prostaglandin E2 (PGE2), and monocyte chemoattractant protein-1 (MCP-1) in rabbits with uveitis [21, 22].

In another study, consuming extracts of this plant could inhibit the progression of cataracts in rats. Total lens proteins glutathione and superoxide dismutase (SOD) levels in the crystalline lens were also significantly preserved. This can be the basis for a new treatment that can prevent cataract progression by suppressing oxidative stress [23]. In addition, it lowers IOP and has anti-oxidant and possible neuroprotective effects. When treated with this extract, IOP was significantly reduced in rabbits with glaucoma, and the concentration of glutathione in the aqueous humor was preserved, proving that the eyes were protected from oxidative damage. So, it has the potential to develop into a drug helpful in the treatment of glaucoma [24].

3. Various effects of alkaloids on the eyes

3.1 Caffeine

In modern society, caffeine ($C_8H_{10}N_4O_2$) is one of the most widely used dietary constituents. Caffeine is an adenosine receptor antagonist and makes a pharmacological effect on various organ systems. The lens progresses to a cataract due to the formation of reactive oxygen species (ROS) by ultraviolet light or diabetes. Caffeine has been shown to protect the lens from oxidative damage in various animal models of cataracts [25–27]. One study has shown that there is a significant negative correlation between coffee consumption and cataract incidence [28]. Given that it reduced the incidence of UV-induced cataracts in animal models, it is thought that caffeine could be an important candidate for future cataract-preventive eye drugs.

It is known that the administration of caffeine induces ocular vasoconstriction in healthy individuals. About 5% of vasoconstriction in the retinal arterioles occurred 1 hour after ingestion of 200 mg of caffeine. How caffeine induces vasoconstriction is not known in detail. Caffeine-induced vasoconstriction may represent autoregulatory myogenic smooth muscle contraction in response to elevated blood pressure. When caffeine was administered, retinal vessel diameter showed a negative correlation with mean arterial pressure, suggesting that it originates from a myogenic response [29]. Caffeine can also induce vasoconstriction by increasing sympathetic tone. Since the choroidal and ciliary circulations receive sympathetic innervation, the increased sympathetic tone may contribute to vasoconstriction of the ocular circulation [30].

Controversy has arisen about the increase in IOP after caffeine intake in normal young people, but it has been found that caffeine intake increases IOP in glaucomatous eyes [31]. Caffeine elevates IOP probably because it antagonizes the actions of adenosine, which reduces IOP. Adenosine receptors A1 and A2 are known to induce vasodilation and decrease IOP [32]. Glaucomatous eyes are known to result from damage to the aqueous humor outflow system. Several studies have shown that patients with glaucoma have abnormal vascular reactivity and peripheral microvascular circulation [33]. The action of caffeine can alter the adenosine signaling pathway, leading to differential vascular effects of caffeine in normal and glaucomatous eyes.

For a long time, studies have shown caffeine to be a potential drug for neurodegenerative diseases because of its adenosine-antagonizing properties. Since the retina is also a neurosensory organ and an extension of the brain, there is an opinion that caffeine may play a role in protecting the retina by blocking the adenosine A_{2A} receptor and controlling the reactivity of microglia [34]. In oxygen-induced retinopathy in the mouse model, caffeine intake attenuated hypoxia-induced pathologic angiogenesis and vascular occlusion without interfering with normal retinal vascular development [35]. There are suggestions that the cellular response to hypoxia is extracellular adenosine production and the markedly induced adenosine receptors, which are thought to be novel targets for pathological angiogenesis. Among them, three adenosine receptor subtypes (A_1R, $A_{2A}R$, and $A_{2B}R$) are expected to play a role [36]. Therefore, it is considered that caffeine can be an important candidate for new drugs for retinal diseases, such as diabetic retinopathy (DR), retinal vascular occlusion, retinopathy of prematurity, and age-related macular degeneration (ARMD), by using the effects of caffeine on the nerve and vascular protection.

3.2 Nicotine

Cigarette smoking is one of the most common and serious health problems today. Chemical toxicity and free radical-related oxidative damage can affect multiple structures in the body. In particular, nicotine ($C_{10}H_{14}N_2$) is known to cause changes in the conjunctival flora, irritation, redness, dry eye, ocular surface inflammation, and meibomian gland dysfunction. Tear film breakup time is known to decrease, indicating an unstable tear film. As a result, dry eye syndrome can become more severe [37–41]. Although it cannot be limited to that caused by nicotine, it is known that cigarettes have various harmful effects on the eyes. It increases the risk of squamous metaplasia of bulbar conjunctiva and conjunctival intraepithelial neoplasia [39, 42], delays corneal wound healing [43], reduces endothelial cell count or hexagonality of endothelial cells [44, 45], and can lead to cataract formation [46]. Smoking is also known to increase the risk of age-related macular degeneration [47], increase IOP [48], and induce non-arteritic anterior ischemic optic neuropathy (NAION) [49].

3.3 Opiates

Morphine ($C_{17}H_{19}NO_3$) causes miosis by acting on opioid receptors [50, 51]. The triad of coma, pupillary constriction, and depressed respiration suggests opioid addiction. Morphine abuse can cause downbeat nystagmus, transient disturbances of eye fixation, saccadic intrusions, and oscillations [52]. Intravenous abuse of this drug may cause embolization of the retinal vasculature and may result in endophthalmitis.

3.4 Quinine

Quinine ($C_{20}H_{24}N_2O_2$) was first isolated in 1820 from the bark of a cinchona tree. It has been used as a remedy for malaria since 1632. Quinine is a flavor component of tonic water and bitter lemon drink mixers. Tonic water was initially marketed as a means of delivering quinine to consumers to offer antimalarial protection. Because of the various complications of quinine and resistance to malaria, as of 2006, the World Health Organization no longer recommends it as a first-line treatment for malaria [53].

Chloroquine ($C_{18}H_{26}ClN_3$) and hydroxychloroquine ($C_{18}H_{26}ClN_3O$), derivatives of quinine, were developed and used as antimalarial drugs, but are now widely used to treat connective tissue disorders, such as systemic lupus erythematosus and rheumatoid arthritis. Retinopathy can be caused by the use of hydroxychloroquine and chloroquine, which is a serious complication. This is largely related to the dose, and it is known that the incidence of retinopathy increases when the hydroxychloroquine dose exceeds 5.0 mg/kg or the chloroquine dose exceeds 2.3 mg/kg. Although the mechanisms of chloroquine and hydroxychloroquine retinopathy have not been clarified, these drugs bind to melanin and deposit in the retinal pigment epithelium. They are thought to increase cell lysosomal pH, thereby preventing autophagosomal attachment to lysosomes, and leading to photoreceptor degradation [54].

3.5 Scopolamine

Scopolamine ($C_{17}H_{21}NO_4$) is an alkaloid used to treat motion sickness and postoperative nausea and vomiting. It was the first drug to be made commercially available in a transdermal therapeutic system delivering alkaloids. It competitively inhibits all four muscarinic receptors (M1, M2, M3, and M4) for acetylcholine and acts as a nonselective muscarinic antagonist, producing both peripheral antimuscarinic properties and central sedative, antiemetic, and amnestic effects [55]. It is used to prevent motion sickness in the form of a transdermal patch. There have been reports of mydriasis and reduced near vision occurring when rubbing the eyes with the hand that touched the patch. There are many reasons for the occurrence of mydriasis, but if there is no specific cause, contamination by scopolamine transdermal patches should also be considered [56].

It was confirmed that continuous systemic administration of scopolamine in rats could induce dry eye due to inflammation of the lacrimal gland by cholinergic blockade induced by scopolamine [57].

4. Alkaloids as candidates for new drugs in ophthalmology

4.1 Piperine

Piperine ($C_{17}H_{19}NO_3$) was discovered by Hans Christian Ørsted in 1819, and piperine was isolated from *Piper nigrum*, the source plant of both black and white pepper. Piperine is known to be able to inhibit free radicals and ROS, thereby protecting apoptotic cell death from oxidative damage. In a steroid-induced chick embryo lens model, it was confirmed that piperine exerted an effect as an antioxidant substance and prevented the development of cataracts by reducing the increase in the level of ROS [58].

The effect of piperine was also confirmed to have a protective effect on the retina in a mouse model with diabetic retinopathy. In a hypoxia-induced DR mouse model, intraperitoneal injection of piperine was found to reduce the expression of hypoxia-inducible factor-1α and vascular endothelial growth factor (VEGF) A, which are known to have an angiogenic effect [59].

4.2 Matrine

Matrine ($C_{15}H_{24}N_2O$) is an alkaloid found in *Leguminosae* plants, *including Sophora flavescens Ait*. It is known to have potent antitumor activity by inhibiting tumor cell proliferation through a variety of mechanisms, including inducing cancer cell differentiation and apoptosis, altering the tumor cell cycle, and inhibiting telomerase activity. Antitumor effects of matrine were found in vincristine-resistant retinoblastoma cells. Retinoblastoma is a malignant tumor of the retina and usually affects children under the age of 6 years. Retinoblastoma is a threat to both a child's vision and life. Treatment for retinoblastoma includes chemotherapy, radiotherapy, surgery, laser treatment, and freezing, among which vincristine is the most commonly used chemotherapy. However, resistance to chemotherapeutic agents can lead to treatment failure. When the drug-resistant retinoblastoma cell line was treated with matrine, it was confirmed that the proliferation of tumor cells was suppressed, apoptosis was suppressed, and the cell cycle was arrested. Matrine appears to induce apoptosis by downregulating the protein Bcl-2, which affects the antiapoptotic process. Matrine was also confirmed to regulate the cell cycle of tumor cells by reducing cyclin D1 expression. Matrine may be a potential treatment for vincristine-resistant retinoblastoma [60].

Matrine has been shown to inhibit optic nerve infiltration and demyelination in optic neuritis. Optic neuritis is a condition in which inflammation, demyelination, and axonal injury occur in the optic nerve, resulting in demyelination leading to temporary or permanent loss of vision. Retinal ganglion cells (RGCs) are known to undergo significant loss during apoptosis in optic neuritis. The death of RGCs has been considered the main cause of vision loss after an episode of optic neuritis. It was confirmed that matrine can promote survival by protecting RGCs from inflammation-induced apoptosis. When matrine was injected intraperitoneally in optic neuritis in the experimental autoimmune encephalomyelitis rat model, it was confirmed that the increased numbers of CD4+ T cells and Iba1+ microglia/macrophages in the optic nerves were reduced. Matrine also inhibits the production of proinflammatory cytokines, such as IFN-γ, TNF-α, and IL-17, and blocks the migration of peripheral immune cells. What causes RGCs apoptosis is a shift toward a more proapoptotic ratio in the Bcl-2 family and reduced phosphorylation of protein kinase B (Akt) proteins. Matrine is thought to protect RGCs from apoptosis by shifting the Bcl-2/Bax ratio back to an antiapoptotic one and promoting Akt phosphorylation. Matrine reduced optic nerve inflammation, demyelination, and axonal loss, and protected retinal ganglion cells from inflammation-induced cell death. Thus, matrine shows promise as a novel treatment of optic neuritis, which can lead to blindness [61].

4.3 Vincamine

Vincamine ($C_{21}H_{26}N_2O_3$) is a monoterpenoid indole alkaloid found in the Apocynaceae *Vinca* plant (lesser periwinkle). It is used as a treatment for primary degenerative and vascular dementia. It can improve the metabolism of ischemic tissue and protect the neuron. A recent study demonstrated that vincamine has a potential neuroprotection effect in NAION. Vincamine can rescue the death of retinal ganglion cells and reduce the number of apoptotic cells. The protection of vincamine might play through the phosphoinositide 3-kinases (PI3K)/Akt/endothelial nitric oxide synthase (eNOS) signaling pathway. Therefore, vincamine can be an effective therapy method NAION [62].

4.4 Papaverine

Papaverine ($C_{20}H_{21}NO_4$) was discovered in 1848 by Georg Merck. Papaverine is a nonselective phosphodiesterase inhibitor and is mainly used for cerebral thrombosis, pulmonary embolism, and arterial spasms by relaxing cardiovascular, respiratory, and gastrointestinal smooth muscles. Recent studies have confirmed evidence that papaverine can protect the optic nerve. Cyclic adenosine 3,5′-monophosphate (cAMP) is known to play an important role in ATP metabolism. It is known that the exogenous addition of cAMP increases the content of synaptic binding protein in axons, promotes the survival of neurons and outgrowth of axons due to nerve injury, and accelerates functional recovery of the central nervous system. Intracellular cAMP levels are regulated by the activity of phosphodiesterase, and phosphodiesterase inhibitors increase cAMP levels by inhibiting the hydrolysis of cAMP. Papaverine regulates the expression of cAMP by inhibiting lipopolysaccharide-induced retinal microglial activation, which plays a role in phagocytosis and secretion of inflammatory mediators by regulating the nuclear factor-kB (NF- kB) and mitogen-activated protein kinase (MEK) /extracellular signal-regulated kinases (ERK) pathways. This was eventually confirmed to induce axonal regeneration of RGCs. This showed potential as a treatment for optic nerve damage, such as glaucoma [63–65].

4.5 Berberine

Berberine ($C_{20}H_{18}NO_4^+$) is a natural bioactive alkaloid derived from a variety of Chinese Medicinal herbs, including *Rhizoma Coptidis*. It has been reported with various pharmacological effects, such as anti-inflammation, anti-oxidation, hepatic protection, and anticancer. In a recent study, berberine was found to be effective in insulin-induced diabetic retinopathy. When Akt/mTOR signaling is activated by insulin, the risk of neovascularization in the retina of diabetic animals may increase due to an increase in hypoxia-inducible factor-1α (HIF-1α)/VEGF in retinal endothelial cells. When insulin-induced neovasculature of retina endothelial cells was treated with berberine, it was found to improve insulin-induced DR by inhibiting Akt/mammalian target of rapamycin (mTOR) activity and reducing the expression of the HIF-1α/VEGF pathway [66].

In addition, studies have shown that berberine can protect the retina from light-induced photoreceptor degeneration. In the light-damaged retina, RPE65 and Mct3 proteins were down-regulated, resulting in photoreceptor damage. It has been shown that the PI3K/AKT/ERK pathway plays a major role in ultraviolet-induced RPE damage. The mice treated with berberine had more photoreceptor nuclei in the outer retina and photoreceptor inner/outer segments and higher RPE65 and Mct3 in the RPE than the control group. Berberine was found to protect against light-induced retinal damage by activating the PI3K/AKT/ERK pathway. This can be considered to show the potential of a drug that can protect photoreceptors from ARMD [67].

4.6 Sanguinarine

Sanguinarine ($C_{20}H_{14}NO_4$) is a type of benzophenanthridine alkaloid extracted from the root of the herbaceous plant *Sanguinaria canadensis*. It is known to have antimicrobial, anti-inflammatory, anti-oxidative, and tumor-suppressing properties. Sanguinarine has been found to be effective in preventing after-cataracts. After-cataract refers to the posterior capsule opacification that occurs after cataract surgery and is caused by the regeneration of residual lens epithelial cells. Sanguinarine significantly reduced the viability of human lens epithelial B-3 cells and induced apoptosis. Apoptotic effects probably induce reactive oxygen species generation and promote phosphorylation of c-Jun N-terminal kinase (JNK) and p38 kinases, suggesting that the mitogen-activated protein Kinase (MAPK) pathway is involved in apoptosis. Sanguinarine may be used as a potential drug for after-cataract prevention [68].

Sanguinarine has been shown to have antiangiogenic effects in wet ARMD. A major feature of wet ARMD is choroidal neovascularization, in which pathological neovascularization originating from the choriocapillaris breaks through Bruch's membrane and creates leakage in the subretinal space, resulting in reduced visual acuity. The treatment of wet ARMD is to suppress angiogenesis by administering intravitreal injections of antibodies against VEGF. Intravitreal injection of sanguinarine chloride was performed in the choroidal neovascularization mouse model, and as a result, the formation of choroidal neovascularization was suppressed and the expression of VEGF was reduced. Sanguinarine inhibited VEGF-induced AKT, ERK, and MAPK signaling pathways. Sanguinarine has been suggested as a potential treatment for wet ARMD [69].

4.7 Galantamine

Galantamine ($C_{17}H_{21}NO_3$) is an alkaloid used as a treatment for Alzheimer's disease, a cognitive disorder. These are the bulbs and flowers of *Galanthus nivalis* (Common snowdrop), *Galanthus caucasicus* (Caucasian snowdrop), *Galanthus woronowii* (Voronov's snowdrop), and some other members of the family *Amaryllidaceae*, such as *Narcissus* (daffodil), *Leucojum aestivum* (snowflake), and *Lycoris,* including *Lycoris radiata* (red spider lily). Galantamine acts as an acetylcholinesterase inhibitor and an allosteric ligand of nicotinic acetylcholine receptors. Recent studies have shown that it also has neuroprotective effects. In one study, galantamine was found to promote the protection of RGCs in a rat glaucoma model. Galantamine-induced ganglion cell survival was caused by the activation of types M1 and M4 muscarinic acetylcholine receptors. This showed the potential of galantamine as a neuroprotectant for glaucoma [70]. A further study by the same authors confirmed that galantamine preserved microvasculature density and improved retinal blood flow in the glaucomatous retina, strengthening the evidence for its neuroprotective effect in glaucoma [71].

5. Conclusions

Since ancient times, alkaloids have been extracted from natural substances and have various effects on the eyes. Several alkaloids have been used medicinally since that time. Atropine induces mydriasis and has been used for diagnosis and treatment. Physostigmine and pilocarpine were first used as treatments for glaucoma because they constrict the pupil and reduce IOP. Cocaine was used as an ophthalmic anesthetic but is not currently used due to toxicity. However, there are cases where existing alkaloids are used for new purposes. Recently, atropine has attracted attention as a therapeutic agent that inhibits myopic progression, and pilocarpine has been recognized and used as a treatment for presbyopia.

Alkaloids also had various effects. Caffeine inhibits cataract progression from oxidative damage and reduces hypoxia-induced angiogenesis, but is known to induce an increase in IOP. Nicotine is known to aggravate dry eye syndrome and blepharitis by influencing the ocular surface and to induce the formation of conjunctival tumors and cataracts. Chloroquine and hydroxychloroquine, derivatives of quinine, are drugs widely used in rheumatic diseases, but can cause retinopathy.

Finally, alkaloids are being studied in some studies as new drugs in the field of ophthalmology. Matrine, vincamine, papaverine, and galantamine were newly found to be able to protect the optic nerve, confirming the possibility of developing a treatment for diseases, such as glaucoma or optic neuropathy. In addition, piperine and sanguinarine have been found to be associated with the formation of cataracts. Matrine is expected to be effective in treating vincristine-resistant retinoblastoma. Piperine, berberine, and sanguinarine are expected to be helpful in treating diseases related to retinal neovascularization. They are expected to become therapeutic agents for various ophthalmic diseases in the future.

Conflict of interest

The authors declare no conflict of interest.

Acronyms and abbreviations

RPE	Retinal pigment epithelium
IOP	intraocular pressure
TNF-α	tumor necrosis factor-α
PGE2	prostaglandin E2
MCP-1	monocyte chemoattractant protein-1
SOD	superoxide dismutase
ROS	reactive oxygen species
DR	diabetic retinopathy
ARMD	age-related macular degeneration
NAION	non-arteritic anterior ischemic optic neuropathy
VEGF	vascular endothelial growth factor
RGCs	Retinal ganglion cells
Akt	protein kinase B
PI3K	phosphoinositide 3-kinases
eNOS	endothelial Nitric Oxide Synthase
cAMP	cyclic adenosine 3,5′-monophosphate
NF- kB	nuclear factor-kB
MEK	mitogen-activated protein kinase
ERK	extracellular signal-regulated kinases
HIF-1α	hypoxia-inducible factor-1α
mTOR	mammalian target of rapamycin
JNK	c-Jun N-terminal kinase
MAPK	mitogen-activated protein Kinase

DOI: http://dx.doi.org/10.5772/intechopen.110257

Author details

Jin-Ho Joo
Department of Ophthalmology, College of Medicine, Uijeongbu St. Mary's Hospital, The Catholic University of Korea, Uijeongbu-si, Gyeonggi-do, Republic of Korea

*Address all correspondence to: oph.jhjoo@gmail.com

References

[1] Luch A. Molecular, clinical and environmental toxicology. Preface. Exs. 2009;**99**:Xi-xiv

[2] Wicks C, Hudlicky T, Rinner U. Morphine alkaloids: History, biology, and synthesis. The Alkaloids Chemistry and Biology. 2021;**86**:145-342

[3] Tran HDM, Tran YH, Tran TD, Jong M, Coroneo M, Sankaridurg P. A review of myopia control with atropine. Journal of Ocular Pharmacology and Therapeutics: the Official Journal of the Association for Ocular Pharmacology and Therapeutics. 2018;**34**(5):374-379

[4] North RV, Kelly ME. A review of the uses and adverse effects of topical administration of atropine. Ophthalmic & Physiological Optics: the Journal of the British College of Ophthalmic Opticians (Optometrists). 1987;7(2):109-114

[5] Li FF, Yam JC. Low-concentration atropine eye drops for myopia progression. Asia-Pacific Journal of Ophthalmology (Philadelphia, Pa). 2019;**8**(5):360-365

[6] Chua WH, Balakrishnan V, Chan YH, Tong L, Ling Y, Quah BL, et al. Atropine for the treatment of childhood myopia. Ophthalmology. 2006;**113**(12):2285-2291

[7] Upadhyay A, Beuerman RW. Biological mechanisms of atropine control of myopia. Eye & Contact Lens. 2020;**46**(3):129-135

[8] Realini T. A history of glaucoma pharmacology. Optometry and Vision Science: Official Publication of the American Academy of Optometry. 2011;**88**(1):36-38

[9] Pinheiro G, Araújo Filho I, Araújo Neto I, Rêgo ACM, Azevedo EP, Pinheiro FI, et al. Nature as a source of drugs for ophthalmology. Arquivos brasileiros de oftalmologia. 2018;**81**(5): 443-454

[10] Holmstedt B, Wassén SH, Schultes RE. Jaborandi: An interdisciplinary appraisal. Journal of Ethnopharmacology. 1979;**1**(1):3-21

[11] Hung L, Yang CH, Chen MS. Effect of pilocarpine on anterior chamber angles. Journal of Ocular Pharmacology and Therapeutics: The Official Journal of the Association for Ocular Pharmacology and Therapeutics. 1995;**11**(3):221-226

[12] Yunard A, Oktariana VD, Artini W, Prihartono J. Comparison of intraocular pressure and anterior chamber angle changes between pilocarpine and laser peripheral Iridotomy. Journal of Current Glaucoma Practice. 2019;**13**(1):32-36

[13] Yoo YJ, Hwang JM, Yang HK. Dilute pilocarpine test for diagnosis of Adie's tonic pupil. Scientific Reports. 2021;**11**(1):10089

[14] Meghpara BB, Lee JK, Rapuano CJ, Mian SI, Ho AC. Pilocarpine 1.25% and the changing landscape of presbyopia treatment. Current Opinion in Ophthalmology. 2022;**33**(4):269-274

[15] Grzybowski A, Ruamviboonsuk V. Pharmacological treatment in presbyopia. Journal of Clinical Medicine. 3 Mar 2022;**11**(5):1385

[16] Markel H. Über coca: Sigmund Freud, Carl Koller, and cocaine. Journal of the American Medical Association. 2011;**305**(13):1360-1361

[17] Ruetsch YA, Böni T, Borgeat A. From cocaine to ropivacaine: The history of

local anesthetic drugs. Current Topics in Medicinal Chemistry. 2001;**1**(3):175-182

[18] Dhingra D, Kaur S, Ram J. Illicit drugs: Effects on eye. The Indian Journal of Medical Research. 2019;**150**(3):228-238

[19] Firth AY. Editorial: Ocular effects of criminal drug use. Canadian Journal of Ophthalmology Journal canadien d'ophtalmologie. 2006;**41**(2):140-146

[20] Malihi M, Turbin RE, Frohman LP. Saturday night retinopathy with Ophthalmoplegia: A case series. Neuro-Ophthalmology (Aeolus Press). 2015;**39**(2):77-82

[21] Kyei S, Koffuor GA, Ramkissoon P, Abokyi S, Owusu-Afriyie O, Wiredu EA. Possible mechanism of action of the Antiallergic effect of an aqueous extract of Heliotropium indicum L. in ovalbumin-induced allergic conjunctivitis. Journal of Allergy. 2015;**2015**:245370

[22] Kyei S, Koffuor GA, Ramkissoon P, Ameyaw EO, Asiamah EA. Anti-inflammatory effect of Heliotropium indicum Linn on lipopolysaccharide-induced uveitis in New Zealand white rabbits. International Journal of Ophthalmology. 2016;**9**(4):528-535

[23] Kyei S, Koffuor GA, Ramkissoon P, Abu EK, Sarpong JF. Anti-cataract potential of Heliotropium indicum Linn on galactose-induced cataract in Sprague-Dawley rats. Current Eye Research. 2017;**42**(3):394-401

[24] Kyei S, Koffuor GA, Ramkissoon P, Owusu-Afriyie O. Anti-glaucoma potential of Heliotropium indicum Linn in experimentally-induced glaucoma. Eye and Vision (London, England). 2015;**2**:16

[25] Varma SD, Hegde KR, Kovtun S. UV-B-induced damage to the lens in vitro: Prevention by caffeine. Journal of Ocular Pharmacology and Therapeutics: the Official Journal of the Association for Ocular Pharmacology and Therapeutics. 2008;**24**(5):439-444

[26] Varma SD, Kovtun S. Protective effect of caffeine against high sugar-induced transcription of microRNAs and consequent gene silencing: A study using lenses of galactosemic mice. Molecular Vision. 2013;**19**:493-500

[27] Kronschläger M, Löfgren S, Yu Z, Talebizadeh N, Varma SD, Söderberg P. Caffeine eye drops protect against UV-B cataract. Experimental Eye Research. 2013;**113**:26-31

[28] Varma SD. Effect of coffee (caffeine) against human cataract blindness. Clinical Ophthalmology (Auckland, NZ). 2016;**10**:213-220

[29] Terai N, Spoerl E, Pillunat LE, Stodtmeister R. The effect of caffeine on retinal vessel diameter in young healthy subjects. Acta Ophthalmologica. 2012;**90**(7):e524-e528

[30] Echeverri D, Montes FR, Cabrera M, Galán A, Prieto A. Caffeine's vascular mechanisms of action. International Journal of Vascular Medicine. 2010;**2010**:834060

[31] Chandrasekaran S, Rochtchina E, Mitchell P. Effects of caffeine on intraocular pressure: The Blue Mountains eye study. Journal of Glaucoma. 2005;**14**(6):504-507

[32] Zhong Y, Yang Z, Huang WC, Luo X. Adenosine, adenosine receptors and glaucoma: An updated overview. Biochimica et Biophysica Acta. 2013;**1830**(4):2882-2890

[33] Pasquale LR. Vascular and autonomic dysregulation in primary open-angle glaucoma. Current Opinion in Ophthalmology. 2016;**27**(2):94-101

[34] Boia R, Ambrósio AF, Santiago AR. Therapeutic opportunities for caffeine and A2A receptor antagonists in retinal diseases. Ophthalmic Research. 2016;**55**(4):212-218

[35] Zhang S, Zhou R, Li B, Li H, Wang Y, Gu X, et al. Caffeine preferentially protects against oxygen-induced retinopathy. FASEB journal: Official Publication of the Federation of American Societies for Experimental Biology. 2017;**31**(8):3334-3348

[36] Chen JF, Zhang S, Zhou R, Lin Z, Cai X, Lin J, et al. Adenosine receptors and caffeine in retinopathy of prematurity. Molecular Aspects of Medicine. 2017;**55**:118-125

[37] Moss SE, Klein R, Klein BE. Prevalence of and risk factors for dry eye syndrome. Archives of Ophthalmology (Chicago, Ill: 1960). 2000;**118**(9):1264-1268

[38] Wang S, Zhao H, Huang C, Li Z, Li W, Zhang X, et al. Impact of chronic smoking on Meibomian gland dysfunction. PLoS One. 2016;**11**(12):e0168763

[39] Satici A, Bitiren M, Ozardali I, Vural H, Kilic A, Guzey M. The effects of chronic smoking on the ocular surface and tear characteristics: A clinical, histological and biochemical study. Acta Ophthalmologica Scandinavica. 2003;**81**(6):583-587

[40] Moon SW, Chung EJ, Jung SA, Lee JH. PDGF stimulation of Müller cell proliferation: Contributions of c-JNK and the PI3K/Akt pathway. Biochemical and Biophysical Research Communications. 2009;**388**(1):167-171

[41] Yoon KC, Song BY, Seo MS. Effects of smoking on tear film and ocular surface. Korean Journal of Ophthalmology: KJO. 2005;**19**(1):18-22

[42] Napora C, Cohen EJ, Genvert GI, Presson AC, Arentsen JJ, Eagle RC, et al. Factors associated with conjunctival intraepithelial neoplasia: A case control study. Ophthalmic Surgery. 1990;**21**(1):27-30

[43] Jetton JA, Ding K, Kim Y, Stone DU. Effects of tobacco smoking on human corneal wound healing. Cornea. 2014;**33**(5):453-456

[44] Ilhan N, Ilhan O, Coskun M, Daglioglu MC, Ayhan Tuzcu E, Kahraman H, et al. Effects of smoking on central corneal thickness and the corneal endothelial cell layer in otherwise healthy subjects. Eye & Contact Lens. 2016;**42**(5):303-307

[45] Sayin N, Kara N, Pekel G, Altinkaynak H. Effects of chronic smoking on central corneal thickness, endothelial cell, and dry eye parameters. Cutaneous and Ocular Toxicology. 2014;**33**(3):201-205

[46] Pekel G, Cetin EN, Acer S, Yagci R, Altintas S, Ongun GT. Effect of chronic smoking on lens nucleus as assessed by Pentacam HR lens densitometry in young adults. Cutaneous and Ocular Toxicology. 2014;**33**(2):145-149

[47] Tan JS, Mitchell P, Kifley A, Flood V, Smith W, Wang JJ. Smoking and the long-term incidence of age-related macular degeneration: The Blue Mountains eye study. Archives of Ophthalmology (Chicago, Ill: 1960). 2007;**125**(8):1089-1095

[48] Mansouri K, Pajic B, Hafezi F. Effect of cigarette smoking on intraocular pressure. Journal of Cataract and Refractive Surgery. 2015;**41**(3):682-683

[49] Chung SM, Gay CA, McCrary JA 3rd. Nonarteritic ischemic optic neuropathy. The impact of Tobacco Use. Ophthalmology. 1994;**101**(4):779-782

[50] Lee HK, Wang SC. Mechanism of morphine-induced miosis in the dog. The Journal of Pharmacology and Experimental Therapeutics. 1975;**192**(2):415-431

[51] Pickworth WB, Welch P, Henningfield JE, Cone EJ. Opiate-induced pupillary effects in humans. Methods and Findings in Experimental and Clinical Pharmacology. 1989;**11**(12):759-763

[52] Rottach KG, Wohlgemuth WA, Dzaja AE, Eggert T, Straube A. Effects of intravenous opioids on eye movements in humans: Possible mechanisms. Journal of Neurology. 2002;**249**(9):1200-1205

[53] Shanks GD. Historical review: Problematic malaria prophylaxis with quinine. The American Journal of Tropical Medicine and Hygiene. 2016;**95**(2):269-272

[54] Doyno C, Sobieraj DM, Baker WL. Toxicity of chloroquine and hydroxychloroquine following therapeutic use or overdose. Clinical Toxicology (Philadelphia, Pa). 2021;**59**(1):12-23

[55] Renner UD, Oertel R, Kirch W. Pharmacokinetics and pharmacodynamics in clinical use of scopolamine. Therapeutic Drug Monitoring. 2005;**27**(5):655-665

[56] Joo JH. Anisocoria after scopolamine transdermal patch contamination: A case report. Medicine. 2021;**100**(46):e27887

[57] Viau S, Maire MA, Pasquis B, Grégoire S, Fourgeux C, Acar N, et al. Time course of ocular surface and lacrimal gland changes in a new scopolamine-induced dry eye model. Graefe's Archive for Clinical and Experimental Ophthalmology = Albrecht von Graefes Archiv fur klinische und experimentelle Ophthalmologie. 2008;**246**(6):857-867

[58] Vurmaz A, Duman R, Sabaner MC, Ertekin T, Bilir A. Antioxidant effects of piperine in in-vivo chick embryo cataract model induced by steroids. Cutaneous and Ocular Toxicology. 2019;**38**(2):182-189

[59] Zhang P, Zhou YD, Tan Y, Gao L. Protective effects of piperine on the retina of mice with streptozotocin-induced diabetes by suppressing HIF-1/VEGFA pathway and promoting PEDF expression. International Journal of Ophthalmology. 2021;**14**(5):656-665

[60] Zhao B, Li B, Liu Q, Gao F, Zhang Z, Bai H, et al. Effects of matrine on the proliferation and apoptosis of vincristine-resistant retinoblastoma cells. Experimental and Therapeutic Medicine. 2020;**20**(3):2838-2844

[61] Kang J, Liu S, Song Y, Chu Y, Wang M, Shi Y, et al. Matrine treatment reduces retinal ganglion cell apoptosis in experimental optic neuritis. Scientific Reports. 2021;**11**(1):9520

[62] Li L, Su Y, Liu J, Chen C. Efficacy of Vincamine treatment in a rat model of anterior ischemic optic neuropathy. European Journal of Ophthalmology. 2021;**31**(6):3442-3449

[63] Ma S, Zhang K, Zhu Y, Cao X, Wang L. Effect of papaverine on axonal outgrowth of primary retinal ganglion cells of Sprague Dawley

rats. Experimental Eye Research. 2021;**212**:108797

[64] Zhou T, Zhu Y. Cascade signals of Papaverine inhibiting LPS-induced retinal microglial activation. Journal of Molecular Neuroscience: MN. 2019;**68**(1):111-119

[65] Dang Y, Xu Y, Wu W, Li W, Sun Y, Yang J, et al. Tetrandrine suppresses lipopolysaccharide-induced microglial activation by inhibiting NF-κB and ERK signaling pathways in BV2 cells. PLoS One. 2014;**9**(8):e102522

[66] Wang N, Zhang C, Xu Y, Tan HY, Chen H, Feng Y. Berberine improves insulin-induced diabetic retinopathy through exclusively suppressing Akt/mTOR-mediated HIF-1α/VEGF activation in retina endothelial cells. International Journal of Biological Sciences. 2021;**17**(15):4316-4326

[67] Song D, Song J, Wang C, Li Y, Dunaief JL. Berberine protects against light-induced photoreceptor degeneration in the mouse retina. Experimental Eye Research. 2016;**145**:1-9

[68] Zhang Y, Huang WR. Sanguinarine induces apoptosis of human lens epithelial cells by increasing reactive oxygen species via the MAPK signaling pathway. Molecular Medicine Reports. 2019;**19**(5):4449-4456

[69] Zhang J, Mao K, Gu Q, Wu X. The antiangiogenic effect of Sanguinarine chloride on experimental choroidal Neovacularization in mice via inhibiting vascular endothelial growth factor. Frontiers in Pharmacology. 2021;**12**:638215

[70] Almasieh M, Zhou Y, Kelly ME, Casanova C, Di Polo A. Structural and functional neuroprotection in glaucoma: Role of galantamine-mediated activation of muscarinic acetylcholine receptors. Cell Death & Disease. 2010;**1**(2):e27

[71] Almasieh M, MacIntyre JN, Pouliot M, Casanova C, Vaucher E, Kelly ME, et al. Acetylcholinesterase inhibition promotes retinal vasoprotection and increases ocular blood flow in experimental glaucoma. Investigative Ophthalmology & Visual Science. 2013;**54**(5):3171-3183